Lecture Notes in Computer Science 14305

Founding Editors

Gerhard Goos
Juris Hartmanis

The series Lecture Notes in Computer Science (LNCS), including its subseries Lecture Notes in Artificial Intelligence (LNAI) and Lecture Notes in Bioinformatics (LNBI), has established itself as a medium for the publication of new developments in computer science and information technology research, teaching, and education.

LNCS enjoys close cooperation with the computer science R & D community, the series counts many renowned academics among its volume editors and paper authors, and collaborates with prestigious societies. Its mission is to serve this international community by providing an invaluable service, mainly focused on the publication of conference and workshop proceedings and postproceedings. LNCS commenced publication in 1973.

Yan Li · Zhisheng Huang · Manik Sharma ·
Lu Chen · Rui Zhou
Editors

Health
Information Science

12th International Conference, HIS 2023
Melbourne, VIC, Australia, October 23–24, 2023
Proceedings

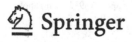

Editors
Yan Li
University of Southern Queensland
Darling Heights, Australia

Zhisheng Huang
Vrije University
Amsterdam, The Netherlands

Manik Sharma
DAV University Jalandhar
Jalandhar, Punjab, India

Lu Chen ⓘ
Swinburne University of Technology
Hawthorn, VIC, Australia

Rui Zhou
Swinburne University of Technology
Hawthorn, VIC, Australia

ISSN 0302-9743   ISSN 1611-3349 (electronic)
Lecture Notes in Computer Science
ISBN 978-981-99-7107-7   ISBN 978-981-99-7108-4 (eBook)
https://doi.org/10.1007/978-981-99-7108-4

This Springer imprint is published by the registered company Springer Nature Singapore Pte Ltd.
The registered company address is: 152 Beach Road, #21-01/04 Gateway East, Singapore 189721, Singapore

Paper in this product is recyclable.

Preface

The International Conference Series on Health Information Science (HIS) provides a forum for disseminating and exchanging multidisciplinary research results in computer science/information technology and health science and services. It covers all aspects of health information sciences and systems that support health information management and health service delivery.

The 12th International Conference on Health Information Science (HIS 2023) was held in Melbourne, Australia, during October 23–34, 2023. Founded in April 2012 as the International Conference on Health Information Science, the conference continues to grow to include an ever broader scope of activities. The main goal of these events is to provide international scientific forums for researchers to exchange new ideas in a number of fields through discussions with their peers from around the world. The scope of the conference includes (1) medical/health/biomedicine information resources, such as patient medical records, devices and equipment, software and tools to capture, store, retrieve, process, analyze, and optimize the use of information in the health domain; (2) data management, data mining, and knowledge discovery, all of which play a crucial role in decision-making, management of public health, examination of standards, privacy and security issues; and (3) development of new architectures and applications for health information systems.

The conference solicited and gathered technical research submissions related to all aspects of the conference scope. All the submitted papers were peer-reviewed by at least three international experts drawn from the Program Committee. After the rigorous peer-review process, a total of 12 papers and 19 short papers among 54 submissions were selected on the basis of originality, significance, and clarity and were accepted for publication in the proceedings. The high quality of the program – guaranteed by the presence of an unparalleled number of internationally recognized top experts – is reflected in the content of the proceedings. The conference was therefore a unique event where attendees were able to appreciate the latest results in their field of expertise and to acquire additional knowledge in other fields. The program was structured to favour interactions among attendees coming from many different areas, scientifically and geographically, from academia and from industry.

Finally, we acknowledge all those who contributed to the success of HIS 2022 but whose names are not listed here.

October 2023

Yan Li
Zhisheng Huang
Manik Sharma
Rui Zhou
Lu Chen

Organization

General Co-chairs

Fernando Martín Sánchez   Instituto de Salud Carlos III, Spain
Uwe Aickelin   University of Melbourne, Australia
Hua Wang   Victoria University, Australia

PC Co-chairs

Yan Li   University of Southern Queensland, Australia
Zhisheng Huang   Vrije Universiteit Amsterdam, The Netherlands
Manik Sharma   DAV University, India

Publicity Co-chairs

Yan Li   University of Southern Queensland, Australia
Zhisheng Huang   Vrije Universiteit Amsterdam, The Netherlands
Manik Sharma   DAV University, India

Coordination Chair

Siuly Siuly   Victoria University, Australia

Publication Co-chairs

Rui Zhou   Swinburne University of Technology, Australia
Lu Chen   Swinburne University of Technology, Australia

Diversity and Inclusion Chair

Juanying Xie   Shaanxi Normal University, China

Website Co-chairs

Mingshan You   Victoria University, Australia
Yong-Feng Ge   La Trobe University, Australia

Local Arrangement Co-chairs

Enamul Kabir   University of Southern Queensland, Australia
Jiao Yin   Victoria University, Australia

HIS Steering Committee Representatives

Yanchun Zhang   Guangzhou University, China, Pengcheng
                                Laboratory, China, Victoria University,
                                Australia
Agma Traina   University of São Paulo, Brazil

Program Committee

Mohammed Eunus Ali   Bangladesh University of Engineering and
                                Technology, Bangladesh
Ashik Mostafa Alvi   Victoria University, Australia
Luciano Baresi   Politecnico di Milano, Italy
Djamal Benslimane   Lyon 1 University, France
Mohamed Reda Bouadjenek   Deakin University, Australia
Jinli Cao   Latrobe University, Australia
Xin Cao   University of New South Wales, Australia
Cinzia Cappiello   Politecnico di Milano, Italy
Sven Casteleyn   Universitat Jaume I, Spain
Richard Chbeir   Univ. Pau & Pays Adour, France
Cindy Chen   UMass Lowell, USA
Lu Chen   Swinburne University of Technology, Australia
Maria Cola   IRCCS Centro Neurolesi Bonino-Pulejo, Italy
Dario Colazzo   Paris-Dauphine University, CNRS, France
Hai Dong   RMIT University, Australia
Yongfeng Ge   Victoria University, Australia
Allel Hadjali   LIAS/ENSMA, France
Tanzima Hashem   Bangladesh University of Engineering and
                                Technology, Bangladesh

Md Rafiul Hassan	King Fahd University of Petroleum and Minerals, Saudi Arabia
Zhisheng Huang	Vrije Universiteit Amsterdam, The Netherlands
Samsad Jahan	Victoria University, Australia
Peiquan Jin	University of Science and Technology of China, China
Enamul Kabir	University of Southern Queensland, Australia
Eleanna Kafeza	Athens University of Economics and Business, Greece
Georgios Kambourakis	University of the Aegean, Greece
Verena Kantere	University of Ottawa, Canada
Epaminondas Kapetanios	University of Hertfordshire, UK
Anne Laurent	Université de Montpellier, France
Xia Li	La Trobe University, Australia
Kewen Liao	Australian Catholic University, Australia
Guanfeng Liu	Macquarie University, Australia
Jiangang Ma	Federation University, Australia
Santiago Melia	Universidad de Alicante, Spain
Sajib Mistry	Curtin University, Australia
Lourdes Moreno	Universidad Carlos III de Madrid, Spain
Vincent Oria	New Jersey Institute of Technology, USA
George Papastefanatos	ATHENA Research Center, Greece
Alfonso Pierantonio	University of L'Aquila, Italy
Werner Retschitzegger	Johannes Kepler University Linz, Austria
Thomas Richter	Rhein-Waal University of Applied Sciences, Germany
Jarogniew Rykowski	Poznan University of Economics, Poland
Harald Sack	FIZ Karlsruhe, Germany
Heiko Schuldt	University of Basel, Switzerland
Wieland Schwinger	Johannes Kepler University Linz, Austria
Manik Sharma	DAV University, India
Siuly Siuly	Victoria University, Australia
Supriya Supriya	Torrens University, Australia
Bo Tang	Southern University of Science and Technology, China
Xiaohui Tao	University of Southern Queensland, Australia
Md. Nurul Ahad Tawhid	Victoria University, Australia
Dimitri Theodoratos	New Jersey Institute of Technology, USA
Markel Vigo	University of Manchester, UK
Hanchen Wang	University of Technology Sydney, Australia
Hongzhi Wang	Harbin Institute of Technology, China
Hua Wang	Victoria University, Australia

Xin Wang	Tianjin University, China
Michael Weiss	Carleton University, Canada
Puti Xu	Victoria University, Australia
Xun Yi	RMIT University, Australia
Jiao Yin	Victoria University, Australia
Mingshan You	Victoria University, Australia
Mariapia Zanghi	IRCCS Centro Neurolesi Bonino Pulejo, Sicily
Nicola Zannone	Eindhoven University of Technology, The Netherlands
Gefei Zhang	HTW Berlin, Germany
Wenjie Zhang	University of New South Wales, Australia
Rui Zhou	Swinburne University of Technology, Australia
Xiangmin Zhou	RMIT University, Australia

Additional Reviewers

Alvi, Ashik Mostafa
Hammoudi, Slimane
Inan, Muhammad Sakib Khan
Jajodia, Sourov
Kelarev, Andrei
Majumder, Shafayat Hossain
Su, Guangxin
Yang, Xuechao

Contents

Depression and Mental Health

Detection of Depression and Its Likelihood in Children and Adolescents:
Evidence from a 15-Years Study 3
   Umme Marzia Haque, Enamul Kabir, and Rasheda Khanam

A Combined Attribute Extraction Method for Detecting Postpartum
Depression Using Social Media 17
   Abinaya Gopalakrishnan, Raj Gururajan, Revathi Venkataraman,
   Xujuan Zhou, and Ka Ching Chan

Network Analysis of Relationships and Change Patterns in Depression
and Multiple Chronic Diseases Based on the China Health and Retirement
Longitudinal Study 30
   Xia Li, Shuo Li, and Ying Liu

Exploring Etiology of Nonsuicidal Self-injury by Using Knowledge Graph
Approach 40
   Zhisheng Huang, Xiyan Zhang, Fazhan Chen, Mengmeng Zhang,
   Haojie Fu, Qianqian Wu, and Xudong Zhao

A Question and Answering System for Mental Health of the Elderly Based
on BiLSTM-CRF Model and Knowledge Graph 50
   Beijia He, Shaofu Lin, Zhisheng Huang, and Chaogui Guo

Data Security, Privacy and Healthcare Systems

Australia's Notifiable Data Breach Scheme: An Analysis of Risk
Management Findings for Healthcare 65
   Martin Dart and Mohiuddin Ahmed

Analysis and Protection of Public Medical Dataset: From Privacy
Perspective 79
   Samsad Jahan, Yong-Feng Ge, Enamul Kabir, and Hua Wang

Enhancing Health Information Systems Security: An Ontology Model
Approach 91
   Raza Nowrozy and Khandakar Ahmed

Developing a Comprehensive Risk Management Framework for E-Health
Care Delivery 101
   Avisen Moonsamy and Mohiuddin Ahmed

Neurological and Cognitive Disease Studies

Knowledge-Based Nonlinear to Linear Dataset Transformation for Chronic
Illness Classification 115
   Markian Jaworsky, Xiaohui Tao, Jianming Yong, Lei Pan, Ji Zhang,
   and Shiva Raj Pokhrel

A Robust Approach for Parkinson Disease Detection from Voice Signal 127
   Sarmad K. D. Alkhafaji and Sarab Jalal

Analysis on Association Between Vascular Risk Factors and Lifestyle
Factors with the Risk of Dementia/Alzheimer's Disease Using Medical
Ontologies 135
   Wenjuan Hong, Can Wang, Chenping Hu, Yanhua Chen, Xiyan Zhang,
   Zhisheng Huang, and Hongyun Qin

COVID-19 Impact Studies

Unveiling the Pandemic's Impact: A Dataset for Probing COVID-19's
Effects on E-Learning Activities and Academic Performance 149
   Yanjun Liu, Daizhong Luo, Kate Wang, and Jiao Yin

Understanding the Influence of Multiple Factors on the Spread of Omicron
Variant Strains via the Multivariate Regression Method 161
   Zhenkai Xu, Shaofu Lin, Zhisheng Huang, and Yu Fu

Analyzing the Impact of COVID-19 on Education: A Comparative Study
Based on TOEFL Test Results 175
   Puti Xu, Wei Hong, Jiao Yin, Kate Wang, and Yanchun Zhang

Advanced Medical Data and AI Techniques

BiblioEngine: An AI-Empowered Platform for Disease Genetic
Knowledge Mining 187
   Mengjia Wu, Yi Zhang, Hua Lin, Mark Grosser, Guangquan Zhang,
   and Jie Lu

Enhancing Clustering Performance in Sepsis Time Series Data Using
Gravity Field 199
    Rui Hao, Ming Sheng, Yong Zhang, Huiying Zhao, Chenxiao Hao,
    Wenyao Li, Luoxi Wang, and Chao Li

Multi-modal Medical Data Exploration Based on Data Lake 213
    Tao Zhao, Nan Hai, Wenyao Li, Wenkui Zheng, Yong Zhang, Xin Li,
    and Gao Fei

Multi-model Transfer Learning and Genotypic Analysis for Seizure Type
Classification 223
    Yue Yang, Kairui Guo, Zhen Fang, Hua Lin, Mark Grosser, and Jie Lu

Requirement Survey in Thai Clinician for Designing Digital Solution
of Pain Assessment 235
    Noppon Choosri, Pattama Gomutbutra, Adisak Kittisares,
    Atigorn Sanguansri, and Peerasak Lettrakarnon

Predictive Analysis and Disease Recognition

A Comprehensive Approach for Enhancing Motor Imagery EEG
Classification in BCI's 247
    Muhammad Tariq Sadiq, Siuly Siuly, Yan Li, and Paul Wen

Image Recognition of Chicken Diseases Based on Improved Residual
Networks 261
    Nan Zhang, Xinqiang Ma, Yi Huang, and Jinsheng Bai

An Adaptive Feature Fusion Network for Alzheimer's Disease Prediction 271
    Shicheng Wei, Yan Li, and Wencheng Yang

A Review on Predicting Drug Target Interactions Based on Machine
Learning 283
    Wen Shi, Dandan Peng, Jinyuan Luo, Guozhu Chen, Hong Yang,
    Linhai Xie, Xiao-Xia Yin, and Yanchun Zhang

KNN-Based Patient Network and Ensemble Machine Learning for Disease
Prediction 296
    Haohui Lu and Shahadat Uddin

Medical Imaging and Dataset Exploration

Optimizing the Size of Peritumoral Region for Assessing Non-Small Cell
Lung Cancer Heterogeneity Using Radiomics 309
    Xingping Zhang, Guijuan Zhang, Xingting Qiu, Jiao Yin, Wenjun Tan,
    Xiaoxia Yin, Hong Yang, Kun Wang, and Yanchun Zhang

Multi-dimensional Complex Query Optimization for Disease-Specific
Data Exploration Based on Data Lake 321
    Zhentao Hu, Kaige Wang, Weifan Wang, Wenkui Zheng, Yong Zhang,
    Xin Li, Gao Fei, Wenyao Li, and Luoxi Wang

Analyzing Health Risks Resulting from Unplanned Land Use Plan
and Structure: A Case Study in Historic Old Dhaka 331
    Nishat Tasnim Manami, Ashik Mostafa Alvi, and Siuly Siuly

Elderly Care and Knowledge Systems

Home Self-medication Question-Answering System for the Elderly Based
on Seq2Seq Model and Knowledge Graph Technology 343
    Baoxin Wang, Shaofu Lin, Zhisheng Huang, and Chaohui Guo

Constructing Multi-constrained Cognitive Diagnostic Tests: An Improved
Ant Colony Optimization Algorithm 354
    Xi Cao, Yong-Feng Ge, and Ying Lin

Health Informatics and Patient Safety in Pharmacotherapy 366
    Antti Rissanen and Marjo Rissanen

Author Index 375

Depression and Mental Health

Detection of Depression and Its Likelihood in Children and Adolescents: Evidence from a 15-Years Study

Umme Marzia Haque[1]([∅]) [iD], Enamul Kabir[1] [iD], and Rasheda Khanam[2] [iD]

[1] School of Mathematics, Physics and Computing, University of Southern Queensland, Toowoomba, Australia
{UmmeMarzia.Haque,enamul.kabir}@usq.edu.au,
marziahaque202@gmail.com
[2] School of Business, University of Southern Queensland, Toowoomba, Australia
rasheda.khanam@usq.edu.au

Abstract.

Purpose The increasing concern over mental health issues, particularly depression in children and adolescents, has prompted research into accurate methods of diagnosis. However, previous studies have been limited in terms of data and age groups, hindering their effectiveness. Therefore, this study aims to use machine learning algorithms with the latest data from Australia to improve accuracy in identifying depression in young people. It also highlights the importance of early detection and explores how depressive symptoms differ across different age groups. Additionally, the study provides insights into the likelihood of depression in individuals of various ages.

Methods Machine learning algorithms were employed to identify the onset, persistence, and development of depression in children and adolescents. Three algorithms, random forest, support vector machine, and logistic regression, have been chosen for their ability to handle complex data, capture correlations, and make accurate predictions. These algorithms were applied to the recent longitudinal dataset from Australia, and their performance was compared.

Results The study found that using the random forest algorithm produced noteworthy results in terms of accuracy, precision, recall, and F1 score for diagnosing depression. The random forest model achieved an impressive accuracy of 94% and weighted precision of 95%. Additionally, logistic regression was employed to measure the likelihood of depression, resulting in an accuracy rate of 89% and a weighted precision of 91%.

Conclusion The study findings suggest that developing a predictive model that comprehends the characteristics and trends linked to mental illness during different stages of children and adolescents' lives has substantial potential for promoting early intervention and identifying individuals who might be at risk of developing mental illness in the future.

© The Author(s), under exclusive license to Springer Nature Singapore Pte Ltd. 2023
Y. Li et al. (Eds.): HIS 2023, LNCS 14305, pp. 3–16, 2023.
https://doi.org/10.1007/978-981-99-7108-4_1

Keywords: Machine learning · random forest · support vector machine · logistic regression

Statements and Declarations

We confirm that all authors declare that they have no competing interests. The paper has been seen and approved by all authors that they agree on the order of authorship. We ensure that this manuscript has not been published elsewhere and is not under consideration by another conference. All authors have read and approved the manuscript and agreed to be accountable for all aspects of the work.

1 Introduction

Mental health disorders have become a growing concern worldwide, with depression being one of the most prevalent disorders among children and adolescents. According to the World Health Organization, depression is the leading cause of disability worldwide among children and adolescents aged 10 to 19 years. In Australia, depression is prevalent in young people, with approximately one in four adolescents suffering from some form of mental illness, highlighting the significance of the issue [1]. However, despite the increasing awareness, early detection of mental health problems remains a challenging endeavour, posing a significant obstacle in addressing the well-being of young Australians.

Over the years, researchers have employed different methods to detect depression in individuals. Recently, machine learning (ML) algorithms have emerged as a promising tool for identifying mental health disorders. These algorithms possess the capability to analyse extensive datasets, identify patterns, and make accurate predictions. Moreover, they can identify individuals who may be at risk of developing mental illness, even before symptoms are evident. The utilization of machine learning algorithms to detect depression in children and adolescents represents a significant advancement in improving mental health outcomes. Summaries of the methods employed in a previous synthesis of related literature and their results are shown in Table 1.

Table 1. Summaries of the methods and outcomes of previous literature reviews

Method/Classifier	Dataset	Performance Metric	Reference
Convolutional neural network	EEG signals from left and right hemispheres of the brain	99.12% and 97.66% classification accuracies for the right and left hemisphere	[2]
Smoothness, significance, and sanction (SS3) supervised learning model	User provided data over social media	55% F1 value and 42%precission	[3]
Support vector machine	EEG, EOG, chin EMG, ECG, oxygen saturation (SpO2), respiration and rectal body temperature from polysomnography data	86.51% accuracy	[4]

(continued)

Table 1. (*continued*)

Method/Classifier	Dataset	Performance Metric	Reference
Logistic regression	I. Age 15 or over adult data from 58 articles of online journal II. <250 sample size of various adverse health outcomes for the mothers III. 57,486 elderly populations from different articles	I. OR = 1.39, P = 0.15 II. Pooled prevalence of perinatal depression was 16.3% (CI = 95%; 14.7% to 18.2%, P < 0.001), with antenatal depression 19.7% (CI = 95%; 15.8% to 24.2%, P < 0.001) and postnatal depression 14.8% (CI = 95%; 13.1% to 16.6%, P < 0.001) III. Pooled prevalence of depression among old age was 31.74% (95% CI 27.90, 35.59)	[5–7]
Multivariate analysis	148 Canadian university students	Strong to moderate impact of several determinants on depression	[8]
Decision tree	Facebook data	73% accuracy	[9]
Linear regression analysis	268 participants	95% confidence level and a 6% margin of error	[10]
Naive Bayes	348 people of aged 20–60	85% accuracy	[11]
Random Forest	I. 153 of individuals from social media data of writings: textual spreading, time gap, and time span II. 250 individuals (18 + age) with criminal record III. Cross-sectional data of 667 different children and adolescents with adolescents where follow-up was not possible	I. Early risk detection error with depression detection 21.67% II. 90% AUC III. 95% accuracy	[12–14]

As depicted in Table 1, ML algorithms have been employed to diagnose depression. However, limited research has been conducted on depression detection in young individuals due to unavailability of data. Despite a small sample size and inter-participant heterogeneity resulting from data collected from many sites, previous studies have demonstrated good utility and accuracy [2–14]. The majority of literature utilize ML algorithms with social media data, MRI images, EEG, EOG, and ECG data to develop an automated diagnosis tool that enables experts to identify depression without relying solely on clinical tests. Previous cross-sectional studies have predominantly focused on mature participants; however, these studies have been limited in terms of data and age groups, limiting their efficacy. There is a notable absence of longitudinal studies tracking the progression of depression symptoms as individuals mature. Currently, there seems to be a lack of research investigating the identification of individuals who may be susceptible to developing mental illness in the future. Therefore, the primary objective of this study is to address this research gap by utilizing a longitudinal dataset of Australian children and adolescents aged 6–15 years. This research focuses on capturing the variations in depressive symptoms throughout different developmental phases and is the first of its kind to provide insights into the likelihood of experiencing depression at specific ages. The dataset includes repeated measurements of the same individuals at two-year intervals, allowing for the detection of depression using popular ML algorithms such as Support Vector Machine (SVM), Logistic Regression (LR), and Random Forest (RF).

Research has consistently demonstrated that early detection and timely treatment of mental health problems in children and adolescents can significantly reduce the risk of long-term complications [15]. By detecting depression in children and adolescents' early stage, this study aims to decrease the likelihood of negative outcomes. Additionally, gaining insights into the variation in symptoms across age groups will facilitate the development of targeted prevention and early intervention strategies. The implications of these findings extend to parents, caregivers, and school authorities, who can benefit from improved monitoring and response to depression risk. Moreover, health professionals can utilize the study's findings to inform the design of effective mental health interventions specially tailored for children and adolescents.

2   Methodology

The proposed study suggests a technique for identifying depression based on longitudinal dataset analysis. The framework of the method is shown in Fig. 1. The methodology is divided into three components: data processing, case selection, and a machine learning-driven approach.

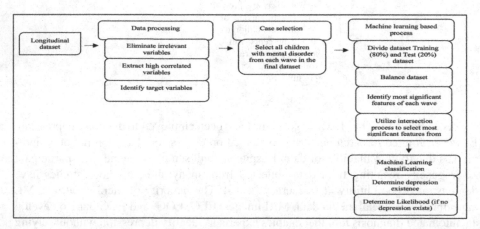

Fig. 1. An overview of the proposed framework

2.1 Data Processing

The longitudinal data processing requires the elimination of irrelevant variables and identification of the response variable. Data extraction is required to remove lower correlated variables. Most importantly, a final dataset is produced to contain all the mental disorder cases from different waves for the evaluation of symptoms over time.

2.2 Case Selection

The main focus of case selection is to include all children with mental disorders from each wave of the study in the final dataset to track the onset, persistence, and evolution of symptoms over time. This approach helps identify potential triggers and risk factors. The depressed and non-depressed cases are selected for each dataset based on the child's mental health status. The selected cases of a particular dataset are considered for instances from other waves, creating a final dataset.

2.3 Machine Learning Based Process

The ML based classification process consists of four sub processes: data extraction, feature selection, handling imbalance dataset and classification.

2.3.1 Data Extraction

Each wave is considered for data extraction. At first, chi-square test is performed to check the association between categorical variables with the response variable. The variables with p-value less than .05 are taken to the next step as these variables are associated with the response variable. Then, correlation is measured. As this dataset contains only binary variables, Point Biserial, Phi coefficient and Tetrachoric correlation method are considered to measure the strongly associated independent variables with response variable. However, the results are same. This happened due to the binary variables which can only take two possible values. This is why, calculating the covariance between them is equivalent to calculating the correlation coefficient. However, for these binary categorical variables, Tetrachoric correlation is selected as this is useful in cases where the underlying continuous variable are not directly observable but can be assumed normally distributed [16].

2.3.2 Feature Selection

To determine the most important features between these highly correlated variables of each dataset, the Boruta method employing the Random Forest (RF) classifier is utilised for its unbiased and stable feature selection.

The Boruta algorithm is a feature selection technique that utilises a Random Forest model as a wrapper. This feature selection is a process that involves the removal of irrelevant or redundant features to determine the significance and relevance of characteristics with respect to the response variable [17, 18]. It is necessary to state that these features set are nearly the same across datasets in different time points. The union operation can be applied for adding up the most significant features from all the datasets. Eventually, a feature which is important in one dataset but absent from another can be replaced with zero. However, it important to note, that this approach may result in a larger feature space than necessary and may also introduce noise or unrelated features that could adversely impact the accuracy of any analysis or modelling performed on the resulting dataset. Some features may have different meanings or interpretations in various datasets, which may impact the validity of any analysis or modelling performed on the combined dataset. For this, it is recommended to thoroughly consider the implications and potential limitations of this strategy. The intersection process has been employed to select complete feature sets when there is variation in features across different time points. This ensures that the common features of the datasets from various time periods have been considered.

2.3.3   Handling Imbalanced Dataset

In machine learning, it is essential to balance these cases to prevent the model from becoming biased towards either class. If one class has substantially more samples than the other, the model may become overfit to the majority class and disregard the minority class. This can lead to poor performance on the minority class, which may be significant for the current issue. By balancing the classes, the model is forced to devote equal attention to both classes and can learn to classify them accurately. This improves overall efficacy of the model and generalisation ability. This motivated the use of the Synthetic Minority Oversampling Technique (SMOTE) whereby a random subset of the majority cases is selected to equal the number of minority cases.

2.3.4   Classification

In this study, these renowned supervised learning models are examined and described below, which are anticipated to yield optimal results for the longitudinal dataset.

Random Forest (RF)
RF is an ensemble learning algorithm that constructs a large number of decision trees and combines their predictions to produce a more accurate and stable result. RF creates decision trees using a bootstrap sample of the training data set and a random subset of features for each split of the tree [19]. The ultimate feature relevance is its average over all trees. Since it predicts random subsets of features and instances, it overfits less than other methods. The total number of trees is divided by the sum of the feature importance values on each tree with the following equation:

$$RFfi_i = \frac{\sum_{j \in alltrees} normfi_j}{T} \tag{1}$$

where $RFfi_i$ = the feature importance, i calculated from all trees in the RF model, $normfi_j$ = the normalized feature importance for i in tree j and T = total number of trees.

Support Vector Machine (SVM)
SVM is an algorithm that identifies hyperplanes in multi-dimensional space to separate data into different classes, with the goal of maximizing the margin between them.

The margin is the distance between the hyperplane and the closest data point of each class [20]. It performs well in high-dimensional feature spaces and datasets with significantly greater number of features than instances. This efficacy extends to both linear and non-linear classification problems, facilitated by the utilisation of various kernels. The following formula is used to measure the probabilities for input values for each class through this equation;

$$f(x) = (\sum_{j=1}^{m} (a_i x_{ij} + a_0) y_j \tag{2}$$

where n = number of data points, m = number of attributes, $x_{ij} = i^{th}$ attribute of jth data point and $y_j = 1$ or, -1.

Logistic Regression (LR)

LR is a binary classification algorithm that predicts the probability of a categorical response variable based on one or more predictor variables, unlike linear regression which predicts a continuous response variable. Logistic Regression is a simple and interpretable algorithm suitable for linear classification problems, that works effectively with binary and multi-class categorisation. The logistic function (sigmoid function) is used to calculate the probability of the outcome variable with this equation [21]:

$$\hat{y} = \frac{e^{(b_0 + b_1 X)}}{1 + e^{(b_0 + b_1 X)}} \tag{3}$$

where x = input value, $\hat{y}$ = predicted output, b_0 = bias or intercept term, b_1 = coefficient for input (x).

Performance Metrics

The performance of the proposed ML algorithms has been evaluated by accumulating True Positive (TP), True Negative (TN), False Positive (FP), and False Negative (FN) results by the confusion matrix. The accuracy, precision, recall, F1 scores in each ML model have been determined following the equations:

$$\text{Accuracy Rate} = \frac{TP + TN}{TP + FP + TN + FN} \tag{4}$$

$$\text{Precision} = \frac{TP}{TP + FP} \tag{5}$$

$$\text{Recall} = \frac{TP}{TP + FN} \tag{6}$$

$$\text{F1 score} = \frac{2 * Precision * Recall}{Precision + Recall} \tag{7}$$

3   Experiments

In order to valid the predictive performance of proposed model, longitudinal data is utilised from the Longitudinal Study of Australian Children (LSAC) dataset. The dataset is briefly described along with its corresponding sample.

3.1 Dataset

Data is collected from LSAC, a comprehensive nationwide study that has been following the development of 10,000 Australian children and their families since 2004. Information has been gathered every two years from parents, carers, and teachers, and children themselves, as they reach the appropriate age to participate. Ethical approval is obtained from Longitudinal Studies Data Access Team of the Department of Social Services. This dataset can be accessed by contacting the Australian Data Archive (ADA) at the provided site (https://dataverse.ada.edu.au).

3.2 Sample

Briefly, LSAC is a national longitudinal data on the maturation of Australian children across their first decade of life. It commenced with 2 cohorts: birth (aged 0–1) and kindergarten (aged 4–5) of 5,000 children each. Extensive data about health, social background, and demographic profile of early childhood, middle school, late adolescent, and early adulthood provide possibilities to understand changes in development of children through time. The LSAC study utilised a two-stage, stratified, clustered design with the Medicare database of the Health Insurance Commission (HIC) as the sampling framework. Details about strategy and methodology of the survey can be found in [22].

This study used data from the LSAC birth cohort collected between 2010 and 2018 to conduct a longitudinal analysis of the same children to monitor changes in mental health symptoms with age (6–15). Although the birth cohort begins with children aged (0–1), this research has started the analysis with 6 years children as the mental health concern became apparent at that time and continue with 15 years aged adolescents. In this research, the focus has been drawn to parenting, family relationship, overall behaviours and mental health outcomes from Waves (4–8) of (6–15) years aged children and adolescents for identifying the potential long-term consequences of depression to highlight the importance of early identification as well as its likelihood. However, mental health evidence is also available in Wave 9 of birth cohort and in the other kindergarten cohort waves, the variables of these datasets differ significantly used previously in Waves (4–8) of birth cohort datasets. Consequently, these datasets have not been considered in this study.

3.3 Result and Analysis

To develop this approach, experiments are conducted using the Python 3.7.3 sci-kit-learn package. The dataset is processed by removing the variables with more than 2000 null values and rows with null values, resulting in 1711 variables. Categorical variables are encoded using one-hot encoding. The whole data extraction procedure is then applied to the dataset, resulting in 165–170 variables out of the total variables of each wave. The variable comprising the question "Would you describe the child's anxiety disorder and depression as mild, moderate, or severe?" was considered as the response variable. The selected cases of 'depressed' and 'non-depressed' cases are combined to produce the final dataset comprising of 1785 individuals. The final dataset is imbalanced, with the percentage of 'non-depressed' class being 74% where the percentage of 'depressed' class is 26%. The dataset is handled using SMOTE. The complete dataset is divided into 80% of training and 20% of test datasets. Then most significant features are extracted using Boruta on RF to identify the most significant features. Table 2 presents a concise description of the most significant features that were identified.

Table 2. Most significant features

Identified sign/symptoms of depression	Description of variables
Medical condition: Nervousness[a,b]	Does the study child have nervous condition?
Coping[a,b]	Does the study child have a difficulty or delay in any of the following areas compared to children of a similar age? Cope with emotions
Social and emotional outcomes: Reacts strongly to disappointment[a,b]	Does the study child react strongly (cries or complains loudly) to a disappointment or failure?
Homework incomplete unless reminded[a,b]	Does the study not complete homework unless reminders are given?
Difficulty completing assignments[a,b]	Has difficulty completing assignments (homework, chores.)?
Complained of headaches etc.[a]	Does the study child complain of headaches etc.?
Often seemed worried[a,b]	Does the study child often seem worried?
Often been unhappy or tearful[a]	Does the study child often seem unhappy?
Easily lose confidence[a]	Does the study child often lose confidence?
Had many fears[a]	Does the study child have many fears?
Temperament[a,b]	Does the study child become angry frequently?
Emotional development: Problems feeling afraid or scared[a]	Has the study child has had a problem with this?
Problems feeling sad[a]	Has the study child has had a problem with this?
Trouble sleeping[a]	Has the study child has had a problem with sleeping?
Social development: Unable to do what other children can[a,b]	Has the study child has had a problem with this?
Problems keeping up with other children[a,b]	Has the study child has had a problem with this?
School readiness: Problems missing days due to illness[a]	Has the study child has had a problem with this?
Parental involvement: Contacted school about attendance[a]	Has the parent contacted the school for various reason?
Parent living elsewhere: Study Child excitement on arrival in home[a]	Does the study child become excited on the parent's arrival?
Social development Helpful if someone is hurt etc.[a,b]	Is the study child helpful if someone gets hurt?

[a] asked to parent (father/mother)
[b] asked to teacher

Data on depression affected victims have been provided by 1785 children and adolescents, 20% (n = 357) of each wave. Among them 26% (n = 464) of them are depression affected. Table 3 shows the classification reports and evaluation metrics used by RF, SVM with linear kernel, LR.

Table 3. Classification report and evaluation metrics with RF

RF Classification Report				
	Precision	Recall	F1-score	Support
Negative	0.96	0.95	0.96	261
Positive	0.88	0.89	0.88	96
Accuracy			0.94	357
Macro avg	0.92	0.92	0.92	357
Weighted avg	0.94	0.94	0.94	357
Accuracy: 94%				
Weighted precision: 95%				
SVM Classification Report				
	Precision	Recall	F1-score	Support
Negative	0.93	0.95	0.94	261
Positive	0.84	0.79	0.82	96
Accuracy			0.90	357
Macro avg	0.88	0.87	0.88	357
Weighted avg	0.90	0.90	0.90	357
Accuracy: 90%				
Weighted precision: 95%				
LR Classification Report				
	Precision	Recall	F1-score	Support
Negative	0.91	0.92	0.92	261
Positive	0.78	0.76	0.77	96
Accuracy			0.88	357
Macro avg	0.84	0.84	0.84	357
Weighted avg	0.88	0.88	0.88	357
Accuracy: 88%				
Weighted precision: 91%				

For ML based classification, performances of the proposed system have been shown in Table 3. Among the three classifiers used, the RF-based classification shows the best overall performance across metrics, achieving an accuracy of 94%. SVM ranks second with an accuracy of 90%, while the LR-based method shows the lowest overall with an accuracy of 88%. To further evaluate the performance, AUC scores of these three classifiers have been plotted Fig. 2. RF scores the highest AUC of 92% indicating super discriminatory power. SVM and LR follow with AUC scores of 87% and 84%, respectively.

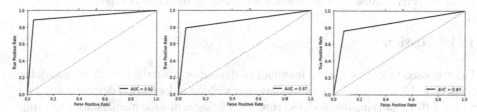

Fig. 2. AUC scores of a) RF, b) SVM and c) LR models

Additionally, the research offers significant perspectives on the probability of experiencing depression among individuals belonging to various age cohorts. The utilisation of LR has been employed to assess the likelihood of depression in the absence of its existence. The LR results for depression likelihood, which demonstrate an accuracy of 89%, have been presented in Table 4. Furthermore, the AUC score of LR for measuring depression likelihood across various age groups is reported as 87% in Fig. 3.

Table 4. Classification with LR for likelihood measuring

LR Classification Report				
	Precision	Recall	F1-score	Support
Negative	0.94	0.91	0.92	261
Positive	0.77	0.83	0.80	96
Accuracy			0.89	357
Macro avg	0.85	0.87	0.86	357
Weighted avg	0.89	0.89	0.89	357
Accuracy: 89%				
Weighted precision: 91%				

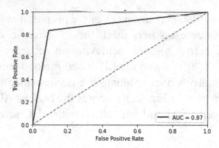

Fig. 3. AUC score of LR model for measuring likelihood of depression

4 Discussion

The proposed technique using a longitudinal dataset of Australian children and adolescents of 6–15 years old with an RF classifier yielded a depression detection accuracy rate of 94%, signifying the model's proficiency in detecting the manifestation of symptoms. The precision and recall rates for the prediction of 'non-depressed' cases are 96% and 95%, respectively. In contrast, the precision and recall rates for the prediction of 'depressed' cases are 88% and 89%, respectively.

These outcomes are notably superior to those reported in prior studies that used user data from social media platforms and cross-sectional data [3, 9, 11–14]. The precision and f1 score of depressed and non-depressed class are 88% and 96% respectively, which is significantly higher than the 55% and 42% values observed in [3]. The accuracy score is 94% which is significantly higher when compared to the accuracy scores of 73% [9], 85% [11], and 78.33% [12]. While the accuracy score exhibits a slight increase to 95% [14], a closer examination of the individual performance metrics, such as precision, recall, and f1 score, reveals that the research demonstrates superior results in the depressed and non-depressed classes. The AUC score has been determined to be 92%, surpassing the findings among mentally disordered offenders [13]. The findings indicate that the model effectively detected instances of depression within the studied population. The macro and weighted averages for precision, recall, and F1-score were all above 0.9, demonstrating the robustness of the model. The likelihood of depression at given ages can be measured with 89% accuracy, precision (depressed: 77%, non-depressed: 94%), recall (depressed: 83%, non-depressed: 91%), f1 score (depressed: 80%, non-depressed: 92%). Overall, the longitudinal analysis provides valuable insights into how symptoms change across diverse age groups. These findings can be utilised to develop focused prevention and intervention approaches.

5 Conclusion

The present investigation employs longitudinal data of children and adolescents from Australia to construct a model aimed at identifying indications of depression. The model has a 94% accuracy rate, with a 96% precision rate and a 95% recall rate for predicting 'non-depressed' instances. However, the prediction of 'depressed' instances outperforms prior efforts, with a precision and recall of 88% and 89%, respectively. Additionally, the study examines the variation of depression symptoms with age and identifies depression risk across different by age groups. The results obtained from this investigation can be utilized to formulate specific strategies for preventing and intervening in cases of depression. The results obtained from this investigation are instrumental in developing a robust depression detection model that can effectively identify depression across different age groups. Additionally, the model can provide an estimation of the likelihood of depression based on specific characteristics within a given age group with 89% accuracy, precision (depressed: 77%, non-depressed: 94%), recall (depressed: 83%, non-depressed: 91%), f1 score (depressed: 80%, non-depressed: 92%). This capability enables the formulation of targeted strategies for preventing and intervening in cases of depression. By utilizing the model's insights, it becomes possible to implement proactive measures and interventions to address depression at any age, thereby improving mental health outcomes.

References

1. AIHW. Mental health: prevalence and impact. In: Mental Health Services in Australia. AIHW, Canberra (2022)
2. Ay, B., et al.: Automated depression detection using deep representation and sequence learning with EEG signals. J. Med. Syst. **43**, 1–12 (2019)
3. Burdisso, S.G., Errecalde, M., Montes-y-Gómez, M.: A text classification framework for simple and effective early depression detection over social media streams. Expert Syst. Appl. **133**, 182–197 (2019)
4. Zhang, B., et al.: Ubiquitous depression detection of sleep physiological data by using combination learning and functional networks. IEEE Access **8**, 94220–94235 (2020)
5. Habtamu, K., et al.: Interventions to improve the detection of depression in primary healthcare: systematic review. Syst. Rev. **12**(1), 1–28 (2023)
6. Nisar, A., et al.: Prevalence of perinatal depression and its determinants in Mainland China: a systematic review and meta-analysis. J. Affect. Disord. **277**, 1022–1037 (2020)
7. Zenebe, Y., Akele, B., Necho, M.: Prevalence and determinants of depression among old age: a systematic review and meta-analysis. Ann. Gen. Psychiatry **20**(1), 1–19 (2021)
8. Othman, N., et al.: Perceived impact of contextual determinants on depression, anxiety and stress: a survey with university students. Int. J. Ment. Heal. Syst. **13**(1), 1–9 (2019)
9. Islam, M.R., et al.: Depression detection from social network data using machine learning techniques. Health Inf. Sci. Syst. **6**(1), 1–12 (2018)
10. Nguyen, M.-H., et al.: A dataset of students' mental health and help-seeking behaviors in a multicultural environment. Data **4**(3), 124 (2019)
11. Priya, A., Garg, S., Tigga, N.P.: Predicting anxiety, depression and stress in modern life using machine learning algorithms. Procedia Comput. Sci. **167**, 1258–1267 (2020)
12. Cacheda, F., et al.: Early detection of depression: social network analysis and random forest techniques. J. Med. Internet Res. **21**(6), e12554 (2019)
13. Pflueger, M.O., et al.: Predicting general criminal recidivism in mentally disordered offenders using a random forest approach. BMC Psychiatry **15**(1), 1–10 (2015)
14. Haque, U.M., Kabir, E., Khanam, R.: Detection of child depression using machine learning methods. PLoS ONE **16**(12), e0261131 (2021)
15. Green, H., et al.: Mental Health of Children and Young People in Great Britain. Palgrave Macmillan, Basingstoke (2005)
16. Kubinger, K.D.: On artificial results due to using factor analysis for dichotomous variables. Psychol. Sci. **45**(1), 106–110 (2003)

17. Kursa, M.B., Jankowski, A., Rudnicki, W.R.: Boruta–a system for feature selection. Fund. Inform. **101**(4), 271–285 (2010)
18. Kursa, M.B.: Boruta for those in a hurry (2020)
19. Breiman, L.: Random forests. Mach. Learn. **45**(1), 5–32 (2001)
20. Cortes, C., Vapnik, V.: Support vector machine. Mach. Learn. **20**(3), 273–297 (1995)
21. Hosmer Jr., D.W., Lemeshow, S., Sturdivant, R.X.: Applied Logistic Regression, vol. 398. Wiley, Hoboken (2013)
22. Soloff, C., Lawrence, D., Johnstone, R.: Sample Design. Australian Institute of Family Studies, Melbourne (2005)

A Combined Attribute Extraction Method for Detecting Postpartum Depression Using Social Media

Abinaya Gopalakrishnan[1,2](✉) , Raj Gururajan[1,2], Revathi Venkataraman[2] ,
Xujuan Zhou[1](✉), and Ka Ching Chan[1]

[1] School of Business, University of Southern Queensland, Springfield, Australia
{Abinaya.Gopalakrishnan,Raj.Gururajan,Xujuan.Zhou,KC.Chan}@usq.edu.au
[2] Department Networking and Communications, School of Computing,
SRM Institute of Science and Technology, Chennai, India
revathin@srmit.edu.in

Abstract. Women's lives change with pregnancy and birth. Pregnancy
and delivery, like other fleeting life events, can have lasting psychological and physiological effects on women. They also increase Postpartum
Depression (PPD) rates. If untreated, PPD can drain a mother's energy
and make it hard to care for her children. Mental diseases are multi-
faceted, making social media identification difficult. Social media like
Instagram, Twitter, Facebook, and others have grown in importance,
changing this study topic. Mothers can communicate to their friends
and share their feelings, images, and videos on social media. Posts let us
see how freshly delivered mothers talk to each other on social networks.
This study identifies postpartum depressive women from Twitter messages that show depressed attitudes. Thus, we use NLP for prediction and
machine learning to evaluate our proposed approach. We list the most
common words used by PPD and control group account holders here.
Our strategy improves performance using integrated attribute extraction. Bigram best detects PPD with 82% accuracy and 0.80 F1 scores
using the Random Forest (RF) classifier and single attribute extraction.
SVM classifiers perform best for PPD detection, with 89% accuracy and
0.91 F1 scores. Our research reveals that effective attribute selections
and their many attribute combinations can boost performance.

Keywords: Postpartum Depression · social networks · behavior ·
emotion · Natural language processing · machine learning

1 Introduction

The birth of a child is a transformative experience for parents. Many women
endure emotional fluctuations after initial elation. Postpartum alterations
include the "baby blues", a period of emotional instability lasting six weeks following childbirth. 12–20% of primi mums experience postpartum depression. Postpartum depression (PPD) symptoms include grief, sleep and dietary changes,

exhaustion, decreased libido, sobbing, and anxiety [1]. It impacts children's growth, moods, and social development [2]. Previous research suggests 50% of PPD cases are unreported [3]. Fear of grief, social isolation, and the belief that new parenthood modifies moods may cause under reporting [4]. Ignorance of risk factors, lack of access to competent treatment and preventative programmes, and a desire for privacy also limit aid [4]. Social media has reduced youth loneliness. Social media users share photos, videos, status updates, and opinions on many topics. Depression is conveyed through social media status posts, photos, films, and articles that depict crimes, partiality, and dictators and provoke uprisings. A Pew Research Centre research found that 97% of people use Instagram, Twitter, YouTube, and Facebook everyday [5]. Over 75% of mothers with PDD do not seek early medical care, exploiting their health [6]. Social media can assist young mothers discover physical and mental health difficulties. Thus, social media data detects PDD. Twitter is great for character research because people are honest in their tweets and retweets [7]. This study examines well-tagged depression and non-depression datasets plus a big Twitter dataset to discover hidden differences in online behaviours between troubled and everyday people. Machine learning and NLP are used to research PPD depression. Some researchers detect writing depression with a single set of features. N-grams [8], BOW [9,10], LDA [11], and LIWC [12] are used to mine these single-set properties. In order to enhance PPD identification, it may be helpful to use specialized attributes and their ensemble combinations, such as Term Frequency - Inverse Document Frequency+ Latent Dirichlet Allocation [13], BOW+Latent Dirichlet Allocation, or N-grams+Linguistic Inquiry and Word Count [14]. Tyshchenko et al. suggested classifying stop words and adding LIWC-like word categories to an existing system (BOW+TFIDF+LIWC).For the purpose of identifying social media tools for mental health, analyzed and compared various data sources, NLP strategies, and computational methods.The overall objective of this study is to dectect the Postpartum Depression of women's share the feelings through Social Media posts. We have come a long way, yet there are still obstacles to overcome. This study investigates if picking the right qualities and combining them in different ways for early PPD detection might improve system performancein long run early detection reduces the risk factors associated with the mother-baby bonding.

- First, to characterize the content of the postpartum depressed mother's postings, we select the linguistic attributes that are the most helpful when applied to the identification of various kinds of depression.
- Second, we compare the word frequencies, topical similarities, and correlations between the posts of those with PPD and those who do not suffer from depression.
- The attribute extraction was carried out by relying on the vectors generated by the TF-IDF method; we use unigrams and bigrams to calculate word frequency to predict correlation, our attention is focused on the LIWC dictionary and its three attributes (Morphological factors, personal concerns and psychological dimensions). And we decided to use the LDA approach as one

of the successful elements in the topic examination that we are using for associating the risk factors to the linguistic words in PPD-related posts.
- We compare the results from analyzing three different single-attribute sets with those obtained from analyzing their corresponding multi-attribute combinations using Text-classifying algorithms.

The paper's remaining parts are organized as follows. Dataset details needed to make the PPD prediction are shown in Sect. 2. The methodology of the proposed framework is presented in Sect. 3, including data pretreatment, attribute extraction, and classification methods. In Sect. 4, we compare the attribute sets and assess the findings, determining the most effective machine learning technique for identifying postpartum depression. In Sect. 5, we provide a conclusion and suggestions for future study.

2 Materials

This section describes the dataset used in this combined attribute extraction framework to predict PPD among the posts shared on Twitter social media. There are eight different Twitter-Self-Reported Temporally-Contextual Mental Health Diagnosis Dataset (STMHD) disorder categories, which map directly to the Diagnostic and Statistical Manual of Mental Disorders(DSM-V) sub types [15]. Major depressive disorder (MDD), Postpartum Depression (PPD), and depression all fall under the umbrella term "depressive disorders". At the same time, Post-Traumatic Stress Disorder (PTSD) is a subset of trauma and stress-related illnesses, and Attention-Deficit/Hyperactivity Disorder (ADIID) is categorized as a neurodevelopmental disorder. Other mental illnesses include anxiety disorders, bipolar disorders, and obsessive-compulsive disorders (OCD). The dataset now includes a ninth grouping, "control-users", who will serve as a reference point for future analyses. Around 8000 healthy individuals served as controls, while 25,860 individuals with at least one of the eight disorders represented in the dataset. Table 1 shows a detailed description of the dataset collected. There are 713 Postpartum Depression (PPD) mothers' tweets initially detected using the loose regex tool; 333 valid ones are recognized using hand annotations, and 263 were identified by pattern matching. The total number of posts in the dataset belonging to the PPD diseases class is 547, which are chosen for our analysis. Posts of standard, depressed mothers' postings within friends and family-related are compiled. Table 2 includes frequent words of PPD depressed mothers' posts and non-depressed control users' posts.

3 Methods

More and more methods are being developed to identify depressive symptoms in posts shared on social media. This section shows how to recognize PPD symptoms through the use of text categorization and Natural Language Processing

Table 1. The final column shows the percentage of users in each disease class whose tweets were used as anchors and how many tweets were identified using a sloppy regex

Disorders	Collected Tweets	Final User count
ADHD	43764	8095
Depression	37149	6803
PTSD	30077	3414
Anxiety	267339	4843
OCD	7558	1325
PPD	713	547
MDD	651	325
Bipolar	5967	1651
Total Counts	152618	27003

Table 2. Frequent words found in both Postpartum Depression-indicative Posts and Major Depressive Disorder

PPD-Indicative Posts	Non depressed control users posts
baby, crying, alone, no sleep, unsuccessful, feeding not good,no breast milk, pressure, too worried, uncomfortable, blame, hopeless, sleeping, isolation, dependent, fatigue,dullness, frustration, critical, melancholy, expectation, discouragement, problems,financial, unsafe, appetite	awesome, too good, text me, uncles, friends, need, better, parents, married, don't care, beautiful, advice, close friends, engaged, discussion, wrong, attention, presented, often, large, recognition, different, online, community, cooperation, concerns, accomplishment

(NLP) methods. Figure 1 depicts the framework, which includes preprocessing of data, attribute extraction, machine learning classifiers, attribute analysis, and experimental outcomes.

3.1 Data Pre-processing

For attribute extraction and training purposes, we utilize natural language processing algorithms. To begin with, we utilize tokenization to break down the depressed postings into smaller units. The next step is eliminating potentially misleading characters, such as URLs, punctuation, and stop words. The next step is stemming, which removes unnecessary letters from words and clusters those that are structurally similar.

3.2 Attributes Extraction

After cleaning the data, we employ methods that extract mothers' linguistic preferences in PPD Twitter posts as inputs to our models. We use combined

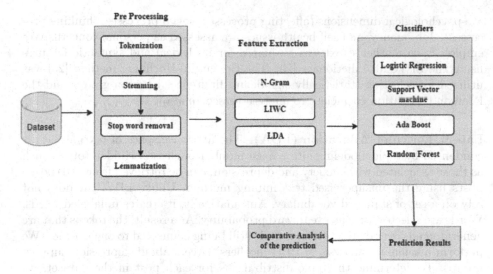

Fig. 1. Postpartum Depression(PPD) detection framework.

attribute extraction methods such as N-gram characteristics, LDA topics, and linguistic inquiry tools like the Word Count (LIWC) lexicon to examine the language patterns of recent mothers.

N-Gram Attributes. PPD Twitter post characteristics are analyzed using N-gram modeling. To diagnose PPD by calculating the likelihood of co-occurrence of each input sentence as a unigram and bigram [16,17]. For the purposes of n-gram modeling, the term frequency-inverse document frequency is a numerical metric that highlights the importance of a word in each document of the corpus. Experimentally less instructive tokens that occur frequently are ignored to make place for the more informative ones that occur infrequently. The TF-IDF value of a term increases if it appears in only one post [18]. We extracted 194,613 unigrams and bigrams using scikit-learn Python's TF-IDF vectorizer [19].

Linguistic Inquiry and Word Count (LIWC). The LIWC dictionary is frequently utilized in the field of linguistic computation as a source of information for analyzing language and mental health [20]. Many studies in the field of mental health present this method, which relies on a correlation between behaviors and words, as its foundation [21,22]. Through a series of experiments, we were able to quantify 68 of the 95 linguistic characteristics of depressive posts and non-depressive PPD posts. That is how we calculate the overall scores for three more abstract classes: common morphological features, psychological dimensions, and individual preferences. The goal of the LIWC psycholinguistic dictionary bundle was to highlight the importance of mothers in fostering harmonious communities. We begin by categorizing mothers' content based on their use of nine different linguistic features: verbs, auxiliary verbs, adverbs, articles, conjunctions, generic and personal pronouns, prepositions, and negations. Then we divide the Morphological criteria define the moms' postings. Social and thinking processes are psychological dimensions (affecting processes, social processes, thinking processes). Job, money, and self health issues are assessed as personal concerns. We employ Each mother's text was evaluated for its lexical and syntactic features using the LIWC2015 dictionary [20]. The Benjamini-Hochberg method [23] was utilized for selecting statistically significant differences between groups and the Pearson correlation coefficient to analyze the correlation.

Latent Dirichlet Allocation (LDA). The attribute space of textual data is condensed by topic modeling into a fixed number of classes. Hidden topics, such as those associated with anxiety and depression, can be retrieved from the chosen posts using the unsupervised text mining method. Unlike LIWC, it does not rely on a set of standard vocabulary. Automatically, it creates unlabeled words. Words are selected with an eye toward probability. As a result, the tokens that are generated all cover distinct themes while still being connected to one another. We perform a semantic analysis of PPD mothers' tweets about depression support groups. To determine the topic distributions for each post in the dataset, we used the LDA module. Finding its topic structures is aided by a probabilistic generative model for exploratory data collection [24]. According to our findings, the LDA model performs best when limited to 70 themes in the validation set. When choosing discussion topics, we only look at terms that have at least 10 comments. Each and every PPD entry is included in a single tokenized and stemmed document. Using this method, we are able to compute themes across the document set and tag them with depression or non-depression classifications. All of the stop words must be eliminated before we can continue on to the subject modeling phase.

3.3   Text Classification Techniques

Predictions of postpartum depression can be made using classification algorithms. This framework is built with the help of several different machine learning techniques, including logistic regression, support vector machine, random forest, and adaptive boosting. Estimating the probability of a binary response from one or more attributes is the goal of Logistic Regression (LR), a linear classification technique. Point-based samples are classified by means of a high-dimensional space in Support Vector Machine (SVM) models. New examples are added to the same space and assigned to a category according to the gap in which they fall [25]. Bagged decision trees are used by Random Forest (RF) to improve performance [26]. If you have numerous weak classifiers, you can combine them into a single robust classifier using the ensemble method Adaptive Boosting (AdaBoost). It is a common method for dividing things into two groups.

4   Experimental Results

This section will first discuss a few quantitative outcomes before analyzing the categorization results. We determine the frequency of the words, then forecast the importance of the connection between the words and the attributes related to Postpartum depression (PPD) depression, and then investigate how well N-grams, Latent Dirichlet Allocation (LDA), Linguistic Inquiry and Word Count (LIWC), and combinations of the above methods' characteristics can predict PPD outcomes.

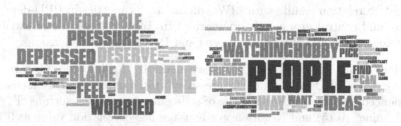

(a) Most frequent N-grams key- (b) Most frequent N-grams key-words in Post Partum Depres- words in non depressed users posts sion(PPD) posts

Fig. 2. Word clouds for the contents of posts PPD, Non depressed users

4.1 Attributes Analysis of Various Methods

Here we have discussed the prediction PPD with extraction of attributes using N-grams, LDA, LIWC attributes by determining the frequency of the words, then forecast the importance of the connection between the words and the attributes related Postpartum depression (PPD) depression.

Extraction of Attributes Using N-Gram. In order to analyze vocabulary shifts, we categorize the full labeled corpus of PPD-related tweets. To understand how PPD depression is, we compare the frequency of individual unigrams and bigrams between posts containing PPD depression indicators and posts non depressed users. In each category, we select the top one hundred unigrams and bigrams. In Figs. 2(a) and 2(b)), we showcase that the most common 100 unigrams and 100 bigrams found in PPD and non-depressed (control group) are examined. On both world cloud, you can see examples of the newly-emerging words associated with high frequency.

We found that words indicative of related baby (asleep, feeding, dullness, crying), the pain felt after delivery(melancholy, pain, hopeless, pressure, discomfort), Angry expressions (crap, angry, hated), social support(Nobody, alone, escape, blame, unsafe, discouragement, isolation), and Notion of denial(no) are all present in PPD depressive-indicative posts. Words like "tired", "I'm exhausted", and "sleep" symbolizes depression-related sensations of fatigue, drowsiness, or restlessness and agitation [27]. It is often verbalized regarding physical discomfort (my head, stomach, and knee hurt). Unigrams and bigrams in typical posts, as opposed to those suggestive of depression, tend to focus on words referring to the distant past (year, month, time), the solicitation of advice (please help, recommendation) and interpersonal connections (mom, friend, husband, family, friendship).

Extraction of Attributes Using LIWC. Out of a possible 95 attributes, we narrowed it down to 72 to examine how they relate to the textual data. The best correlation results with LIWC dictionary properties in PPD-depressed mothers and control groups are summarized in Table 3 under three attributes Morphological factors, Personal concerns and Psychological dimensions.

- In light of the Morphological factors are again divided into the sub-categories that express PPD predominantly are shown to be more inwardly focused, as evidenced by their increased usage of self-centred pronouns such as "I", "me", and "mine" (0.15) and Negation words usage has correlation value as 0.16.
- The personal concerns for conversation follow the linguistic factors attributes that can be summed up by their top three personal circumstances: (0.15) Job, (0.16) finances, and (0.17) self-health, respectively.
- The psycholinguistic attributes resulting in correlation described in the attributes extraction, we quantified all posts classified as either PPD depression or non-depressive. We looked at the Affecting processes (happy, cry, hurt, hate) that showed the strongest association (0.19) within the Psychological dimensions, positive (0.07) and negative (0.39) feelings. Findings from the social processes (0.18) (spouse, friend, mother) are similar to those from the thinking processes components (0.15).

Table 3. Highest correlation values obtained with LIWC attributes in PPD posts

LIWC attributes	Sub categories	Example words from PPD posts	P value
Morphological factors	Negations	no, not, never, ever, lack	0.16***
	Personal Pronoun	I, them, her, his	0.14*
	Singular (mother/baby)	I, me, mine, baby, we(mom & child),	0.15**
Personal concerns	Job	concentration, full time, unwilling	0.15*
	Money	cash, expenses, salary	0.16**
	self health	obese, asleep, appetite	0.17***
Psychological dimensions	Affecting processes	happy, cry, hurt, hate	0.19***
	Social processes	alone, discomfort, isolated	0.18**
	Thinking processes	feel, always, at times, blame	0.15*

Note *** P < 0.001, **P < 0.01 Al most all correlation coefficients meet the P value < 0.05

Our research shows that incorporating LIWC into design tools can improve the performance of data detection models.

Extraction of Attributes Using LDA. Using a topic model, we can determine the depression expressed in the posts, which served as an early warning system for signs of PPD. The number of generated topics is input into LDA and must be specified. The precision of the classification may shift depending on how the parameter is adjusted. As a result, it's essential to settle on a reasonable number. When limiting the validation set size, as described in Sect. 3.2, 70 different subjects become valid.

Table 4. Example of risk factors with LDA attributes in PPD depression-related texts.

Domain	PPD risk factors	Most representative words
challenges in life	Causes of Workplace Stress	unempolyed, company, broke, jobless, work pressure
	Fear of returning to the workforce	boss, pronlonged time, boring, unhappy, fired, leave
Obstetric	Bond Between Parents	best, insecure, happy, no friends, worthless, help, request, not close, no relationship
	Mode of delivery	induced, c section, normal
Maternal tolerance	Feeding	Very unsatisfied, unsatisfied, very satisfied
	Ready to leave hospital	satisfied, lone, boring, yes , no
	Planned conception	not exactly at this time, no definitely not
Socio demographic	Age	aged, middle age
	Education	un educated, immature, illiterate, graduate, school or less
	Ability to mange income	easy, Always difficult, not bad, sometimes difficult

Based on the previous research's [28] the temporal analysis, we narrowed our focus with certain words in a tweet to predict depression was top listed in Table 4 leads to data classification. In this case, we use t-SNE to reduce the number of dimensions and create a two-dimensional visualisation of our data [29]. Words that are highly linked with postings' respective topics are shown in Table 4.

There is a shared vocabulary of depressing terms in the cases. Words associated with disclosure, such as unemployed, "broke", "insecure", "no friends", "worthless", "broke", and "tired", convey the anguish, suffering, or PPD-depressed symptoms of the mothers. Other users suffer from low self-esteem and an unhealthy preoccupation with themselves, among other negative emotions. Other themes also represent hatred, aggression, or their relationships with friends.

4.2 Classification Results

This section explains the evaluation metrics used to assess the performance of the proposed method. In order to determine Postpartum depression, We obtain the Twitter-STMHD data set's attribute space and start text classification. We train our baseline attributes from Twitter PPD posts by integrating N-gram probabilities, LIWC categories, an LDA model, and other attributes. Combining these NLP approaches is intended to investigate which attributes improve performance accuracy when screening for PPD in posts by depressed new mothers. The four significant classifiers estimate posting PPD prevalence by measuring the accuracy(Acc), F1 score(F1), precision(P) and recall(R) among the various classifiers such as Logistic regression(LR), Support Vector Machine(SVM), Random Forest(RF) and Ada Boost respectively. Five classification models using the NLP characteristics are shown in Table 5 along with their corresponding accuracy values. Each categorized corpus has values for accuracy, F1-score, precision, and recall. Much research on depression identification utilizes accuracy as a metric, but we also show precision, recall, and F1-score to further dig into the results. We can see a performance improvement when we compare the classifiers' use of individual attributes (LIWC, LDA, unigram/bigram) to their own. With an LR learning method, bigrams achieve 81% accuracy and 0.83 F1 score, which is higher than the SVM attribute (80% accuracy, 0.80 F1) and the RF with LR text classification algorithm (71% accuracy, 0.81 F1). Whereas bigram handles well on its own, it has significant limitations when combined with other attributes. The predictive power of LIWC as a single attribute is higher than that of LDA. Compared to SVM (74%, 0.74), and RF model yields higher accuracy (78%, 0.84). It is identical to prior studies [23], where LDA is superior to LIWC. Our goal in comparing the effectiveness of several attribute combinations is to identify one that is particularly helpful in correctly classifying PPD posts. In addition to

Table 5. Performance results of the classification models.

attribute	LR				SVM				RF				Ada Boost			
	Acc	F1	P	R	Acc	F1	P	R	Acc	F1	P	R	Acc	F1	P	R
LIWC	69%	.80	.95	.69	72%	.74	.75	.72	68%	.84	.77	.95	66%	.74	.61	.95
LDA	77%	.83	.82	.84	74%	.80	.75	.88	78%	.66	.62	.62	67%	.81	.68	.99
unigram	68%	.80	.93	.79	70%	.81	.70	.85	72%	.82	.79	.96	71%	.68	.75	.63
Bigram	81%	.83	.87	.80	80%	.80	.76	.81	71%	.81	.74	.92	73%	.68	.74	.68
LIWC+LDA+Unigram	82%	.82	.87	.80	79%	.84	.82	.83	80%	.84	.82	.87	73%	.72	.87	.62
LIWC+LDA+Bigram	80%	.78	.82	.79	**90%**	**.91**	**.89**	**.87**	85%	.83	.87	.85	89%	.88	.87	.79

N-grams, we apply LIWC and LDA in this analysis. According to our findings, the LIWC+LDA+bigram performs best for PPD identification. Accuracy-wise, SVM (90%), is superior to AdaBoost (89%), RF (85%), and LR (80%), with a 0.91, 0.88, 0.83, and 0.87 F1 score, respectively. Ada Boost is also superior to another combined attribute set that uses bigrams (LIWC, LDA, bigram) (89%). Our findings indicate that the key to improved performance lies in the careful selection of attributes and the careful combination of those attributes.

5   Conclusion and Future Work

We used Twitter data to identify PPD signs and improve PPD depression screening tools. Using natural language processing and text classification, a more direct connection between PPD and linguistic practice discovered. Shared vocabulary in the postings is identified by comparing PPD and non-PPD accounts. Statements about the present or future, melancholy, worry, rage, violence, or suicide ideation indicate PPD, according to our research. We compared text classification methods that predict PPD symptoms using one or more attributes. We found that careful attribute selection and multiple attribute utilization can improve prediction performance. Twitter profiles of new moms were analyzed for signs of postpartum depression, and the SVM classifier found 0.91 F1 score and 90% accuracy (the optimal performance) for this task. Using the LR classifier, Bigram can accurately foretell PPD with an 81% success rate (accuracy) and an F1 score of 0.83. LDA topic models outperformed LIWC. Our experiment showed that our approaches work well, but the high absolute values of the measures suggest that this is a difficult subject that needs more exploration. This work should support emerging methods used in healthcare settings to assess depression and related characteristics. Mental health patients may benefit from taking more extraordinary steps to get healthy faster. We will investigate whether individuals' personalities affect their online depressed behavior.

References

1. Beck, C.T.: Predictors of postpartum depression: an update. Nurs. Res. **50**(5), 275–285 (2001)
2. Halligan, S.L., Murray, L., Martins, C., Cooper, P.J.: Maternal depression and psychiatric outcomes in adolescent offspring: a 13-year longitudinal study. J. Affect. Disord. **97**(1–3), 145–154 (2007)
3. De Choudhury, M., Counts, S., Horvitz, E.J., Hoff, A.: Characterizing and predicting postpartum depression from shared Facebook data. In: Proceedings of the 17th ACM conference on Computer Supported Cooperative Work & Social Computing, Portland, Oregon, pp. 626–638 (2014)
4. Dennis, C.L., Chung-Lee, L.: Postpartum depression help-seeking barriers and maternal treatment preferences: a qualitative systematic review. Birth **33**(4), 323–331 (2006)
5. Holleran, S.: The early detection of depression from social networking sites. The University of Arizona (2010)

6. Elliott, R., Greenberg, L.: Humanistic-experiential psychotherapy in practice: emotion-focused therapy. In: Comprehensive Textbook of Psychotherapy: Theory And Practice, pp. 106–120 (2017)
7. Shrivatava, A., Mayor, S., Pant, B.: Opinion mining of real time twitter tweets. Int. J. Comput. Appl. **100**(19) (2014)
8. Benton, A., Mitchell, M., Hovy, D.: Multi-task learning for mental health using social media text (2017). https://arxiv.org/abs/1712.03538
9. Nadeem, M.: Identifying depression on twitter (2016). https://arxiv.org/abs/1607.07384
10. Paul, S., Jandhyala, S.K., Basu, T.: Early detection of signs of anorexia and depression over social media using effective machine learning frameworks. In: Proceedings of the CLEF, pp. 1–9 (2018)
11. Maupomés, D., Meurs, M.: Using topic extraction on social media content for the early detection of depression. In: Proceedings of the CLEF (Working Notes), vol. 2125 (2018). https://CEUR-WS.org
12. Coppersmith, G., Dredze, M., Harman, C., Hollingshead, K.: From ADHD to SAD: analyzing the language of mental health on twitter through self-reported diagnoses. in Proceedings of the 2nd Workshop on Computational Linguistics and Clinical Psychology: From Linguistic Signal to Clinical Reality, pp. 1–10 (2015)
13. Tyshchenko, Y.: Depression and anxiety detection from blog posts data. Nature Precision Science, Institute of Computer Science, University of Tartu, Tartu, Estonia (2018)
14. Wolohan, J., Hiraga, M., Mukherjee, A., Sayyed, Z.A., Millard, M.: Detecting linguistic traces of depression in topic-restricted text: Attending to self-stigmatized depression with NLP. In: Proceedings of the 1st International Workshop on Language Cognition and computational Models, pp. 11–21 (2018)
15. Singh, A.K., Arora, U., Shrivastava, S., Singh, A., Shah, R.R., Kumaraguru, P.: Twitter-STMHD: an extensive user-level database of multiple mental health disorders. In: Proceedings of the International AAAI Conference on Web and Social Media, vol. 16, pp. 1182–1191 (2022)
16. Preotiuc-Pietro, D., et al.: The role of personality, age, and gender in tweeting about mental illness. In: Proceedings of the 2nd Workshop on Computational Linguistics and Clinical Psychology: From Linguistic Signal to Clinical Reality, pp. 21–30 (2015)
17. Coppersmith, G., Dredze, M., Harman, C., Hollingshead, K., Mitchell, M.: Clpsych 2015 shared task: depression and PTSD on twitter. In: Proceedings of the 2nd Workshop on Computational Linguistics and Clinical Psychology: From Linguistic Signal to Clinical Reality, pp. 31–39 (2015)
18. Salton, G., Buckley, C.: Term-weighting approaches in automatic text retrieval. Inf. Process. Manage. **24**(5), 513–523 (1988)
19. Pedregosa, F., et al.: Scikit-learn: machine learning in Python. J. Mach. Learn. Res. **12**, 2825–2830 (2011)
20. Pennebaker, J.W., Booth, R.J., Boyd, R.L., Francis, M.E.: Linguistic inquiry and word count: LIWC2015. In: Pennebaker Conglomerates, Austin, TX, USA (2015). https://www.LIWC.net
21. Schwartz, H.A., et al.: Towards assessing changes in degree of depression through Facebook. In: Proceedings of the Workshop on Computational Linguistics and Clinical Psychology: From Linguistic Signal to Clinical Reality, pp. 118–125 (2014)
22. Tsugawa, S., Kikuchi, Y., Kishino, F., Nakajima, K., Itoh, Y., Ohsaki, H.: Recognizing depression from twitter activity. In: Proceedings of the 33rd Annual ACM Conference on Human Factors in Computing Systems, pp. 3187–3196 (2015)

23. Resnik, P., Garron, A., Resnik, R.: Using topic modeling to improve prediction of neuroticism and depression in college students. In: Proceedings of the 2013 Conference on Empirical Methods in Natural Language Processing, pp. 1348–1353 (2013)
24. Blei, D.M., Ng, A.Y., Jordan, M.I.: Latent Dirichlet allocation. J. Mach. Learn. Res. **3**, 993–1022 (2003)
25. Noble, W.S.: What is a support vector machine? Nature Biotechnol. **24**(12), 1565 (2006)
26. Xu, B., Ye, Y., Nie, L.: An improved random forest classifier for image classification. In: Proceedings of the IEEE International Conference on Information and Automation, pp. 795–800(2012)
27. Buyukdura, J.S., McClintock, S.M., Croarkin, P.E.: Psychomotor retardation in depression: biological underpinnings, measurement, and treatment. Progr. Neuro-Psychopharmacol. Biol. Psychiatry **35**(2), 395–409 (2011)
28. Gopalakrishnan, A., Venkataraman, R., Gururajan, R., Zhou, X., Zhu, G.: Predicting women with postpartum depression symptoms using machine learning techniques. Mathematics **10**(23), 4570 (2022)
29. van der Maaten, L., Hinton, G.E.: Visualizing data using T-SNE. J. Mach. Learn. Res. **9**, 2579–2605 (2008)

Network Analysis of Relationships and Change Patterns in Depression and Multiple Chronic Diseases Based on the China Health and Retirement Longitudinal Study

Xia Li[1]([✉]) [iD], Shuo Li[2] [iD], and Ying Liu[3] [iD]

[1] La Trobe University, Melbourne, Australia
x.li2@latrobe.edu.au
[2] Shandong Experimental High School, Jinan, China
[3] China Academy of Chinese Medical Sciences, Beijing, China

Abstract. This study aims to explore the relationships and change patterns between depression and multiple chronic diseases using network analysis techniques applied to the China Health and Retirement Longitudinal Study (CHARLS) data. Depression and chronic diseases often coexist and have a significant impact on individuals' health and well-being. However, the complex interplay and dynamic nature of these conditions remain poorly understood. By utilizing network analysis on longitudinal data, we aim to uncover the underlying network structure and identify key variables associated with depression and multiple chronic diseases. Specifically, we employed Mixed Graphical Model (MGM) networks to estimate the relationships among selected items and investigated network interconnectedness, stability, temporal differences, community structure, and bridge nodes. Our network analyses were conducted on a large cohort sample of middle-aged participants, revealing central items and strong associations. These findings contribute to a better understanding of the complex relationships between depression and chronic diseases, offering insights for the development of targeted interventions to improve health outcomes.

Keywords: Network analysis · Chronic disease · Depression · Multimorbidity

1 Introduction

Adults who have many chronic diseases or ailments concurrently are said to have multimorbidity, which is the most prevalent chronic condition. For instance, only 17% of patients with coronary disease had it as their only ailment 3 in 4 folks over 65 years old who get healthcare numerous have chronic diseases [1]. Depression is the emotional expression of a state of ego-helplessness and ego-powerlessness to live up to certain strongly maintained [2]. It is also the single most commonly co-morbid disease in older adults and was paired with 8 different diseases (Sinnige J, et al., 2013) [3]. Domestic studies show that the middle-aged and old people are not only the main population

Y. Li et al. (Eds.): HIS 2023, LNCS 14305, pp. 30–39, 2023.
https://doi.org/10.1007/978-981-99-7108-4_3

of chronic diseases, but also the high incidence population of depression and network analysis can be used to investigate the complicated patterns of multiple relationships (David Hevey, 2018) [4, 5]. A network analysis which is conducted in 2019 using data of the 1995 Nova Scotia Health Survey shows that the prevalence of depression is 8.2%; the prevalence of Arthritis is the highest (28.4%), and the prevalence of hypertension, ischemic heart disease and diabetes are 23.7%, 3.7%, 3.5%, respectively [6]. Southern California study also showed the relationships between morbidity and depression, especially in men and woman respectively [7]. Using a sizable, nationally representative, and longitudinal sample of Americans over the age of 50, the connection between disease and depressed symptoms is investigated in research carried out by Jason Schnittker in 2004 [11]. Seven illnesses, including cancer, heart condition, diabetes, high blood pressure, stroke, and arthritis, and three forms of disability, activities in daily living, mobility, chronic obstructed pulmonary disease, and strength, substantially increase the depressive symptoms (Heeringa et al., 1999) [10]. After a univariate analysis and a multivariate logistic regression analysis of data from the 2015 CHARLS in 2020, it was discovered that there is a correlation between the occurrence of depression in elderly patients with chronic diseases, regardless of whether they are men or women. However, the influence of chronic diseases became insignificant due to the impact of many other factors. It should be mentioned here that according to community research conducted on 257 elderly chronic disease patients in Beijing, the main influencing factor of depression in elderly patients with chronic diseases is self-rated health status [8]. Research on meta-analyses reveals that depression is a substantial risk marker for the subsequent development of ischemic heart disease and Type 2 diabetes [9, 14]. Two additional meta-analyses discovered a significantly higher risk of coronary heart disease, and a higher risk of ventricular tachycardia/ventricular fibrillation associated with ischemic heart disease [12]. The studies above show that there is a correlation with statistical significance between chronic diseases and depressive symptoms. Chronic pulmonary and renal diseases, arthritis, stroke, cancer, diabetes is some of the multi-morbidity that are most related to depression. However, the cause-and-effect relationship between chronic disease and depression is not fully understood. In different research, researchers obtain different results from various dataset of different population and different years. According to analysis of 2011 CHARLS, the correlation between chronic diseases and depression is significant despite of the impact of other factors, but the analysis based on 2015 CHARLS makes known that the correlation became insignificant under the influence of diverse factors. As a result, a more comprehensive analysis based on data of several years is required. Network, which can better present the relationships should be used as the major analytical method.

2 Methods

2.1 Study Population and Measurements

The data used in our research was drawn from CHARLS study, which collected information on a variety of health, social, family, and financial characteristics through face-to-face interviews in respondents' homes. CHARLS survey started from year 2011, followed by another three waves in year 2013, 2015 and 2018. Higher response rates (above 80%) of all samples were obtained across all waves (Zhao Y, et al., 2020) [16].

The CHARLS survey questionnaire included the chronic diseases items based on a physician's diagnosis. Fourteen chronic diseases questions were included as follows: chronic lung diseases, diabetes, hypertension, cancer or malignant tumor, liver disease, dyslipidemia, kidney disease, heart problems, stroke, stomach diseases, emotional problems, memory-related disease, arthritis or rheumatism and asthma. The 10-items Center for Epidemiologic Studies Depression (CESD-10) scale short form was used to assess depression. All the items in this short form were 4-point Likert scales. Each participant was evaluated based on this form. The total score was summed up after reversing the scores of items 5 (felt hopeful about the future) and 8 (happy). As we know, CESD-10 total score has a range of 0–30, and higher depressive with higher scores. The CESD-10 has been validated for the community-dwelling older population in China [17].

2.2 Statistical Analyses

We used the statistical software R (version 4.1.2) to complete all the statistical analyses. Apart from descriptive analysis, network analysis was used in this study. In our study, Fruchterman and Reingold (1991) [18] algorithm was used to plot the network graph. Gaussian Graphical Model (GGM) and regularized based on Least Absolute Shrinkage and Selection Operator (LASSO, Tibshirani, 1996) [19] was used to get an undirected weighted network. According to one recent literature, our network model be estimated without any regularization (Williams et al., 2019) [20] whilst still controlling for the false-positive rate. Centrality indices including node strength, betweenness, and closeness were also provided to detect the most central item. Once the network was obtained, R package "Bootnet" then help to check the network accuracy and stability to gain further insight on the precision of network estimates through the confidence intervals based on 1000 bootstrapping. Then the stability of the centrality indices was checked from a subsample with a percentage participant missing. Finally, the edge and centrality indices difference tests were performed. Network Comparison Test (NCT) was used to assess the difference between two temporal networks via several invariance measures. The R functions NCT in package Network Comparison Test was used in this study, testing if this difference is significant based on a permutation test.

3 Results

3.1 Characteristics of the Study Population

This study used all the four waves (Year 2011, 2013, 2015 and 2018) in CHARLS cohort survey. The first baseline wave (Year 2011) includes 17,594 respondents, with a mean age of 59 years (standard deviation 10.1 years), 52.1% female and 47.9% male. Among all the fourteen chronic diseases we included, "Arthritis or rheumatism" and "Hypertension" are most prevalent which is 32.8% and 24.3% respectively. The most recent wave (Year 2018) included 19,717 respondents, with a mean age of 61.8 years (standard deviation 10.4 years), and 52.9% female and 47.1% male. "Hypertension" and "Dyslipidemia" are most prevalent which is 11.1% and 9.6% respectively. The higher depression score indicates greater depression. According to CES-D cutoff values (16 or greater), the average depression levels from the four waves are all above 16, ranging from 17.8 (Year 2013 and 2015) to 19.7 (Year 2018). The White Blood Cell (WBC) count and C-reactive protein (CRP) are only from wave 1 baseline participants. The participants characteristics are showed in Table 1.

Table 1 Characteristics of study population

Variables	Year 2011 (N = 17,594)	Year 2013 (N = 18,448)	Year 2015 (N = 20,965)	Year 2018 (N = 19,717)
Hypertension	4284 (24.3%)	598 (3.2%)	137 (0.7%)	2181 (11.1%)
Dyslipidemia	1595 (9.1%)	320 (1.7%)	83 (0.4%)	1901 (9.6%)
Diabetes	993 (5.6%)	190 (1.0%)	48 (0.2%)	1048 (5.3%)
Cancer/malignant tumor	180 (1.0%)	44 (0.2%)	11 (0.1%)	259 (1.3%)
Chronic lung diseases	1781 (10.1%)	255 (1.4%)	29 (0.1%)	990 (5.0%)
Liver disease	676 (3.8%)	124 (0.7%)	23 (0.1%)	632 (3.2%)
Heart attack	2093 (11.9%)	327 (1.8%)	62 (0.3%)	1367 (6.9%)
Stroke	413 (2.3%)	60 (0.3%)	11 (0.1%)	973 (4.9%)
Kidney disease	1106 (6.3%)	171 (0.9%)	38 (0.2%)	760 (3.9%)
Stomach or other digestive diseases	3902 (22.2%)	616 (3.3%)	94 (0.4%)	1549 (7.9%)
Emotional Problem	251 (1.4%)	32 (0.2%)	4 (0.0%)	228 (1.2%)
Memory-related disease	277 (1.6%)	48 (0.3%)	8 (0.0%)	445 (2.3%)
Arthritis or rheumatism	5773 (32.8%)	762 (4.1%)	90 (0.4%)	1513 (7.7%)
Asthma	637 (3.6%)	79 (0.4%)	9 (0.0%)	409 (2.1%)
Male	8421 (47.9%)	8792 (47.7%)	9972 (47.6%)	9294 (47.1%)
Age (Mean (SD))	59.0 (10.1)	59.9 (10.2)	59.4 (10.7)	61.8 (10.4)
CES-D (Mean (SD))	18.4 (6.35)	17.8 (5.78)	17.8 (6.36)	19.7 (8.65)

3.2 Depression, Chronic Diseases Network

The four waves' networks with "tuning = 0" were carried out for all these network estimations. Firstly, the networks consisting of age, gender, depression, and chronic Diseases were estimated. The network was displayed in Figs. 1, 2, 3 and 4, which showed the estimated graphical LASSO network and centrality measures among the fourteen chronic diseases (1: Yes, 0: No) and CES-D score from year 2011 to year 2018. We only used the complete cases for the network estimations and the final valid case numbers were showed without doing any missing data imputations. As we noticed, wave 1 and wave 4 have the largest valid sample size with 14,669 and 6,478 participants respectively. Therefore, the networks estimated based on these two waves were assumed to be much more reliable than the other two waves which have less valid sample size with 2,193 and 411. In this network analysis, the central items including the strength, closeness, and betweenness were also displayed in Figs. 1, 2, 3 and 4.

From all four estimated networks, the edge between the two nodes "Chronic Lung Diseases" and "Asthma" has been identified consistently strong across all the four waves; "age" consistently and positively correlates to "Memory-Related Disease" which means older people getting more likely to have "Memory-Related Disease". As showed in the Fig. 1, depression was positively correlated with "Emotional Problems", "Stroke" and "Arthritis" which means people with more depression tend to more likely to have "Emotional Problems", "Stroke" and "Arthritis" disease. Depression was also found positively correlated to gender (Male 0, Female 1) which means females are more likely have depression. There are not clear correlations with depression in the network estimated from wave 2, 3 and 4. The strength of "Chronic Lung Diseases" was almost consistently high across the four networks. In Fig. 1, "Depression" and "Heart Attack" were found having the large betweenness values. In Fig. 4, only "Heart Attack" was found having the largest betweenness values.

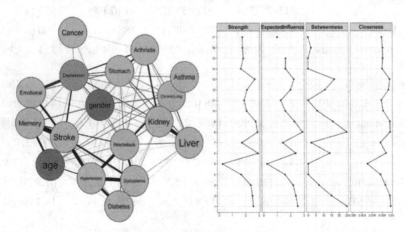

Fig. 1. Network structure (left) and centrality indices (right) for year 2011 (valid N = 14,669). Note: the node order is the same in Fig. 1 which follows from 1 to 17 "Depression", "Hypertension", "Dyslipidemia", "Diabetes", "Cancer", "Chronic Lung Diseases", "Liver Disease", "Heart Attack", "Stroke", "kidney disease", "Stomach Disease", "Emotional Problems", "Memory-Related Disease", "Arthritis", "Asthma", "gender", "age"

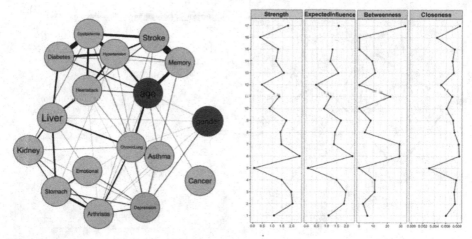

Fig. 2. Network structure (left) and centrality indices (right) for year 2013 (Valid N = 2193) (Color figure online)

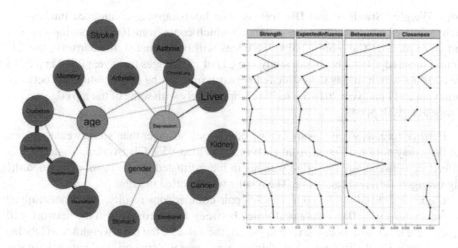

Fig. 3. Network structure (left) and centrality indices (right) for year 2015 (valid N = 411)

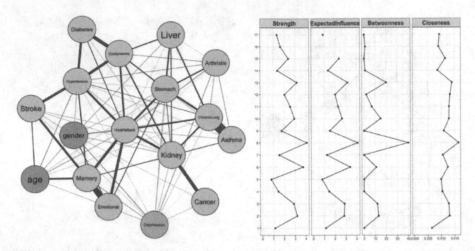

Fig. 4. Network structure (left) and centrality indices (right) for year 2018 (valid N = 6478)

3.3 Network Stability and Accuracy

Edge Weights Stability and Difference. The bootstrapping confidence intervals of each estimated edge weights were estimated which come from 1000 bootstrap samples and were plotted. The more reliable the edges will be estimated, the narrower the CIs around these edges will be. In our study, the CIs of most edges from year 2013 and 2015 are overlap, which means the estimated network may not be stable, while the network form year 2011 and year 2018 are stable comparatively with some of the top edge weight hardly get overlapped.

Furthermore, as we are aware certain edges look stronger than some weaker edges, but they may not be different from each other as their 95% CIs overlap. To detect this difference between any two edge weights in the estimated network, we performed the edge weights different test using. The results were plotted in Fig. 2.

Figure 2 showed all the edge weights pair comparisons results. The Bootstrapped difference tests (p = 0.05) were performed between non-zero edges in the network. All edges were labeled on both x-axis and y-axis, the value of the edge weights was labeled in the diagonal with different color which is consistent with the original network figures colors; black color means significant difference between these two edges while grey color means non-significant. Each row in the graph indicates one edge. As the pairwise test does not control for multiple comparisons, the results should be interpreted with caution. As we observed from Fig. 3, most of the edges differ from each other in wave 1.

Centrality Stability and Difference. The centrality measures stability was then accessed via case-dropping bootstrap method. Correlation-Stability Coefficient (CS-Coefficient) can be used to acquire the mean percentage of our sample that can be dropped and still preserve a correlation of 0.7 between our sample's centrality measures and our case-dropped bootstraps' centrality measures. The strength centrality result shows a relatively stable in wave 1, 2, 3 and 4, with a centrality strength stability coefficient

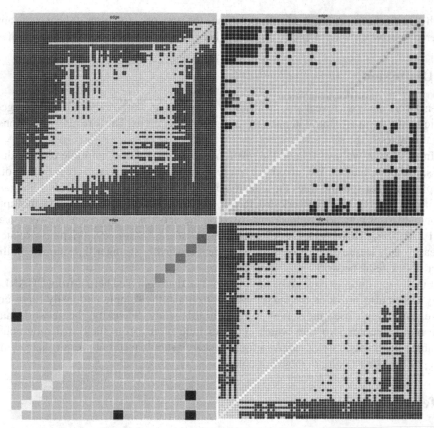

Fig. 5. Edge weight difference test (top left: year 2011, top left: year 2013, bottom left: year 2015, bottom right: year 2018)

(CS-coefficient) of 0.67, 0.36, 0.59, and 0.44, respectively. Epskamp et al. suggest that the "CS-coefficient should not be below 0.25, and preferably above 0.5" [21]. According to this rule, the strength measure from wave 1 and 4 networks can be acceptable. Finally, just as we did in the edge weight pairwise difference comparisons, we can also check whether centrality measures differ from each other. The centrality difference test results were showed in Fig. 5. As showed in Fig. 5, we found the first five central nodes "Chronic Lung Diseases", "Heart Attack", "Stroke" and "Memory-Related Disease" are equally central in wave 1 network.

3.4 Network Comparisons Test (NCT)

As network from wave 1 and 4 both showed higher edge weight and centrality indices stability, the network comparison tests will be only carried out between these two networks. From the NCT analyses, we observed that the two networks seem to be the same as the test for network structure invariance was not significant M = 0.65 with p = 0.26. Similarly, network global strength comparison for wave 1 and 4 networks also failed to reach significance with S = 1.15, p = 0.8. Since the network structures did not show any difference between wave 1 and 4, no further between-wave analyses were carried out.

4 Discussion

Our network analyses reveal among a variety of factors in a large cohort of middle-aged participants, the most central items, and strongest associations. These results were robust to stability tests.

In this study, we investigated the relationships of depression, multiple chronic diseases, and other factors. We aimed to explore if the networks diverge across time in our sample and what specific roles these factors have in these networks. we didn't find any significant differences in network structure or global strength across depression, multiple chronic diseases network comparisons based on the network comparisons between year 2011 and 2018. "Heart Attack", "Chronic Lung Diseases", "stroke", "Memory-Related Disease" and "Depression" have showed to be statistically stronger than almost all the other nodes in the network.

Finally, our findings have some limitations. The data analyzed here is from CHARLS study which also provided the survey weight to make the sample nationally representative. We haven't used the survey weights in this study. Secondly, the network may have more complex structure which could include more items such as demographic variables and lifestyle styles etc. Additional research should test if our results here could be replicated after taking in more variables.

References

1. Bibring, E.: The mechanism of depression. In: Greenacre, P. (ed.) Affective Disorders; Psychoanalytic Contributions to Their Study, pp. 13–48. International Universities Press, New York (1953)
2. Tinetti, M.E., Fried, T.R., Boyd, C.M.: Designing health care for the most common chronic condition multimorbidity. JAMA 307(23), 2493–2494 (2012). https://doi.org/10.1001/jama.2012.5265
3. Sinnige, J., Braspenning, J., Schellevis, F., Stirbu-Wagner, I., Westert, G., et al.: The prevalence of disease clusters in older adults with multiple chronic diseases – a systematic literature review. PLoS ONE 8(11), e79641 (2013). https://doi.org/10.1371/journal.pone.0079641
4. Hevey, D.: Network analysis: a brief overview and tutorial. Health Psychol. Behav. Med. 6(1), 301–328 (2018). https://doi.org/10.1080/21642850.2018.1521283
5. Zhao, Y., Hu, Y., Smith, J.P., John, S., Yang, G.: Cohort profile: the China health and retirement longitudinal study (CHARLS). Int. J. Epidemiol. (1), 61. https://doi.org/10.1093/ije/dys203
6. Shaffer, J.A., et al.: Depressive symptoms are not associated with leukocyte telomere length: findings from the Nova Scotia Health Survey (NSHS95), a population-based study. PLoS ONE 7(10), e48318 (2012)
7. Palinkas, L.A., Wingard, D.L., Barrett-Connor, E.: Chronic illness and depressive symptoms in the elderly: a population-based study 43(11), 1131–1141 (1990). https://doi.org/10.1016/0895-4356(90)90014-G
8. Zhang, S., Du, L., Jin, G., et al.: Investigation of depression status and cognitive situation of depressive mood among elderly patients with chronic diseases in the community. Chin. General Pract. Med. 2011(16). https://doi.org/10.3969/j.issn.1007-9572.2011.16.026

9. Chen, L., Wu, C., Peng, C., Li, W.: A study on the association between chronic diseases and depressive symptoms in Chinese middle-aged and elderly individuals over 45 years old. Med. Soc. **2021**(10), 90–94+99

10. Heeringa, S.G., Connor, J.H.: Technical Description of the Health and Retirement Survey Sample Design. Institute for Social Research, University of Michigan, Ann Arbor (1999)

11. Schnittker, J.: Chronic illness and depressive symptoms in late life **60**(1), 13–23 (2005). https://doi.org/10.1016/j.socscimed.2004.04.020

12. Birk, J.L., Kronish, I.M., Moise, N., Falzon, L., Yoon, S., Davidson, K.W.: Depression and multimorbidity: considering temporal characteristics of the associations between depression and multiple chronic diseases. Health Psychol. **38**(9), 802–811 (2019). https://doi.org/10.1037/hea0000737

13. Meng, L., Chen, D., Yang, Y., Zheng, Y., Hui, R.: Depression increases the risk of hypertension incidence: a meta-analysis of prospective cohort studies. J. Hypertens. **30**, 842–851 (2012). https://doi.org/10.1097/HJH.0b013e32835080b7

14. Patten, S.B., Williams, J.V., Lavorato, D.H., Modgill, G., Jetté, N., Eliasziw, M.: Major depression as a risk factor for chronic disease incidence: longitudinal analyses in a general population cohort. Gen. Hosp. Psychiatry **30**, 407–413 (2008). https://doi.org/10.1016/j.genhosppsych.2008.05.001

15. Zhao, Y., Hu, Y., Smith, J.P., Strauss, J., Yang, G.: Cohort profile: the China health and retirement longitudinal study (CHARLS). Int. J. Epidemiol. **43**(1), 61–68 (2014)

16. Zhao, Y., et al.: China Health and Retirement Longitudinal Study Wave 4 User's Guide. National School of Development, Peking University, Beijing (2020)

17. Chen, H., Mui, A.C.: Factorial validity of the center for epidemiologic studies depression scale short form in older population in China. Int. Psychogeriatr. **26**, 49–57 (2014)

18. Fruchterman, T.M., Reingold, E.M.: Graph drawing by force directed placement. Software **21**, 1129–1164 (1991). https://doi.org/10.1002/spe.4380211102

19. Tibshirani, R.: Regression shrinkage and selection via the lasso. J. R. Stat. Soc. Ser. B (Methodol.) **58**, 267–288 (1996)

20. Williams, D., Rhemtulla, M., Wysocki, A.C., Rast, P.: On nonregularized estimation of psychological networks. Multivar. Behav. Res. **54**, 719–750 (2019)

21. Epskamp, S., Borsboom, D., Fried, E.I.: Estimating psychological networks and their accuracy: a tutorial paper. Behav. Res. **50**, 195–212 (2018). https://doi.org/10.3758/s13428-017-0862-1

Exploring Etiology of Nonsuicidal Self-injury by Using Knowledge Graph Approach

Zhisheng Huang[1,2,3,6], Xiyan Zhang[1], Fazhan Chen[1(✉)], Mengmeng Zhang[4], Haojie Fu[5], Qianqian Wu[6], and Xudong Zhao[1]

[1] Clinical Research Center for Mental Disorders, Shanghai Pudong New Area Mental Health Center, Tongji University School of Medicine, Shanghai, China
develop909@163.com, zhaoxd@tongji.edu.cn
[2] Department of AI, VU University Amsterdam, Amsterdam, The Netherlands
huang@cs.vu.nl
[3] Deep Blue Technology Group, Shanghai, China
[4] Department of Psychosomatic Medicine, Shanghai East Hospital, School of Medicine, Tongji University, Shanghai, China
chinaykcat@tongji.edu.cn
[5] Shanghai Research Institute for Intelligent Autonomous Systems, Tongji University, Shanghai, China
fuhaojie@tongji.edu.cn
[6] Haoxinqing Health Industry Group, Beijing, China

Abstract. Non-suicidal Self-Injury (NSSI) refers to the intentional destruction of one's own body tissue without suicidal intent and for purposes not socially sanctioned. Although many scholars have done a lot of research on NSSI, and there exist large literature on the research of NSSI. But there still lacks a comprehensive picture on the etiology of NSSI. Knowledge Graphs have become an important AI approach to integrating various types of complex knowledge and data resources. We have constructed Knowledge Graphs of NSSI. It integrates a wide range of knowledge resources related to NSSI, including metadata of medical literature, and their semantic annotations with well-known medical terminologies/ontologies such as SNOMED CT and UMLS. It provides a basic integration foundation of knowledge and data concerning NSSI for a comprehensive analysis. In this paper, we will show that Knowledge Graphs are useful for integrating multiple medical knowledge sources, and how Knowledge Graphs can be used for exploring the etiology of NSSI and gain a comprehensive analysis on the targeted problems.

1 Introduction

Nonsuicidal Self-Injury (NSSI) refers to the intentional destruction of one's own body tissue without suicidal intent and for purposes not socially sanctioned [1]. Common behaviours of NSSI include cutting, burning, scratching and banging

Y. Li et al. (Eds.): HIS 2023, LNCS 14305, pp. 40–49, 2023.
https://doi.org/10.1007/978-981-99-7108-4_4

or hitting, and most people who self-injure have used multiple methods [2]. Etiology refers to the study of the causes of a particular disease or condition [3]. In other words, it is the study of the factors or events that lead to the development of a disease or condition. Etiology can involve a wide range of factors, such as genetic, environmental, lifestyle, and psychological factors, and it can vary depending on the particular disease or condition being studied. Understanding the etiology of a disease is important for developing effective prevention, diagnosis, and treatment strategies. Although many scholars have done a lot of research on NSSI, and there exist large literature on the research of NSSI. But there still lacks a comprehensive picture on the etiology of NSSI [4].

The study of etiology in the context of self-injury behavior involves examining the factors or causes that contribute to the development and maintenance of self-injurious behaviors. This can include various factors such as psychological, social, environmental, and biological factors. The research on the etiology of self-injury behavior has identified a range of potential risk factors, such as past trauma or abuse, impulsivity, negative self-image, and difficulty regulating emotions [5]. It has also identified potential protective factors, such as social support, positive coping skills, and effective emotion regulation strategies.

Overall, the study of etiology in the context of self-injury behavior is important for developing a better understanding of this complex behavior and for improving treatment outcomes for those who engage in self-injury. Thus, it is meaningful to study the etiology of NSSI. In this paper, we will propose an approach of knowledge graph to exploring the etiology of NSSI.

The term "Knowledge Graph" is widely used to refer to a large scale semantic network consisting of entities and concepts as well as the semantic relationships among them, using representation languages such as RDF and RDF Schema [6]. Such knowledge graphs are used in the construction of many knowledge-based applications in medicine, such as extracting information from patient records [7], support for co-morbidity analysis [8], data integration on drugs and their interactions [9], and many others.

We have constructed Knowledge Graphs of NSSI, or alternatively called NSSI Knowledge Graphs (NSSIKG). The NSSIKG integrates a variety of knowledge resources related to NSSI, including medical literature, and clinical ontology knowledge bases such as SNOMED CT in clinical medical concept terminology, etc. By constructing Knowledge Graphs of NSSI, comprehensive knowledge can be effectively transformed into well-structured knowledge. It enables us to adopt a knowledge base method and obtain corresponding knowledge quickly and accurately through semantic queries. It provides well-structured data infrastructure for clinical decision support.

In this paper, we describe how Knowledge Graphs of NSSI can be constructed, investigate how we can use Knowledge Graphs of NSSI to explore various aspects of NSSI. In particular we will show how to explore the relations between a mental state and a NSSI behavior to detect an etiology of NSSI. The main contributions of this paper are: (i) We show how to construct Knowledge Graphs of NSSI, ii) We present that Knowledge Graphs can provide a more efficient way on the literature retrieval for the study of NSSI, iii) We show that Knowledge Graphs can be used to explore the etiology of NSSI, in particular, for the analysis of NSSI which is related with mental states of the patients.

The rest of paper is organized as follows: First We illustrate the general ideas of Knowledge Graphs in Sect. 2. In Sect. 3, we introduce the general architecture of Knowledge Graphs of NSSI to show how to integrate various knowledge/data resources about the knowledge and data-sources about NSSI. In Sect. 4 we show a case study how to use Knowledge Graphs for the literature retrieval and semantic analysis on the etiology of NSSI which is related with mental states of patients, before concluding the paper in Sect. 5.

2   Knowledge Graphs

We construct our knowledge graph as an RDF graph. Formally, an RDF graph is a collection of triples $\langle s, p, o \rangle$, each consisting of a subject s, a predicate p and an object o. Each triple represents a statement of a relationship p between the things denoted by the nodes s and o that it links. Identifiers for both p, s and o are URI's (Uniform Resource Identifier), allowing triples in one knowledge graph to refer to elements in another knowledge graph that resides in a physically different location.

The languages RDF and RDF Schema [6] assign a fixed semantics to some of the predicates p. Examples of these are the predicates `rdf:type` to denote membership of a type, `rdfs:subClassOf` to denote (transitive) containment of subclasses, `rdfs:domain` and `rdfs:range` to denote membership of any subject resp. object of a given predicate to a specified type.

A knowledge graph $KG(T)$ is a set of connected triple set T. Here is a simple example which states some semantic relations concerning the concepts in SNOMED CT:

```
snomed:307578000 rdfs:subClassOf snomed:248073004.
snomed:248073004 rdfs:subClassOf snomed:248062006.
snomed:307578000  sct:hasEnglishLabel "Cutting own wrists".
snomed:248073004  sct:hasEnglishLabel "Cutting self".
snomed:248073004  sct:hasEnglishLabel "Cuts self".
snomed:248073004  sct:hasEnglishLabel "Cutting self (finding)".
......
```

These triples state that the concept `cutting own wrists` is a sub-concept `Cutting self`, and the concept `Cutting self` is a `Self-injurious behaviour`, and the concept `Self-injurious behaviour` has multiple synonyms such as `Self-harm`, `Deliberate self-harm`, and others.

3   Knowledge Graphs of NSSI

In the present version (version0.5) of Knowledge Graphs of NSSI, we focus on the following knowledge/data resources:

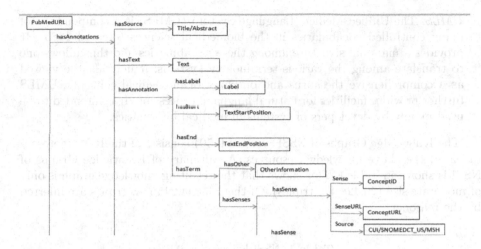

Fig. 1. Structure of Semantic Annotation

- *PubMed.* We used the keyword "NSSI" to search for publications in PubMed[1] obtained the 6440 publications. Removing those publications without the abstract results in the first groups of publications (3679 articles). Furthermore, we use MeSH term "self-injury behaviour/etiology" search for the publications in PubMed obtained 2236 publications. Removing those publications without an abstract results in the second group publications (1617 articles). There are 351 redundant articles on those two groups of articles. Those PubMed data set contains the meta data of a publication, which includes the information about author, title of paper, journal name, publication date, abstract of the paper, PubMed ID (PMID), DOI, and its MeSH Terms. We converted the XML meta-data of PubMed which are downloaded from the PubMed website into RDF Ntriple Data.
- *Semantic Annotations of the articles with NLP.* We used the NLP tool developed by Ztone and XMedlan [10, 11] for semantically annotating medical text (both concept identification and relation extraction) with medical terminologies such as SNOMED CT and UMLS.
  The triple structure of the semantic annotation is shown in Fig. 1.
- *SNOMED CT.* SNOMED CT integrates key terminology, classification and coding standards. SNOMED CT or SNOMED Clinical Terms is a systematically organized computer-processable collection of medical terms providing codes, terms, synonyms and definitions used in clinical documentation and reporting. SNOMED CT is considered to be the most comprehensive, multilingual clinical healthcare terminology in the world.
  SNOMED CT provides the core general terminology for electronic health records. SNOMED CT comprehensive coverage includes: clinical findings, symptoms, diagnoses, procedures, body structures, organisms and others.

---

[1] https://www.ncbi.nlm.nih.gov/pubmed/?term=NSSI.

– *UMLS.* The Unified Medical Language System (UMLS) is a compendium of many controlled vocabularies in the biomedical sciences (created 1986). It provides a mapping structure among these vocabularies and thus allows one to translate among the various terminology systems; it may also be viewed as a comprehensive thesaurus and ontology of biomedical concepts. UMLS further provides facilities for natural language processing. It is intended to be used mainly by developers of systems in medical informatics.

The Knowledge Graphs of NSSI (version 0.50) consists of the RDF representation of the above knowledge resources. A summary of Knowledge Graphs of NSSI is shown in Table 1. This shows that the resulting knowledge graph is only of moderate size (20,428,470 triples). Of them 3,844,245 new triples are inferred by the reasoner.

Table 1. NSSI KG version 0.5

Knowledge Resource	Number of Data Item	Number of Triple
PubMed on NSSI	4,945 papers	276,066
Semantic Annotation on NSSI	4,945 papers	385,934
SNOMED CT		4,291,226
UMLS (partial)		5,045,225
Total (Explicit)		**16,584,225**
Total (Inferred)		**3,844,245**
Total		**20,428,470**

4   Case Study: Semantic Analysis on the Etiology of NSSI Related with Mental States

There are various Etiology of NSSI, which cover emotional dys-regulation, trauma. interpersonal difficulties, dysfunctional family, and many others. Of them, emotional dys-regulation is a common underlying factor in NSSI [12]. It means the difficulties in managing and regulating intense emotions, such as anger, sadness, or anxiety [13]. People who struggle with emotional dys-regulation may experience emotions more intensely than others, and they may have difficulty coping with these emotions in healthy ways [14].

For example, if someone is feeling overwhelmed by anxiety or distress, they may turn to NSSI as a way to cope with the emotional pain. The physical pain of self-injury can provide a temporary distraction from emotional distress and can even release endorphins, which can have a calming effect on the body. However, this relief is often temporary, and the underlying emotional distress remains [15,16].

It is trivial to know that NSSI is relevant with various mental states such as anger and sadness. However, there are many different concepts concerning mental states and many different concepts concerning self-injury behaviors. For example, there are 1,994 different concepts of mental states, and 82 different concepts concerning self-injury in SNOMED CT. We want to gain more exact relevance measure on those various relations concerning mental states and concrete self-injury behaviours. That would be helpful for us to detect the etiology of NSSI due to emotional dys-regulation. That can be achieved by using the knowledge graph approach with the exploration of the concept co-occurrence of two kinds of concepts.

First we are interested in which self-injury behaviour are most frequently occurrence in NSSI. The semantic query is designed as follows:

```
PREFIX ......
select distinct  (COUNT(?t1s1) AS ?count) ?selfinjury ?label
where {?selfinjury rdfs:subClassOf snomed:248062006.
?t1s1 ztonekg:SenseURL ?selfinjury.
?selfinjury sct:hasEnglishPreferredLabel ?label.
FILTER (?selfinjury!=snomed:248061004)}
GROUP BY ?selfinjury  ?label
ORDER BY DESC(?count)
```

We obtain the following results:

```
?count ?selfinjury ?label
88 SCT_248072009 Biting self (finding)
55 SCT_43954004 Head-banging
8 SCT_248069002 Biting own hand (finding)
6 SCT_248070001 Head-hitting (finding)
6 SCT_284756003 Hitting self (finding)
3 SCT_248073004 Cutting self (finding)
2 SCT_225048008 Jumping from height
```

By the semantic query on SNOMED CT, we know that there are 1,991 mental states in that medical ontology. We also know that there are 244 mental related concepts which are used in the semantic annotation of the NSSI literature. Furthermore, we are interested in those top 100 mental states which have been used in the semantic annotations of the NSSI literature. We can make a semantic query as follows:

```
PREFIX ...
select distinct  (COUNT(?t1s1) AS ?count) ?mentalRelated ?label
where {?mentalRelated rdfs:subClassOf snomed:384821006.
?t1s1 ztonekg:SenseURL ?mentalRelated.
?mentalRelated sct:hasEnglishLabel ?label.
FILTER (?mentalRelated!=snomed:106126000)}
GROUP BY ?mentalRelated  ?label
ORDER BY DESC(?count) LIMIt 100
```

The first triple pattern states that we try to obtain all sub-concepts of the mental related concept with the top ID snomed:384821006. The second triple pattern states that we are interested in those have been used in the semantic annotations. The third triple pattern is used to the corresponding concept labels. The fourth line in the semantic query is used to remove the trivial answer. The query result is sorted with the decreasing order on the counts of the occurrences in the NSSI literature. We obtain the following result:

```
?count ?MentalState
1475 Depression, 545 Anxiety
509 Autism, 444 Stress
269 Motivation finding, 227 Victim of abuse
...
100 Phobia
...
```

From the query results we know that depression is the most relevant mental states wich NSSI, followed with the mental states Anxiety, Autism, and Stress, and others.

We are much more interested in the relevance between a mental state and a self-injury behavior. That semantic query can be designed as follows to check the co-occurrence of mental states and self-injury, which is achieved by the tracking on the structures of the semantic annotations with the co-occurrence of two kinds of concept classes (i.e., mental states and self-injury).

```
PREFIX ......
select  ?selfinjuryid ?mentalstateid (COUNT(distinct ?pubmed) as ?count)
where {?selfinjuryid rdfs:subClassOf snomed:248062006.
?t1s1 ztonekg:SenseURL ?selfinjuryid.
?t1 ztonekg:hasSense ?t1s1. ?s7 ztonekg:hasSenses ?t1.
?s ztonekg:hasTerm ?s7. ?s1 ztonekg:hasAnnotation ?s.
?pubmed ztonekg:hasAnnotations ?s1.
?pubmed ztonekg:hasAnnotations ?s1b.
?s1b ztonekg:hasAnnotation ?sb.
?sb ztonekg:hasTerm ?s7b. ?s7b ztonekg:hasSenses ?t1b.
?t1b ztonekg:hasSense ?t1s1b.
?t1s1b ztonekg:SenseURL ?mentalstateid.
?mentalstateid rdfs:subClassOf snomed:384821006.}
GROUP BY ?selfinjuryid ?mentalstateid
ORDER by DESC(?count)
```

The result of the semantic query is shown as follows:

```
?selfinjury ?mentalstate ?count
Self-harm (finding) Depression 348
Self-harm (finding) Morose mood 348
Self-harm (finding) Sad 348
Self-harm (finding) Suicidal thoughts 241
Self-harm (finding) Suicidal behaviour 208
......
```

In particular we are more interested in non-trivial relation between a concrete self injury behavior and a mental state as follows:

```
Biting self  Anxiety 5,  Biting self  Autism 5
Head-banging Autism 5, Biting self  Depression 3
Biting self Stress 3, Biting self  Sad 3
Head-banging Anxiety 2, Hitting self  Anxiety 2
......
```

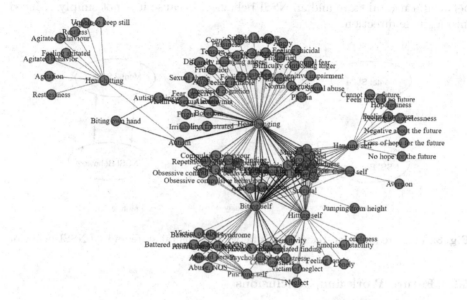

Fig. 2. Relevance between mental state and NSSI

From the query result above we know that the anxiety and autism are the most relevant mental state which would lead to biting self, an NSSI behaviour. The main reason for head banging is also Autism. Depression and Stress would lead to biting self. Those relations are shown in Fig. 2.

5   Discussion and Conclusion

5.1   Discussion

Causality Versus Relevance. Etiology is the study of the causes or origins of a particular disease, condition, or disorder, whereas Causality is the relationship between a cause and an effect. In other words, causality is concerned with identifying whether one variable (the cause) has a direct influence on another variable (the effect). In the semantic analysis of this paper, we just explore the co-occurrence of a mental state and a self-injury behavior. Namely we just use the relevance checking approach, rather than the causality approach.

There are three readings of the relations between a mental state and an NSSI behavior: (a) Relevance, namely, the relevance relation between a mental state and an NSSI behavior. (b) Causality, namely, a mental state would lead to an NSSI behavior, and (c) Mutual causality. Namely, a mental state has some impact on an NSSI behavior and an NSSI behavior may also have an impact on a mental state. Those three relations are shown in Fig. 3. We consider the third relation (i.e. mutual causality) is more meaningful to explore the relation between a mental state and an NSSI behavior, because it is not simply reduced into a single direction.

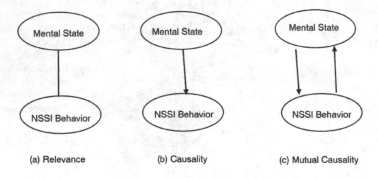

Fig. 3. Three readings on the relations between a mental state and an NSSI behavior

5.2   Future Work and Conclusions

In the future work we will justify the detected relations between mental states and an NSSI behavior with clinical data and patient data. We will extend the Knowledge Graphs of NSSI with more knowledge/data resources such as clinical trial data and the drug data. Furthermore, we will explore other types of Etiology concerning NSSI behaviors.

In this paper We have introduced a method for constructing a Knowledge Graphs of NSSI. Through the knowledge/data integration technology based on semantic technology, we can integrate various knowledge/data resources of NSSI that have been loosely connected into a well-structured ones, thereby providing a data infrastructure for exploring various aspects of NSSI. We have shown a case study to support the idea how Knowledge Graphs of NSSI can be used for efficient semantic analysis.

References

1. Hamza, C., Stewart, S., Willoughby, T.: Examining the link between nonsuicidal self-injury and suicidal behavior: a review of the literature and an integrated model. Clin. Psychol. Rev. **32**(6), 482–495 (2012)

2. Garisch, J.A., Wilson, M.S.: Prevalence, correlates, and prospective predictors of non-suicidal self-injury among New Zealand adolescents: cross-sectional and longitudinal survey data. Child Adolesc. Psychiatry Ment. Health **9**, 28 (2015)
3. Karp, I., Miettinen, O.S.: On the essentials of etiological research for preventive medicine. Eur. J. Epidemiol. **29**(7), 455–457 (2014). https://doi.org/10.1007/s10654-014-9928-x
4. Cipriano, A., Cella, S., Cotrufo, P.: Nonsuicidal self-injury: a systematic review. Front. Psychol. **8**, 1946 (2017)
5. Horváth, L.O., et al.: Nonsuicidal self-injury and suicide: the role of life events in clinical and non-clinical populations of adolescents. Front. Psychiatry **11**, 370 (2020)
6. Cyganiak, R., Wood, D., Lanthaler, M.: RDF 1.1 concepts and abstract syntax (2014)
7. Goodwin, T., Harabagi, S.M.: Automatic generation of a qualified medical knowledge graph and its usage for retrieving patient cohorts from electronic medical records. In: IEEE Seventh International Conference on Semantic Computing (2013)
8. Zamborlini, V., Hoekstra, R., Silveira, M.D., Pruski, C., ten Teije, A., van Harmelen, F.: Inferring recommendation interactions in clinical guidelines. Semant. Web **7**(4), 421–446 (2016)
9. Jovanovik, M., Trajanov, D.: Consolidating drug data on a global scale using linked data. J. Biomed. Semant. **8**(1), 3 (2017)
10. Ait-Mokhtar, S., Bruijn, B.D., Hagege, C., Rupi, P.: Intermediary-stage IE components, D3.5. Technical report, EURECA Project (2014)
11. Khiari, A.: Identification of variants of compound terms, master thesis. Technical report, Université Paul Sabatier, Toulouse (2015)
12. Adrian, M., et al.: Emotional dysregulation and interpersonal difficulties as risk factors for nonsuicidal self-injury in adolescent girls. J. Abnorm. Child Psychol. **39**(3), 389–400 (2011)
13. Faraone, S.V., et al.: Practitioner review: Emotional dysregulation in attention-deficit/hyperactivity disorder - implications for clinical recognition and intervention. J. Child Psychol. Psychiatry **60**(2), 133–150 (2019)
14. Johnstone, J.M., et al.: Development of a composite primary outcome score for children with attention-deficit/hyperactivity disorder and emotional dysregulation. J. Child Adolesc. Psychopharmacol. **30**, 166–172 (2020)
15. Wang, X., Huang, X., Huang, X., Zhao, W.: Parents' lived experience of adolescents' repeated non-suicidal self-injury in china: a qualitative study. BMC Psychiatry **22**(1), 70 (2022)
16. Zhang, Y., et al.: A heterogeneous multi-modal medical data fusion framework supporting hybrid data exploration. Health Inf. Sci. Syst. **10**(1), 22 (2022)

A Question and Answering System for Mental Health of the Elderly Based on BiLSTM-CRF Model and Knowledge Graph

Beijia He[1], Shaofu Lin[1(✉)], Zhisheng Huang[2,3,4], and Chaogui Guo[1]

[1] Faculty of Information Technology, Beijing University of Technology, Beijing 100124, China
linshaofu@bjut.edu.cn
[2] Department of Computer Science, Vrije University Amsterdam, Amsterdam, Netherlands
[3] Clinical Research Center for Mental Disorders, Shanghai Pudong New Area Mental Health Center, Tongji University School of Medicine, Shanghai, China
[4] Deep Blue Technology Group, Shanghai, China

Abstract. Currently, the aging population in China is becoming increasingly severe. Research has shown that 85% of the elderly have varying degrees of psychological problems, and 27% of the elderly have obvious psychological disorders such as anxiety and depression. The demand for offline and online consultation and intervention services is becoming increasingly urgent. However, there is currently a lack of systematic mental health intervention strategies targeting the elderly in relevant research and application practices. In order to explore new intervention services such as online consultation and chat with the elderly on mental health, a prototype system of question and answering for the elderly mental health has been designed, focusing on providing the elderly and related caregivers with daily psychological counseling services for the elderly. Firstly, a public mental health Q&A dataset has been collected, and then the data have been manually screened to obtain mental health Q&A dataset for the elderly. Based on this dataset, combined with the semantic data related to neurology for the elderly, the knowledge graph of mental health of the elderly has been constructed. Then, the problem matching module has been used to determine and analyze the types of problems faced by the elderly and generate corresponding answers to the questions. For the questions related to psychological counseling of the elderly, the BERT and BiLSTM-CRF network have been used to calculate the question template closest to the user's question in the system, and find the corresponding answer matching the question in the knowledge graph. The experimental results show that the system can effectively understand the intention of elderly users to ask questions, and has good accuracy and reliability in answering elderly mental health related questions, which helps to address the mental health service needs of the elderly.

Keywords: The Elderly Mental Health · Deep Learning · Knowledge Graph · Question and Answering System

1 Introduction

The global population is aging, and life expectancy is on the rise. With the increasing growth rate of the global elderly population (aged 60 and above), the mental health issues of the group need to be given sufficient attention [1]. The huge incidence rate of mental health in the aged population has led to a higher number of mental health care service consumers. Therefore, the demand for mental health care is also increasing. The Sustainable Development Goals adopted by the Member States of the United Nations emphasize the health and well-being of everyone, including the elderly [2].

People have many misunderstandings, stigmatization, and discrimination towards mental illnesses and structural barriers such as a lack of personal and financial resources, which make them unwilling to seek help from mental health professionals [3]. Therefore, it is of great significance to construct and develop a prototype of a question and answering method for the mental health of the elderly.

The knowledge graph was proposed by Google in 2012 and is a structured semantic knowledge base used to describe concepts and their interrelationships in the physical world in symbolic form. Its basic unit of composition is the "entity-relationship-entity" triplet, as well as entities and their related attribute value pairs [4]. At present, there are many researches on question and answering. Philip Indra Prayitno et al. [5] made a Chatbot system using NLP (Natural Language Processing), which could understand and answer the questions raised by users. Cosine similarity was used to find the similarity between query words (user raised questions) and documents, and then return the answer of the document with the highest similarity. Ziming Wu [6] proposed a text matching method based on pre-training BERT (Bidirectional Encoder Representation from Transformers) model and enhanced tree model, which achieved good results in Chinese medicine question and answer tasks. Research on question and answering based on knowledge graph has gradually changed from previous research based on semantic analysis to research on knowledge graph question and answering based on in-depth learning of information extraction [7]. Document [8] proposed to apply the representation learning method of word vector to question and answering based on knowledge graph.

In this paper, crawler technology is used to crawl online public questions and answers related to mental health of the elderly. At the same time, psychological counseling related questions and answers have been collected and screened to extract question and answer data specific to the elderly. For the knowledge graph question and answering method with weak dependency information, the BERT and BiLSTM-CRF (Bi-directional Long Short-Term Memory-Conditional Random Field) networks have been used to extract the named entity in the question, and the triple group information related to the entity is located in the knowledge graph. By using an answer matching network, the similarity score of the answers in the triplet set is marked, and a threshold selection strategy has been used to select answers that meet the requirements.

The rest content of this article is organized as follows. The second section describes the data sources and data processing process, the third section describes the research methods, the fourth section displays and analyzes the experimental results, and the fifth section makes the conclusion.

2 Data Resources and Data Processing

2.1 Data Resources

Using information crawler technology, we have crawled the dada on the introduction of mental health diseases of the elderly in the psychiatry and neurology departments in the "https://www.dxy.cn/", and also crawled the question-answer pairs of disease descriptions of the neurology department and the psychiatry department in the "Dr. Dingxiang". There are 358 pairs of question and answering data in the dataset. After standardized processing, the obtained data have been converted into RDF format and stored in the knowledge graph of mental health of the elderly (Table 1).

Table 1. Dataset 1

ID	Question	Answer
1	What is Alzheimer's disease?	Alzheimer's disease (AD) is a slowly onset and progressive neurodegenerative disorder of the nervous system. More common in the elderly, it is the primary cause of dementia in the elderly, clinically characterized by decreased memory, decreased intelligence, and changes in personality and behavioral patterns. In the later stage, one may completely lose the ability to live independently
2	Which department should I visit for Alzheimer's disease?	Internal Medicine-Neurology
...	...	...
358	What is delirium in old age?	Senile delirium refers to a state of delirium or blurred consciousness that occurs in the elderly, resulting in a decrease in the patient's ability to recognize and respond to objective environments, inattention, disorientation, increased speech, incoherent thinking

In addition, Q&A data on psychological counseling have been also collected. After removing duplicate and unusable data, a total of 71739 pairs of question and answering data have been obtained. Then the obtained data have been converted into RDF format after standardizing (Table 2).

Table 2. Dataset 2

ID	Question	Answer
1	What should I do if I have a tendency towards depression?	It is necessary to seek medical attention from the hospital's psychological department. Psychological and medication treatment is necessary, which can be taken with sertraline hydrochloride or amitriptyline hydrochloride tablets. This can control the disease, and it can be treated under the guidance of a psychologist
2	What is the impact of a pregnant woman's bad mood on the fetus?	poor mood can lead to decreased appetite, insomnia, and other problems, which may have some indirect effects. Therefore, it is still important to pay attention to adjusting emotions through some interests and hobbies
...	...	...
71739	Hello doctor, I have been experiencing frequent insomnia recently. Often feeling tired	your situation is considered to be related to neurasthenia and autonomic dysfunction. It is recommended to take orally oryzanol, vitamin B1, and Anshen Buxin Pills

2.2 Data Processing

The collected question and answer data have been manually screened, for example, the question and answering data such as "What's the impact of a pregnant woman's bad mood on the fetus?", "Typical signs of adolescent depression?" have been deleted, and 35168 pairs of question and answering data for the elderly have been obtained and stored in the "knowledge graph of Mental Health for the Elderly". The processed data is shown in the table below (Table 3):

Table 3. Dataset 3

ID	Question	Answer
1	What should I do if I have a tendency towards depression?	It is necessary to seek medical attention from the hospital's psychological department. Psychological and medication treatment is necessary, which can be taken with sertraline hydrochloride or amitriptyline hydrochloride tablets. This can control the disease, and it can be treated under the guidance of a psychologist
2	What does panic and depression mean?	The term 'panic depression' is actually very imprecise, and depression belongs to a mental illness. The state of depression caused by this emotion is actually not only manifested as palpitations, but also discomfort from head to toe
...	...	...
35168	Hello doctor, I have been experiencing frequent insomnia recently. Often feeling tired	your situation is considered to be related to neurasthenia and autonomic dysfunction. It is recommended to take orally oryzanol, vitamin B1, and Anshen Buxin Pills

3   Research Methods

3.1   The Elderly Mental Health Question and Answering System

Question and answering system includes question input module, named-entity recognition module, knowledge graph module and answer matching module. The structure of the question and answering system is shown in Fig. 1:

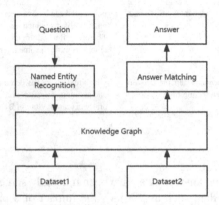

Fig. 1. Framework of question and answering system

The BERT network + BiLSTM-CRF network model is used to conduct named-entity recognition. First, the BERT pre-training language model converts unstructured text data about mental health problems of the elderly and related psychological counseling questions into vector form. Then the BiLSTM model further extracts the context features in the questions. Finally, constraints are added through CRF to reduce the generation of error sequences, and the final marking sequence is output.

3.2   Named-Entity Recognition

Named-entity recognition is a classic task in natural language processing and a sub-task of sequence tagging [9]. It achieves entity extraction by marking the corresponding entity information for each position of the input text. The entity is marked with BIO and BIOES modes [10]. This article adopts the BIO pattern for entity labeling. B-x represents the beginning of entity x, I-x represents the middle or end of entity x, and O represents non entity content. Since the question and answering of the mental health studied in this paper only involves a single entity, only one entity type ENT is defined.

The network model of named-entity recognition is shown in Fig. 2, which mainly includes feature extraction and entity annotation. In the process of feature extraction, the input psychological counseling question with a length of mm is divided into word sequences $\{m_1, m_2, ..., m_w\}$ and sent to the BERT network to obtain w word vectors after word segmentation and word embedding. After feature extraction of transform encoder in T layer, feature matrix with sequence length of w and hidden layer width of d is obtained to complete feature extraction [11]. Firstly, the feature matrix is input into the BiLSTM layer, with t neurons in each direction to further extract the semantic association information of the context. The feature vector passes through a layer of feedforward neural network, and the vector with length and width of w is obtained through linear transformation as the number of types to be marked, which is used as the input of CRF layer.

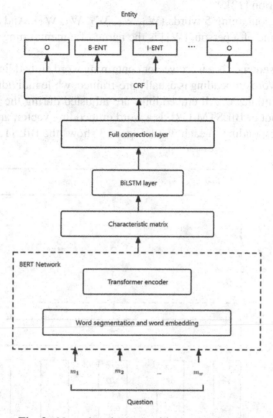

Fig. 2. Named-entity recognition network model

Since this article only defines one entity type, the vector width is 3, representing the state scores of B, I, and O, respectively. At the CRF level, the random field statistical model of the linear chain part calculates the output tag sequence with the maximum conditional probability through the input feature sequence. By analyzing the output annotation sequence, the start and end positions of entities can be located. In the BiLSTM-CRF network, for the input vector i, the corresponding output is j, and its score calculation is as follows:

$$S(i,j) = \sum_x b_x[j_x] + U[j_{x-1}, j_x] \tag{1}$$

where b denotes the 3D vector output from the BiLSTM layer, U denotes the transfer feature matrix, and $U[j_{x-1}, j_x]$ denotes the output label from j_{x-1} to j_x the transfer score.

3.3 BiLSTM-CRF Model

BiLSTM lacks feature analysis at the whole sentence level, so it needs the help of CRF. However, CRF has the problem of difficulty in extracting features and insufficient applicability. Therefore, CRF and BiLSTM can be combined to ensure that sufficient whole sentence features can be extracted while using effective sequence annotation methods for annotation [12].

L is a sentence containing 5 words (W_0, W_1, W_2, W_3, W_4). And in this sentence, [W_0, W_1] is the name of a person, [W_3] is the name of a mental illness, and all others are 'O'.

Each word in a sentence is a word vector containing word embedding and individual word embedding. Word embedding is usually pre-trained, while individual word embedding is randomly initialized. All embeddings are adjusted during the iterative process of training. The input of BiLSTM-CRF is a word embedding vector, and the output is a prediction tag corresponding to each word. Figure 3 shows the BiLSTM-CRF model.

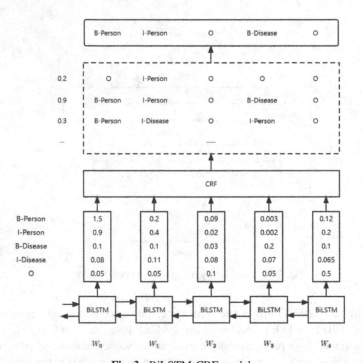

Fig. 3. BiLSTM-CRF model

The input of the BiLSTM layer represents the scores corresponding to each category of the word. These scores are input to the CRF layer. All scores output through the BiLSTM layer are used as inputs to the CRF layer, and the category with the highest score in the category sequence is the final predicted result.

3.4   Answer Matching

After the completion of named-entity recognition, the extracted entity name is used as the key to generate the query statement of the knowledge graph, and then the triple set containing the entity is retrieved and returned to the knowledge graph of mental health for the elderly to prepare for the answer matching. In KBQA (Knowledge-based Question Answering), semantic matching is usually performed between questions and predicates in triples, but semantic match requires the original question pairs contained in training data and specific triplet information [13]. However, task-specific question and answering datasets typically do not have such additional information, requiring extensive manual annotations or special preprocessing methods. The answer matching method proposed in this paper directly matches the question with the answer information, relying only on the original question pair data during training, and calculates the matching degree between the triple answer and the question in the knowledge graph when answering the question. Firstly, the questions are preprocessed by removing named entities to avoid interference from long questions and redundant information in answer matching. Then, the preprocessed questions are matched with the answers in each triplet set, with each answer marked with a similarity score. The similarity score is a value between 0 and 1. Therefore, during the training process, if the input is the correct answer, the corresponding similarity score is marked as 1. Otherwise, the similarity score is marked as 0.

The answer matching network model is shown in Fig. 4. The Q&A begins with the [CLS] notation. In each match, the preprocessed questions and answers are separated by the [SEP] symbol and connected into a sequence.

The feature extraction process of answer matching network is similar to that of named-entity recognition network. After the BERT network process, a feature matrix with a length of (w + t) and a width of d is obtained. Since the last layer of the network is the S-shaped layer, it is a typical output layer of the classful network. Therefore, it is necessary to down sample the feature matrix. Firstly, the most important information in the feature matrix is extracted by using pooling layers. Then, the first column (length d) of the feature matrix is extracted as input for the S-shaped layer. Finally, the activation function of the sigmoid layer is used to output, ensuring that the output of this unit is always between 0 and 1, which is the similarity score.

4   Experimental Results Display and Analysis

4.1   Experimental Setup

This experiment implementation is based on the TensorFlow framework with a 12 layer encoder. The output dimension of each layer's implicit state is 768, and the maximum length of the Chinese problem is 60. Adam algorithm has been used to update and fine tune the parameters of the model, and the initial learning rate is 2E−5. Batch training has been used during the training, with a batch size of 32. The default discard rate is 0.1, the maximum number of iterations is 100, and the model has been saved and the development set is validated every 50 steps during training.

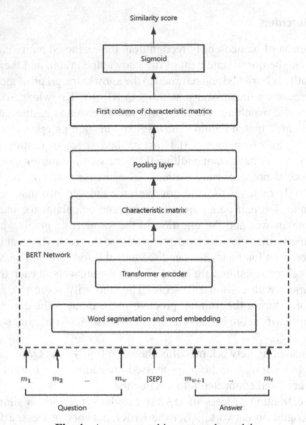

Fig. 4. Answer matching network model

4.2 Implementation and Verification of Question and Answering System

In order to make the operation of question and answering system simpler and more convenient, the front-end interface of the system is developed with Python's standard GUI library to obtain the content of the text box through the Entry in Tkinter, and the content is the questions raised by the users. And then the Button is used to call the function to obtain the answers and display them in the text box.

The question and answering interface in the prototype system is shown in the following figure (Fig. 5):

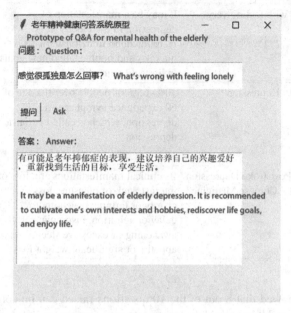

Fig. 5. Display of Q&A system prototype interface

In order to verify the application effect of the designed question and answering system on the elderly mental health, 10 elderly people and their caregivers have been randomly simulated as application objects [14]. Users input their psychological consultation problems into the system, and then investigate and analyze whether their doubts have been solved, so as to judge the actual effect of the system. The following table shows the questions raised by 10 users and the answers returned by the system (Table 4):

Table 4. User Q&A display

ID	Question	Answer	Match or not
1	What's wrong with feeling very lonely?	It may be a manifestation of depression in the elderly. It is recommended to cultivate one's own interests and hobbies, find new goals in life, and enjoy life	Match
2	What is Elderly Depression?	30%–65% of people over the age of 60 experience symptoms of depression, which is called geriatric depression	Match
...	...	...	...
10	How to Treat Poststroke Depression with Traditional Chinese Medicine?	Its clinical manifestations are: loss of interest, lack of pleasure, loss of energy or fatigue, psychomotor delay or agitation, insomnia, early awakening or excessive sleep, loss of appetite or significant weight loss	Match

The results showed that 8 out of the 10 questions raised can be correctly matched with the answers, and it has a high accuracy rate.

The question and answering system combines BERT and BiLSTM-CRF networks to extract named entities in questions, and locate entity related triples in the knowledge graph. Through an answer matching network, the answers in a triplet set are marked as similarity scores [15]. In many application scenarios, question answering tasks require returning a single answer, and threshold selection strategies are used to select the answer that meets the requirements, presenting the answer with the highest similarity to the user. Compared to the Q&A methods in other articles, Literature [7] relies on some manual rules to ensure the performance of Q&A, Literature [16] is not very accurate in certain homogeneous problems. However, the system in this article reduces the need for manual annotation and preprocessing, and has good performance.

5   Conclusion

In order to explore new intervention services such as online consultation and chat with the elderly, we propose a question and answering system for elderly mental health based on BiLSTM-CRF algorithm model. Firstly, the proposed system uses the named-entity recognition network to extract the entities in the problem, and obtains the related triplet set based on the entity name keywords. It then uses an answer matching network to mark the similarity score of each answer. Finally, it filters alternative answers through threshold selection and output the results. The experimental results show that the designed question and answering system protype on elderly mental health weakens the dependence on predicates and other prior information in question and answering data, and has good generalization performance. In the future, the quality of Q&A will be evaluated, benchmark test sets will be standardized, and dialogue history analysis and contextual understanding will be used to determine user intentions, in order to further improve the quality of Q&A.

References

1. Soto, C.S., Ramirez, M.R., Rojas, E.M., Cañas, R.V., Caro, M.S., Moreno, H.B.R.: Mental health of the elderly: towards a proposal for a social simulator based on the complexity approach. In: Chen, YW., Tanaka, S., Howlett, R.J., Jain, L.C. (eds.) Innovation in Medicine and Healthcare. Smart Innovation, Systems and Technologies, vol. 308, pp. 107–115. Springer, Singapore (2022). https://doi.org/10.1007/978-981-19-3440-7_10
2. Pandey, N.M., Tripathi, R.K., Kar, S.K., et al.: Mental health promotion for elderly populations in World Health Organization South-East Asia Region: needs and resource gaps. World J. Psychiatry **12**(1), 117 (2022)
3. Turana, Y., Tengkawan, J., Chia, Y.C., et al.: Mental health problems and hypertension in the elderly: review from the HOPE Asia Network. J. Clin. Hypertens. **23**(3), 504–512 (2021)
4. Wu, Y., Yin, A., Lin, K., et al.: Research on the construction method of knowledge graph based on multiple data sources. J. Fuzhou Univ. (Nat. Sci. Ed.) **45**(03), 329–335 (2017)
5. Prayitno, P.I., Leksono, R.P.P., Chai, F., et al.: Health chatbot using natural language processing for disease prediction and treatment. In: 2021 1st International Conference on Computer Science and Artificial Intelligence (ICCSAI), vol. 1, pp. 62–67. IEEE (2021)
6. Wu, Z., Liang, J., Zhang, Z., et al.: Exploration of text matching methods in Chinese disease Q&A systems: a method using ensemble based on BERT and boosted tree models. J. Biomed. Inform. **115**, 103683 (2021)
7. Tianbo, D.: Implementation and application of intelligent Question answering based on Knowledge graph. Digit. Technol. Appl. **40**(03), 165–167 (2022)
8. Xu, K., Li, C., Tian, Y., et al.: Representation learning on graphs with jumping knowledge networks. In: International Conference on Machine Learning, pp. 5453–5462. PMLR (2018)
9. Xi, Q., Ren, Y., Yao, S., Wu, G., Miao, G., Zhang, Z.: Chinese named entity recognition: applications and challenges. In: Jia, Y., Gu, Z., Li, A. (eds.) MDATA: A New Knowledge Representation Model. LNCS, vol. 12647, pp. 51–81. Springer, Cham (2021). https://doi.org/10.1007/978-3-030-71590-8_4
10. Xu, L., Li, S., Wang, Y., Xu, L.: Named entity recognition of BERT-BiLSTM-CRF combined with self-attention. In: Xing, C., Fu, X., Zhang, Y., Zhang, G., Borjigin, C. (eds.) WISA 2021. LNCS, vol. 12999, pp. 556–564. Springer, Cham (2021). https://doi.org/10.1007/978-3-030-87571-8_48
11. Yan, R., Jiang, X., Dang, D.: Named entity recognition by using XLNet-BiLSTM-CRF. Neural Process. Lett. **53**(5), 3339–3356 (2021)
12. Sarki, R., Ahmed, K., Wang, H., et al.: Convolutional neural network for multi-class classification of diabetic eye disease. EAI Endorsed Trans. Scalable Inf. Syst. **9**(4), e5–e5 (2022)
13. Xiong, H., Wang, S., Tang, M., et al.: Knowledge graph question answering with semantic oriented fusion model. Knowl.-Based Syst. **221**, 106954 (2021)
14. Rehman, O., Al-Busaidi, A.M., Ahmed, S., et al.: Ubiquitous healthcare system: architecture, prototype design and experimental evaluations. EAI Endorsed Trans. Scalable Inf. Syst. **9**(4), e6 (2022)

15. Singh, R., Zhang, Y., Wang, H., et al.: Investigation of social behaviour patterns using location-based data–a Melbourne case study. EAI Endorsed Trans. Scalable Inf. Syst. **8**(31) (2020)
16. Chen, Z., Yin, S., Zhu, X.: Research and implementation of QA system based on the knowledge graph of Chinese classic poetry. In: 2020 IEEE 5th International Conference on Cloud Computing and Big Data Analytics (ICCCBDA), pp. 495–499. IEEE (2020)

Data Security, Privacy and Healthcare Systems

Australia's Notifiable Data Breach Scheme: An Analysis of Risk Management Findings for Healthcare

Martin Dart[✉] ⓘD and Mohiuddin Ahmed ⓘD

School of Science, Edith Cowan University, Joondalup, WA 6027, Australia
m.dart@ecu.edu.au

Abstract. This paper provides an overview of the first five years of data published via the Australian Governments' Notifiable Data Breach (NDB) scheme, operated by the Office of the Australian Information Commissioner (OAIC). Applying investigative techniques including descriptive and inferential statistics, Pareto analysis, distribution analysis, and bivariate correlations it is discovered that 80% of data breach incidents are substantively caused by fives forms of human error, particularly failures in email management. A deeper investigation across each of the periods studied reveals significant correlations often involve insider-based threats, suggesting these can be an indicative predictor for other events such as phishing and ransomware attacks. The included summary of increasing privacy concerns from the public and government-led legislative amendments in Australia, further illustrates the urgency and importance of applying this knowledge to the critical infrastructure of healthcare.

Keywords: Healthcare · Data breach · Cyber security

1 Introduction

There have been many media and industry reports claiming healthcare is the most breached, attacked, or vulnerable industry in Australia [1–3], but seeking confirmatory data beyond the headlines is challenging given the stigma attached to such events. However, learning from data breach mistakes of the past is an important risk management technique [4], and very relevant in the complex field of assuring the digital transformations currently underway in many large Australian healthcare providers (LAHPs).

Khan [5] defines a data breach as, "*a security incident in which sensitive, protected, or confidential data are copied, transmitted, viewed, stolen, or used by an unauthorised individual*", and a similar definition was arrived at by Hendee [6], "*…a confirmed incident in which sensitive, confidential or otherwise protected data has been accessed and/or disclosed in an unauthorised fashion*". Previous analyses of healthcare data breaches [7–9] have tended to rely on figures from the United States due to their 1996 adoption

Y. Li et al. (Eds.): HIS 2023, LNCS 14305, pp. 65–78, 2023.
https://doi.org/10.1007/978-981-99-7108-4_6

of the *Health Insurance Accountability and Portability Act* (HIPAA), which introduced a mandatory data breach reporting scheme. Since implementation began via the Department of Health and Human Services (DHHS) that scheme has recorded 5,501 healthcare incidents over fourteen years, leading to breaches of 435 million patient records [10]. Reviewers of this data include Collins [11] who concluded that the Federal Government legislated approach was essential in ensuring compliance and transparency, and Raghupathi [12] who used a variety of charting and mapping techniques that showed these breach events occurring in every US state.

The United Kingdom also enacted a similar scheme via the *Data Protection Act 2018 (UK)*, with breaches recorded and published by the Information Commissioners Office (ICO). Between 2019–2022 there were 15,629 healthcare breaches recorded in the UK, making it the second most impacted sector in the UK after education [13].

In Australia the *Privacy Act 1988 (Cth)* defines data breaches as, "an act or practice… contrary or inconsistent with any of the Australian Privacy Principles" [14]. Since being amended in 2018 the Act has required many organisations to report such breaches via a mandatory Notifiable Data Breach (NDB) scheme, administered by the Office of the Australian Information Commissioner (OAIC), and this has recorded 929 such incidents occurring in healthcare [15]. Yet while this requirement applies to all private LAHPs in Australia it is not enforceable against all state government agencies delivering public services. This is an important issue to note as it means there is still no single mandatory national scheme, and those exclusions include some of the largest healthcare systems treating millions of patients. This was noted by Hile [16], who concluded that while the Privacy Act and NDB scheme creates in theory an effective liability attribution framework to identify data breaches, it does little to empower impacted individuals with subsequent access to court action or compensation. However, this is a rapidly changing situation and other laws have been tightened (and penalties increased) in response to millions of Australians having their privacy breached via incidents at Optus (telecommunications) and Medibank (health insurance) in 2022 [17]. The most recent major change occurred in 2022 when the Australian Government amended the *Security of Critical Infrastructure Act 2018 (Cth)* to apply to healthcare for the first time, demanding greater risk governance and reporting from LAHP executives including all state entities previously excluded from the Privacy Act [18, 19]. The small sample of media-reported incidents shown at Table 1 illustrates a range of impacts and causes, but to fully understand and manage the risk from data breach events LAHPs need a deeper understanding. This paper uses detailed techniques to analyse the first five years of data from the NDB scheme, to seek conclusions that can practically assist with this.

Table 1. Select Australian healthcare data breaches 2018–2022.

Provider	Incident	Cause	Year
Health Engine	59,600 items of 'patient feedback' accessed [20]	Website misconfiguration	2018
Cabrini Hospital Melbourne Heart Group	15,000 patient records encrypted by malware. Attempts to pay the ransom failed to recover the data [21]	Unpatched systems and malware	2019
Victoria Health	Multiple sites attacked, and numerous systems impacted over several weeks. Multiple surgeries cancelled [22]	Emotet malware	2019
Tasmanian Ambulances	Unencrypted radio transmissions intercepted and posted online [23]	Legacy communications	2021
Eastern Health	Elective surgeries cancelled across 4 Melbourne hospitals [24]	Ransomware	2021
Medibank	A 200Gb database containing approx. 9.7 million customer records stolen [25]	Phishing attack (stolen privileged credentials)	2022

2   Methods

To date the OAIC has recorded NDB scheme data for all industries across 12 periods. This commenced from April 2018 with 5 quarterly reports, and from July 2019 a further 7 reports have been issued covering 6-month intervals [15]. Healthcare data was extracted from this full set to identify the following measures:

1. Descriptive and inferential statistics:
   a. Total occurrences of 4 high-level breach cause categories
   b. Total occurrences of 22 detailed breach cause categories
2. Temporal trends (for 5 x annually aggregated and 12 individual periods):
   a. 2018–2022 trend of 4 high-level breach cause categories
   b. 2018–2022 trend of 22 detailed breach cause categories
3. Analysis:
   a. A Pareto distribution evaluation to establish the most impactful causes
   b. A Pearsons correlation of the top-10 causes to establish r & P values

2.1   Descriptive Statistics for High Level Data Breach Causes

Between 2018–2022 there were $N = 929$ data breaches reported by eligible Australian healthcare entities, using the four high-level classifications shown in Fig. 1.

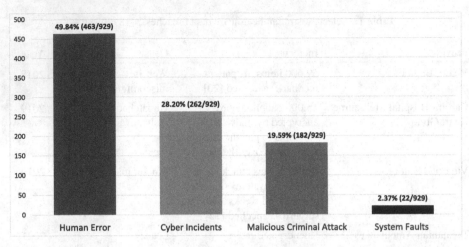

Fig. 1. Australian healthcare data breaches by high level cause, 2018–2022 ($N = 929$).

2.2 Descriptive Statistics for Detailed Data Breach Causes

Within the four high-level classifications (represented by the first 2 letters of each code) further detail is captured to provide 22 specific data breach causes, detailed at Table 2. While the high-level descriptions capture overall risk categories, these detailed causes show exactly how those risks are materialising and this is where LAHPs can begin to extract specific lessons from the data.

Table 2. Data breach causes - detailed categories with definitions.

Category	Detailed Cause	Definition (as per OAIC)
1. (CI) Cyber incidents	CI1: Brute force	Automated software used to generate a large number of consecutive guesses as to the value of the desired data, for example, passwords
	CI2: Hacking (other means)	Unauthorised access to a system or network (other than by phishing, brute-force, or malware), to exploit system data or manipulate its behaviour
	CI3: Ransomware	A type of malicious software designed to block access to data or a computer system until a sum of money is paid or other conditions are met

(continued)

Table 2. (*continued*)

Category	Detailed Cause	Definition (as per OAIC)
	CI4: Compromised/stolen credentials (method unknown)	Credentials are compromised or stolen by methods unknown
	CI5: Phishing (credentials compromised)	Untargeted mass messages asking users for information, to open a malicious attachment, or visit a fake website
	CI6: Malware (malicious software)	Software used to gain unauthorised access to computers, steal information and disrupt or disable networks (i.e., trojans, viruses and worms)
	CI7: Other	-
2. (HE) Human error	HE1: Failed to use BCC	Sending a group email with all recipient email addresses in the 'To' field, thereby disclosing all email addresses to all recipients
	HE2: Loss or insecure disposal of paperwork or devices	Disposing of information in a manner that could lead to its unauthorised disclosure (i.e., using a public rubbish bin to dispose of customer records)
	HE3_Email incorrectly sent	Personal information sent to the wrong recipient via email (i.e., as a result of a misaddressed email or having a wrong address on file)
	HE4: PI incorrectly faxed	Personal information sent to the wrong recipient via fax (i.e., a result of an incorrectly entered fax number or having a wrong fax number on file)
	HE5: PI incorrectly mailed	Personal information sent to the wrong recipient via postal mail (i.e., as a result of a transcribing error or having a wrong address on file)

(continued)

Table 2. (*continued*)

Category	Detailed Cause	Definition (as per OAIC)
	HE6: PI incorrectly sent (other)	Personal information sent to the wrong recipient via channels other than email, fax or mail (i.e., delivery by hand or uploading to a web portal)
	HE7: Failure to redact	Failure to effectively de-identify a record before disclosing it
	HE8: Unauthorised release or publication	Unauthorised disclosure of personal information in a written format, including paper documents or online
	HE9: Unauthorised verbal disclosure	Disclosing personal information verbally without authorisation (i.e., calling it out in a waiting room)
	HE10: Other	-
3. (MC) Malicious or criminal attack	MC1: Rogue employee	Employee or insider/contractor acting against the interests of their employer
	MC2: Social engineering or impersonation	An attack that exploits human interaction to manipulate people into breaking normal security procedures to gain access to systems, networks or locations
	MC3: Paperwork/device theft	Theft of paperwork or data storage device
4. (SF) System faults	SF1: Unintended access	Business or technology process errors not caused by direct human error
	SF2: Unintended release or publication	

Figure 2 presents the data from all 12 periods and shows the 22 detailed breach reasons arranged in order, from the most regularly reported at the furthest peak. This illustrates the differing scale of occurrences stemming from prevalent causes such as email being incorrectly addressed or phishing, as opposed to much rarer threats from unintended access or brute force attacks. The same data is also presented in descending order of frequency at Table 3 and includes the mean occurrence for each incident reason per year (μ), and its representative percentage across all five years of incidents.

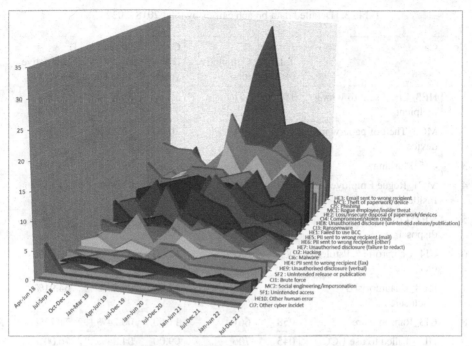

Fig. 2. Detailed data breach causes for 12 periods 2018–2022.

The inclusion of cumulative totals at columns B and E of Table 3 reveals the majority of incidents (751/929, 80.84%) were attributed to a minority of detailed cause categories (10/22, 45%). The most frequently occurring specific cause is shown as 'HE3_Email sent to wrong recipient', responsible for 151/929 (16.25%, $\mu = 30.20$) of all incidents over 5 years.

2.3 Pareto Analysis

The data from Table 3 is further investigated using a Pareto analysis, shown at Fig. 3, which seeks to verify if there is any pattern of "predictable imbalance [26]" present in the data set. Using a standard Pareto approach the dataset shown at Fig. 3 is arranged in descending order of frequency, using annual μ, with an overlay line (in blue) showing the cumulative % of N as each new breach cause is introduced. Also depicted are two boundary zones: k_0, where $n \leq 50\%$ of N, and k_1 where $n \leq 80\%$ of N. The mapping of the k_1 zone achieves the goal of this Pareto analysis, being the identification of those "vital few [27]" items which represent 80% of the data breach risk. To calculate the threshold values for these zones, formulae (1) and (2) were applied to Column C of Table 3:

$$k_0 = \sum_{i=1}^{5} x_i \tag{1}$$

$$k_1 = \sum_{i=1}^{10} x_i \tag{2}$$

Table 3. Detailed data breach causes by total 2018–2022.

No	Cause	A: Total (/929)	B: Cumulative total	C: μ (Per year)	D: % of all breaches	E: Cumulative %
1	HE3_Email sent to wrong recipient	151	151	30.20	16.25%	16.25%
2	MC3_Theft of paperwork/ device	100	251	20.00	10.76%	27.02%
3	CI5_Phishing	087	338	17.40	09.36%	36.38%
4	MC1_Rogue Employee/ Insider threat	072	410	14.40	07.75%	44.13%
5	HE2_Loss/insecure disposal	065	475	13.00	07.00%	51.13% (k_0)
6	CI4_Compromised/stolen creds	064	539	12.80	06.89%	58.02%
7	HE8_Unauthorised disclosure	064	603	12.80	06.89%	64.91%
8	CI3_Ransomware	058	661	11.60	06.24%	71.15%
9	HE1_Failed to use BCC	045	706	09.00	04.84%	76.00%
10	HE5_PI sent to wrong recipient (mail)	045	751	09.00	04:84%	80.84% (k_1)
11	HE6_PI sent to wrong recipient (other)	031	782	06.20	03.34%	84.18%
12	HE7_Unauthorised disclosure (unredacted)	021	803	04.20	02.26%	86.44%
13	CI2_Hacking	020	823	04.00	02.15%	88.59%
14	CI6_Malware	018	841	03.60	01.94%	90.53%
15	HE4_PI sent to wrong recipient (fax)	018	859	03.60	01.94%	92.47%
16	HE9_Unauthorised disclosure (verbal)	018	877	03.60	01.94%	94.40%
17	SF2_Unintended Release or publication	016	893	03.20	01.72%	96.12%
18	CI1_Brute force	014	907	02.80	01.51%	97.63%
19	MC2_Social engineering/impersonation	010	917	02.00	01.08%	98.71%
20	SF1_Unintended Access	006	923	01.20	00.65%	99.35%
21	HE10_Other	005	928	01.00	00.54%	99.89%
22	CI7_Other	001	929	00.20	00.11%	100.0%

This analysis shows that $k_0 = 51.13\%$ (475/929), and is comprised of just five specific causes, being in descending order: 1) incorrect emailing, 2) physical theft, 3) phishing attacks, 4) rogue employees or insider threats, and 5) insecure disposal. Where $k_1 = 80.84\%$ (751/929), an additional five causes contribute to the effect, bringing the total number of causes to ten: 6) compromised credentials, 7) unauthorised publication or release of data, 8) ransomware attacks, 9) failure to use BCC fields in email, and 10) PI data being posted incorrectly.

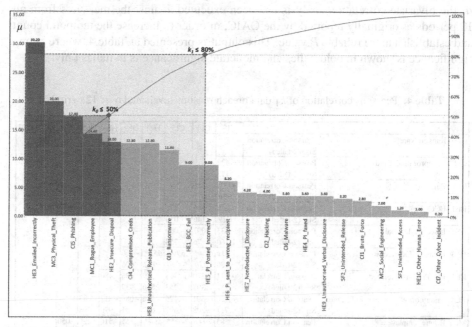

Fig. 3. Pareto analysis of μ 2018–2022 (highlighting k_0 & k_1 boundaries). (Color figure online)

The Pareto analysis provides the detail confirming the ten specific data breach causes (the "vital few", or the k_1 breach threshold) which accounts for 751/929 (80.84%) of all incidents. Within k_1 370/751 (49.26%) of incidents are attributable to elements of 'human error', 209/751 (27.82%) were identified as 'cyber incidents', and 172/751 (22.92%) 'malicious criminal acts'.

2.4 Correlation of Data Breach Causes

To establish if there are any temporal linear relationships occurring within the k_1 data, each of the contributing causes from that region was assessed using a bivariate correlation analysis within SPSS[1]. This analysis was intended to measure the strength of relationship between each pair within the k_1 threshold (using the Pearsons correlation, or r value), and the significance of that relationship (the P value).

---

[1] Software used for analysing results and creating charts was Microsoft Excel V2301 Build 16.0.16026.20196, and IBM SPSS Statistics V29.0.0.0 (241).

The default, or null hypothesis (H_0) for this evaluation was that one type of data breach would not be significantly correlated to any other another ($P = 0$). In this case, for example, increases in phishing data breaches would not lead to regular increases in physical theft incidents within the same reporting period. If such relationships could however be demonstrated via an alternative hypothesis (H_a or $P \neq 0$), they could further increase the power of the Pareto analysis findings by offering a refinement in defining the most problematic data breach cause reasons from within k_1.

While the Pareto analysis was evaluated using total annual figures (x5) to obtain μ, the bivariate correlation analysis has been executed against the measures from all 12 periods as originally reported by the OAIC, in order to increase the temporal count and establish a more reliable P value. This output is presented at Table 4, where strong significance is shown in bold italics and moderate significance is in italics only.

Table 4. Pearsons correlation of k_1 data breach reasons (evaluated over 12 periods).

		CI3	CI4	CI5	HE1	HE2	HE3	HE5	HE8	MC1	MC3
CI3 Ransomware	Pearson Correlation	--									
	Sig. (2-tailed)										
CI4 Compromised_Creds	Pearson Correlation	.422	--								
	Sig. (2-tailed)	.172									
CI5 Phishing	Pearson Correlation	*741**￼*	.539	--							
	Sig. (2-tailed)	*.006*	.071								
HE1 BCC_Fail	Pearson Correlation	*.628**	.446	.576	--						
	Sig. (2-tailed)	*.029*	.146	.050							
HE2 Insecure_Disposal	Pearson Correlation	-.433	.092	-.099	-.397	--					
	Sig. (2-tailed)	.160	.776	.758	.201						
HE3 Emailed_Incorrectly	Pearson Correlation	.415	*624**	*.599**	*652**	-.166	--				
	Sig. (2-tailed)	.180	*.030*	*.040*	*.022*	.606					
HE5 PII_Posted_Incorrectly	Pearson Correlation	-.111	.270	.358	.049	.026	.480	--			
	Sig. (2-tailed)	.732	.397	.253	.880	.937	.114				
HE8 Unauthorised_Release_Publication	Pearson Correlation	.120	.391	.126	-.126	-.086	-.012	-.083	--		
	Sig. (2-tailed)	.711	.208	.697	.697	.791	.970	.798			
MC1 Rogue_Employee	Pearson Correlation	.385	*704**	*746**￼*	*594**	.355	.516	.290	.050	--	
	Sig. (2-tailed)	.217	*.011*	*.005*	*.042*	.257	.086	.361	.877		
MC3 Physical_Theft	Pearson Correlation	.503	-.260	.397	.375	-.062	.113	-.107	-.565	.169	--
	Sig. (2-tailed)	.095	.414	.201	.230	.849	.726	.740	.056	.600	
* Correlation is significant at the 0.05 level (2-tailed).											
** Correlation is significant at the 0.01 level (2-tailed).											

The relationships considered relevant by this analysis include the finding of both strong and moderately positive associations, and these are detailed further in Table 5.

Table 5. Evaluation of significant linear correlations.

1st Measure	2nd Measure	r value	P value
Strong positive associations (H_a is proven)			
MC1_Rogue_Employee →	**CI5_Phishing**	**.746**	**.005**
The strongest correlation uncovered in this analysis shows the danger in rogue employees, who are more likely to engage in reckless online behaviour and are more likely to be targeted in phishing attacks			
CI5_Phishing →	**CI3_Ransomware**	**.741**	**.006**
This strong correlation is strongly supported by real world experience, where users interacting with phishing emails are likely to execute malicious code that initiates a ransomware attack			
Moderate positive associations (H_a is accepted)			
HE1_BCC_Fail →	**CI3_Ransomware**	**.628**	**.029**
A strong association with average significance, but the implications of poor BCC use as shown here as a means by which compromised emails expose large BCC lists to subsequent ransomware attackers			
HE3_Emailed_Incorrectly →	**CI4_Compromised_Credentials**	**.624**	**.030**
Another strong association and average significance, but yet another means by which bad email practice can be exploited to initiate scam conversations that lead to compromised credentials			
HE3_Emailed_Incorrectly →	**CI5_Phishing**	**.599**	**.040**
A strong association and average significance, this suggests bad email practices can lead to 'replay' attacks when incorrect recipients leak valid email addresses to malicious attackers who can then target organisations			
HE3_Emailed_Incorrectly →	**HE1_BCC_Fail**	**.652**	**.022**
On the border of a very strong association, this further demonstrates the need to be mindful of good email usage behaviours, as seen in other associations above this is an association that can lead to ransomware attacks			
MC1_Rogue_Employee →	**CI4_Compromised_Credentials**	**.704**	**.011**
A near very strong correlation, suggesting that rogue employees can have a devastating impact on an organisation, particularly if they are the holder of privileged credentials that are breached			
MC1_Rogue_Employee →	**HE1_BCC_Fail**	**.594**	**.042**
While moderate in its association, this relationship is indicative of how a de-motivated or malicious insider can make mistakes (or deliberately misuse) process in order to cause an incident to 'get back' at their employer			

3 Principal Results

The analysis undertaken by this paper has shown that in Australia the most significant data breach risk for LAHPs stems from 'human error' based incidents with a mean annual occurrence of $\mu = 92.60$, which over 5 years has resulted in 463/929 (49.84%) of all reported data breaches to the NDB scheme. The most persistent threat within this category that has caused the largest number of data breaches across all periods (151/929, 16.25%, $\mu = 30.20$) is sensitive data being emailed to the wrong recipient.

The Pareto analysis has shown that the classic 80:20 rule holds true for this data set, with 751/929 (80.84%) of all data breaches triggered by a "vital few" of 10 repeated data breach causes. Within this priority set (k_1) the strongest contributor was again confirmed as coming from five different forms of 'human error' which between them caused 370/751 (49.26%) of those incidents.

Finally, the linear correlation analysis has shown that for this sample, there are strong indicators that increases in rogue employee associated data breaches can lead to increases in phishing attack breaches ($r = .746$, $P = .005$), and that successful phishing attacks are associated with ransomware data breaches ($r = .741$, $P = .006$).

4 Discussion

The phased approach undertaken for the analysis of this data set supports the hypothesis that human factors are contributing a significant degree to data breaches in LAHP environments. Not only are human factors the single largest contributor, but they are also embedded and persistent in their re-occurrence so cannot be dismissed as only "a few bad apples" doing the wrong thing.

In looking beyond the statistics focussed only the volume of data breaches, the Pareto and linear correlation analyses confirm that LAHPs should consider a holistic approach to learning the lessons from this data. This includes developing a greater awareness of those relationships which can make one type of data breach an enabler, or amplifier, of others. For example, the Pareto chart (Fig. 3) shows that while 5 of the top 10 data breach reasons are human error generated, relative positions 2–4 on the X axis also generate significant events due to malicious targeted attacks and other cyber incidents. The correlation analysis further confirms the power of these linkages with repeated insider threats and email-related failures in particular leading to incidents of phishing, compromised credentials, and ransomware which have all been shown to have had repeated and devastating effects on healthcare providers across Australia (as shown at Table 1).

Worthy of note at the opposite end of the scale is the dearth of data breaches resulting from system faults. This puts some doubt on users who may claim "I never touched anything" when things go wrong in the event of a data breach. Very rarely (only in 22/929, or 2.37% of cases over 5 years) has faulty software or hardware resulted in data breaches, which again supports the fact that systems are unlikely to do bad things unless directed to do so by a human operator.

4.1 Limitations and Future Work

The data breach statistics produced by the OAIC contain inherent limitations, due to restraints in the *Privacy Act 2018 (Cth)* which still do not require all large government-run LAHPs to report all data breach events. It should be noted that legislative review is currently underway by the Australian Government, with amendments already enacted to the *Security of Critical Infrastructure Act 2018 (Cth)* which will require greater board-level risk management and reporting of cyber security incidents by LAHPs from 2023 onwards. A new *Privacy Legislation Amendment (Enforcement and Other Measures) Act 2022 (Cth)* has also been enacted, which greatly increases the financial penalties for privacy data breaches [28]. A Privacy Act Review Report, published in 2023 by the Attorney-General's Department [29], is also seeking public feedback on further proposals to strengthen the Commonwealth's Privacy Act, including enhanced data breach reporting requirements. As these amendments come into effect and provide extended data sets to the research community, this work can be re-visited and expanded to examine if the trends identified in this paper continue or diverge.

It should also be noted that the correlations undertaken at Table 3 are only representative of the currently sampled population within the scope of this paper, and further analysis of related data sets (such as those provided by the UK or USA) could explore the correlations identified there to great benefit.

5 Conclusions

This paper has shown there is significant and urgently needed value to be gained from analysing the NDB scheme data for Australia's healthcare industry. Not only does this allow them to learn from the mistakes and bad fortune of others, but it can also contribute significantly to avoiding future public distrust and legal implications as the national governance environment matures. For LAHPs this has highlighted the need to accept that the highly diverse nature of their very large workforces, which can number in the tens of thousands of employees per organisation, represents a significant risk vector as healthcare adopts ever more digital ways of working. By focussing on improving risk governance, staff awareness and training, incident reporting, and daily monitoring of systems there is great potential to halt the rising tide of healthcare privacy breaches which the first five years of NDB data have evidenced.

References

1. Australian Broadcasting Corporation (ABC). Healthcare industry continues to be main target of data breaches, with 79 reported in six months (2022). https://www.abc.net.au/news/science/2022-11-10/data-breach-medibank-healthcare-system/101612056. Accessed 07 Jan 2023
2. Australian Cyber Security Magazine. Cyberattacks on Australian Healthcare Doubles. Australian Cyber Security Magazine (2022)
3. Landi, H.: Relentless cyberattacks are putting financial pressure on hospitals: Fitch Ratings. Fierce Healthcare (2022). https://www.fiercehealthcare.com/tech/relentless-cyber-attacks-are-putting-pressure hospital-finances-fitch-ratings. Accessed 10 Dec 2022
4. Fleury-Charles, A., Chowdhury, M.M., Rifat, N.: Data breaches: vulnerable privacy. In: 2022 IEEE International Conference on Electro Information Technology (eIT), Minnesota State University, USA. IEEE (2022)
5. Khan, F., Kim, J.H., Mathiassen, L., Moore, R.: Data breach management: an integrated risk model. Inf. Manag. **58**(1), 103392 (2021)
6. Hendee, L.A.: The data breach epidemic: a modern legal analysis. J. Technol. Law Policy **24**(1), 3 (2021)

7. She, A.H., et al.: Healthcare data breaches: insights and implications. Healthcare **8**(2), 133 (2020)
8. Kruse, C.S., Frederick, B., Jacobson, T., Monticone, D.K.: Cybersecurity in healthcare: a systematic review of modern threats and trends. Technol. Health Care **25**, 1–10 (2017). https://doi.org/10.3233/THC-161263
9. Chernyshev, M., Zeadally, S., Baig, Z.: Healthcare data breaches: implications for digital forensic readiness. J. Med. Syst. **43**(1), 7 (2018). https://doi.org/10.1007/s10916-018-1123-2
10. U.S. Department of Health and Human Services. Breach Portal: Notice to the Secretary of HHS Breach of Unsecured Protected Health Information (2023). https://ocrportal.hhs.gov/ocr/breach/breach_report.jsf. Accessed 5 Aug 2023
11. Collins, J.D., Sainato, V.A., Khey, D.N.: Organizational data breaches 2005–2010: applying SCP to the healthcare and education sectors. Int. J. Cyber Criminol. **5**(1), 794–810 (2011)
12. Raghupathi, W., Raghupathi, V., Saharia, A.: Analyzing health data breaches: a visual analytics approach. AppliedMath. **3**(1), 175–199 (2023)
13. UK Information Commissioner's Office (ICO). Data security incident trends (2023). https://ico.org.uk/action-weve-taken/data-security-incident-trends/. Accessed 02 Aug 2023
14. Australian Government. Privacy Act 1988 (Cth) (1988). https://www.legislation.gov.au/Details/C2022C00361. Accessed 14 Jan 2023
15. Office of the Australian Information Commissioner (OAIC). Notifiable data breaches publications (2023). https://www.oaic.gov.au/privacy/notifiable-data-breaches/notifiable-data-breaches-publications. Accessed 14 Aug 2023
16. Hile, J.: Dude, where's my data?: The effectiveness of laws governing data breaches in Australia. J. Telecommun. Digit. Econ. **9**(2), 47–68 (2021)
17. Petkauskas, V.: Hackers were interested in Australia long before Medibank and Optus breaches (2022). https://cybernews.com/security/hackers-australia-medibank-optus/
18. Australian Government. Security Legislation Amendment (Critical Infrastructure Protection) Act 2022 (No. 33, 2022)
19. Australian Government. Security Legislation Amendment (Critical Infrastructure) Act 2021
20. IT News. HealthEngine reveals data breach (2018). https://www.itnews.com.au/news/healthengine-reveals-data-breach-496175. Accessed 14 May 2019
21. Healthcare IT News. Medical records at Victorian hospital get hacked (2019). https://www.healthcareitnews.com/news/anz/medical-records-victorian-hospital-get-hacked
22. The West Australian. Limited delays after Vic hospital hacks (2019)
23. Clarke, P.: Significant data breach from Ambulance Tasmania (2021). http://www.peteraclarke.com.au/2021/01/08/significant-data-breach-from-ambulance-tasmania-through-interception-of-its-paging-service-with-data-of-patients-who-contact-ambulances-published-on-line/
24. Cunningham, M.: Staff unable to access patient files after Eastern Health cyber attack (2021). https://www.theage.com.au/national/victoria/staff-unable-to-access-patient-files-after-eastern-health-cyber-attack-20210329-p57eyj.html
25. Kost, E.: What Caused the Medibank Data Breach? (2022). https://www.upguard.com/blog/what-caused-the-medibank-data-breach
26. Powell, T., Sammut-Bonnici, T.: Pareto analysis (2014)
27. Karuppusami, G., Gandhinathan, R.: Pareto analysis of critical success factors of total quality management: a literature review and analysis. TQM Mag. **18**, 372–385 (2006)
28. Paltiel, M.: Recent amendments to the Australian privacy act. J. Bioethical Inq. **20**, 161–167 (2023)
29. Attorney-General's Department (Australia). Privacy Act Review Report (2023)

Analysis and Protection of Public Medical Dataset: From Privacy Perspective

Samsad Jahan[1], Yong-Feng Ge[1(✉)], Enamul Kabir[2], and Hua Wang[1]

[1] Institute for Sustainable Industries and Liveable Cities, Victoria University, Melbourne 3011, Australia
samsad.jahan@live.vu.edu.au, {yongfeng.ge,hua.wang}@vu.edu.au
[2] School of Mathematics, Physics and Computing, University of Southern Queensland, Toowoomba, Australia
enamul.kabir@usq.edu.au

Abstract. High-quality medical treatment is unattainable without protecting patients' medical records and other sensitive information. One of the most critical challenges in the medical industry is patient privacy in light of medical systems' widespread digitization and networking. What we call "health data" includes a plethora of information on individuals, including their medical records, treatment records, genetic data, and demographic information. In this paper, we review existing methods to keep patients' health records private and compare their advantages and limitations. We then analyze the public medical dataset from the perspective of privacy protection, utilizing the k-anonymity and l-diversity models, and compare the impact of quasi-identifier attributes on privacy protection. Furthermore, we conduct experiments to investigate the trade-off between privacy and utility. Based on the analysis results, this paper provides data owners with a guide on how to choose attributes for medical data publication and how to select the appropriate techniques for preserving privacy in medical data publication.

Keywords: Medical data · Data privacy · k-anonymity · l-diversity

1 Introduction

Healthcare analytics ethics and patient privacy depend on the security of medical datasets. Medical databases contain personal identifying information (PII) such as personal information, medical history, diagnosis, and treatment records. If these datasets are not handled adequately, they pose serious privacy risks [21,40]. Re-identification or unauthorized access to such data can compromise patient confidentiality, trust, and legal liability [41–43]. Therefore, healthcare organizations must develop efficient privacy-preserving algorithms to secure patient privacy while analyzing medical data. Sensitive information includes demographic data, medical history, diagnostic codes, medications, treatment plans, hospitalization records, insurance information, immunization dates, allergy information,

Y. Li et al. (Eds.): HIS 2023, LNCS 14305, pp. 79–90, 2023.
https://doi.org/10.1007/978-981-99-7108-4_7

and laboratory and test results. The availability of large volumes of data has made it feasible to improve healthcare services, particularly patient care outcomes, and medical treatment costs. So, protecting patient data is crucial as healthcare organizations collect and analyze vast amounts of information [2].

Big datasets are valuable for science and technology [14,39], but mishandling them can lead to privacy breaches, compromise patient confidentiality, cause distrust, and invite legal consequences. Unauthorized access or re-identification of such data poses risks. To balance patient privacy and enable insightful medical data analysis, healthcare providers must implement strict privacy-preserving measures [18,20,31,35]. Alnemari et al. employed an adaptive differential privacy (DP) approach for range queries to address the privacy problem in healthcare data. The effectiveness of the suggested strategy was assessed using various workloads across multiple variables. The findings demonstrate that while splitting the vector based on the workload increases privacy, partitioning the vector based on the data may result in more accurate responses [1]. Belsis et al. described a sensor-based system that effectively transmits messages, including patients' vital statistics, to a medical database. Their work offers a comprehensive clustering technique that efficiently maintains connections and routes messages to a medical database. The suggested anonymity-based solutions are compared to existing cryptography-based solutions in terms of energy usage and network performance [5]. Although the publication of healthcare data often has benefits, it may sometimes unintentionally expose personal information. Another potential solution is the utilization of k-anonymity and l-diversity approaches to protect medical datasets [13,27,36]. By employing these privacy-preserving techniques, organizations can minimize the risk of re-identification [13], protect individual privacy [10], and facilitate valuable analysis and research.

The benefit of the k-anonymity model is that it provides protection against identity disclosure. However, it is often vulnerable to attribute disclosure, homogeneity attack, and background knowledge attack [2,9]. On the other hand, l-diversity offers protection against attribute disclosure and ensures a better distribution of sensitive attributes (SA) within groups [29]. However, one limitation of l-diversity is its inability to prevent skewness attacks and similarity attacks [23,26]. DP provides flexible privacy protection for sensitive data, and the level of privacy protection is quantifiable [11]. However, adding noise in the dataset causes lacking of transparency. Also, the trade-off between privacy preservation and data utility maintenance in DP still remains an open problem [15,17,19].

In this paper, firstly, we review some existing anonymization methods for the privacy protection of public medical dataset. Secondly, we employ two privacy models to compare the impact of quasi-identifier (QID) attributes on privacy protection. Finally, we conduct experiments to investigate the trade-off between privacy and utility.

The organization of this paper is as follows. Section 1 provides an introduction and discusses related work. Sections 2 and 3 cover the methods and analysis. Finally, in Sect. 4, we present our conclusions.

2   Method

Our research focuses on analyzing the privacy protection mechanisms of publicly accessible medical data by calculating the distribution of k and l for specific combinations of QID and SA. To investigate the privacy problem, we modify the QID attribute combinations and derived the corresponding l and k values, then analyze their distribution. By examining the distribution of k and l, we estimate their averages and compare them across different QID attribute combinations. Our objective is to identify which characteristics are more susceptible to privacy disclosure, observing that smaller l and k values increase the likelihood of identification.

2.1   Anonymization Approaches in Medical Data

k-anonymity is a concept and technique used to protect the identity and sensitive data of individuals in a dataset. It ensures that each record in the dataset is indistinguishable from at least $k - 1$ other records based on certain identifying attributes or quasi-identifiers [36].

Definition 1 (k-anonymity). *A dataset satisfies k-anonymity if, for every combination of QID attributes, there are at least k records.*

Samarati demonstrated the use of k-anonymity to preserve data accuracy through techniques like generalization and suppression. The concept of minimum generalization, which maintains the properties of the published data while preserving k-anonymity, was also introduced by the authors. They proposed a method for achieving this generalization [30]. The k-anonymity model, developed by Sweeney in 2002, has gained widespread adoption due to its simplicity and effectiveness in preserving individual privacy [36]. Literature also presents different variants of k-anonymity, such as the k-join-anonymity model [33], cluster-based anonymity [6], k-anonymity in DP [32], and the microaggregation sorting framework [24], among others.

Although k-anonymity is a popular anonymization approach, it is not without drawbacks. Issues such as membership disclosure, identity disclosure [3], and attribute disclosure [2, 7] have been identified.

To address the issues of homogeneity and background knowledge, a stronger concept of privacy known as l-diversity is needed. The l-diversity model focuses solely on SA. It achieves privacy protection by forming l-distinct groups and considering QID, thereby reducing privacy violations related to SA. However, creating l-well SA groups can be impractical, and public data may still be vulnerable to similarity attacks [27].

Beyond k-anonymity, the concept and method of l-diversity enhance the security of sensitive data in a dataset [27]. According to the definition:

Definition 2 (l-diversity). *A dataset satisfies l-diversity if, for every QID group, there are at least l well-represented SA.*

l-diversity ensures that each indistinguishable group of data contains a sufficient variety of SA values. It reduces the risk of attribute disclosure attacks, where an adversary deduces specific sensitive information by leveraging patterns in a dataset. By reducing the likelihood of re-identification and enhancing the privacy of individual data, *l*-diversity provides an additional layer of privacy protection.

Table 1. 3-anonymous and 2-diverse patient microdata

No.	Quasi-identifier			Sensitive Attribute
	Age	Zip Code	Gender	
1	<30	860**	Male	Heart Disease
2	<30	860**	Female	Heart Disease
3	<30	860**	Female	Cancer
4	3*	863**	Male	Heart Disease
5	3*	863**	Male	Diabetes
6	3*	863**	Male	Diabetes
7	>40	865**	Female	Diabetes
8	>40	865**	Male	Cancer
9	>40	865**	Female	Cancer

As an illustration, consider Table 1, which represents a 3-anonymous and 2-diverse table. It ensures that each QID group consists of at least three indistinguishable records, and within each group, there are at least two unique values for the SA. However, it is essential to note that the effectiveness of *l*-diversity depends on the range of values for the SA. Skewness attacks and similarity attacks still pose risks of revealing the SA values in the context of *l*-diversity [26, 34]

2.2   Differential Privacy in Medical Data

While the *k*-anonymity model provides protection against identity disclosure, it falls short in preventing attribute disclosure. On the other hand, *l*-diversity focuses on protecting the SA, but it is often susceptible to similarity attacks [2]. In such cases, another approach that can be employed for protecting medical data is DP, which is well-known for its approximation protection techniques. DP is a methodology that enables the analysis of data while preserving users' anonymity. It allows for effective analysis of sensitive data by providing a mathematical framework for privacy guarantees [11]. By utilizing DP strategies, it is possible to protect patients' privacy while enabling analysis and research on healthcare data.

Definition 3 (ϵ-DP). *For all data sets P and Q that only differ by one element, and for every S subset of Range(f),*

$$P[f(P) \in S] \leqslant e^\epsilon P[f(Q) \in S]$$

is the ϵ-DP for a randomized function f.

Here, the parameter ϵ controls the amount of privacy protection. In DP, the commonly used mechanisms are Laplace, Exponential, and Gaussian. Laplace mechanisms are typically applied to numeric output, while the Exponential mechanism is suitable for non-numeric queries [38]. The Gaussian mechanism is often utilized for aggregating sensitive statistics, private data analysis (such as regression analysis or clustering), and machine learning applications [22].

Medical data contains highly sensitive and private information, including diagnoses, genetic information, location data, and other health-related data [25]. DP is employed to protect the privacy of medical data through randomized response combined with the expectation-maximization technique. This integration enhances the model's resistance against security attacks, preventing accurate answers from being obtained in response to fabricated inquiries. Performance assessment of this approach typically focuses on accuracy and precision. However, the expectation-maximization approach has inherent disadvantages, such as slow convergence and a lack of maximum likelihood estimation guarantees [37].

In a separate study comparing DP to other privacy mechanisms for big data, including healthcare data, it was determined that DP is the most suitable technique for privacy applications in large datasets [4]. DP serves as a valuable tool in mitigating re-identification attacks by adding noise to the data, making it difficult to identify individual records in a dataset. It ensures long-term privacy protection even when multiple analyses and queries are performed on the same dataset. Various individuals or attributes within medical data may require different levels of privacy protection. DP allows for personalized privacy levels, where the amount of added noise can be adjusted based on the data sensitivity or patient preferences [12].

3   Analysis

We have chosen the publicly accessible hospital inpatient discharge datasets released by the New York State Department of Health[1] for our investigation. We selected 1,020 observations from this dataset. Our first selected QID combination is QID 1: health service area, hospital county, operating certificate number, facility ID, facility name, age group, and zip code. In addition, the SA is referred to as "CCS diagnosis description". The distribution of k and l for this combination has an average value of 24.238 and 8, respectively.

Then, we choose the second QID attribute combination, QID 2: health service area, hospital county, age, zip code, gender, and race. The sensitive characteristic

---

[1] https://health.data.ny.gov/Health/Hospital-Inpatient-Discharges-SPARCS-De-Identified/82xm-y6g8.

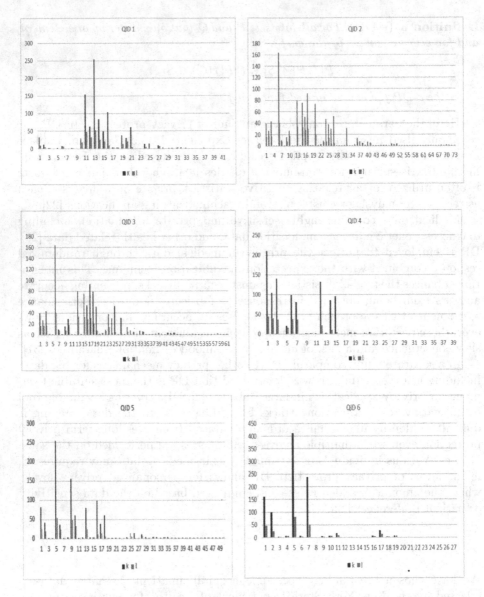

Fig. 1. Distribution of k and l for QID 1, QID 2, QID 3, QID 4, QID 5, and QID 6

remains unchanged. QID 2 includes the most common QID attributes. For QID 2, the mean of k and l is 13.9589 and 5.41, respectively. So, it is clear from the average of the k and l distributions of QID 1 and QID 2 that QID 1 has better privacy protection than QID 2 (see Fig. 1). We consider QID 2 as the combination with the most common QID attributes, as it includes age, gender, zip code, and race. Now we observe the impact by removing one QID at a time. First, we remove the attribute race from QID 2. The new combination becomes QID 3: health service area, hospital county, age, zip code, gender. We can now observe the distribution of k and l by eliminating race. The average values obtained are 16.70492 and 6.295082, respectively. The average values of k and l show a small improvement once the race is removed. Therefore, race serves as a key QID in this dataset.

If we remove the zip code from the second combination, the new combination is QID 4: health service area, hospital country, age, gender, race. The average values of k and l for this combination are 26.12821 and 7.564103, respectively (Fig. 1). We can infer from this result that the zip code is a significant QID because the averages increased after removing this attribute compared to the distribution of k and l of QID 2.

Next, if we remove gender from QID 2, we obtain QID 5: health service area, hospital country, age, zip code, race. After removing gender, the average values of k and l are 20.38 and 6.74, respectively. This indicates that the dataset becomes more private when gender is not included in the list. Now, let's consider what happens if we remove age from QID 2. The new combination becomes QID 6: health service area, hospital country, zip code, gender, race. When the age attribute is removed from the QID 2 combination, the average values of k and l change to 37.74074 and 10.40741, respectively (Fig. 1). This analysis suggests that age is the most influential quasi-identifier (QID) for the hospital inpatient discharge data. Therefore, publishing age information should be approached with greater caution, as it has a significant impact as identifiable information.

3.1   Improving k and l

Although some de-identification has been performed in this dataset, we have identified that it is still not adequately protected. It is possible for an attacker to easily identify unique information. Therefore, we need to improve the values of k and l for better protection. The value of k and l can be enhanced through attribute generalization and record suppression techniques [16,20]. We will demonstrate attribute generalization through a simple example, and record suppression will be conducted through a small experimental study.

Attribute Generalization. Generalization is a technique used to represent attribute values in a table that simplifies tuple identification. This method involves using a general domain where the attribute values become more generic. To generalize the values without compromising the integrity of the data, we can map QID, such as zip codes from Z0 (e.g., 04123, 04126) to Z1 (e.g., 04120, 04120). This mapping is defined by a "domain generalization hierarchy". If the table already satisfies k-anonymity, k-minimum generalization can be applied to maintain privacy while retaining specific values in private tables [30,36]. However, this approach requires a higher degree of generalization when there are outliers or tuples that occur fewer than k times [29].

For example, let's consider a case where an 18-year-old female from Allegany with a zip code of 86040 has a mental illness, and her family does not want her information to be publicly disclosed. Since her information is unique in the dataset (see Table 2), she can be easily identified. In this scenario, performing attribute generalization can help improve the values of k and l. By hiding the zip code, gender, and age, her information becomes less easily identifiable from the published data. The example of attribute generalization by improving k and l is shown in Table 2.

Table 2. Data with the attribute generalization

No.	Quasi-identifier			Sensitive Attribute
	Age	Zip Code	Gender	
1	<30	860**	Person	Heart Disease
2	<30	860**	Person	Heart Disease
3	<30	860**	Person	Cancer
4	<30	860**	Person	Mental illness
5	3*	863*	Person	Heart Disease
6	3*	863*	Person	Diabetes
7	3*	863*	Person	Diabetes
8	>40	865**	Person	Diabetes
9	>40	865**	Person	Cancer
10	>40	865**	Person	Cancer

Here attribute generalization is conducted on age, zip code, and gender. Age is generalized as less than 30, 3*, and greater than 40. Zip code is generalized by suppressing the last two digits, and gender is generalized as the person.

Record Suppression. In this method, the primary objective is to conceal the entire tuple t from the public data, as it may contain both sensitive and non-sensitive information. However, removing certain records from the data can compromise its accuracy [8].

In our study, we attempted to improve the values of k and l through record suppression techniques. Higher values of k and l indicate that the information is less identifiable. Therefore, in order to enhance the privacy of the data, we need to improve the values of k and l. Smaller values of k and l suggest that the record is unique and easily identifiable from the published data. By removing tuples that contain single instances of information, the values of k and l for the hospital inpatient data increase to 2. Thus, the privacy of this data can be enhanced. To preserve privacy, we conducted a small-scale study to estimate the record suppression ratio for different levels of k-anonymity and l-diversity. We removed all the information for which the value of both k and l was 1 in the attribute combination of QID 2. This was done to improve the values to $k=2$ and $l=2$. We then estimated the record suppression ratio. Furthermore, we repeated the process for k values ranging from 3 to 10 and l values ranging from 2 to 8.

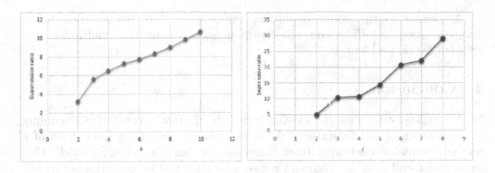

Fig. 2. Record suppression ratio for different k and l

The variation of the record suppression ratio shown in Fig. 2 represents this dataset's trade-off between privacy and utility. As shown in this figure, it is evident that a higher record suppression ratio leads to a higher privacy degree. Accordingly, the number of records in the dataset decreases, which causes a decrease in the dataset's utility. Therefore, when given a privacy requirement, it is crucial to optimize the anonymization solution that can achieve the highest utility maintenance [20]. Formally, we can define this optimization problem as follows:

Definition 4 (Optimal anonymization with privacy requirement). *For a given dataset T, an optimal anonymization solution can be achieved if it satisfies the privacy requirement $(AD(T) \geq k)$ and also achieves the highest UD.*

where AD represents the anonymity degree measured by the k-anonymity privacy model and UD represents the utility degree of the anonymous dataset.

On the other hand, when given a utility requirement, we can also optimize the anonymization solution that can achieve the highest privacy preservation. Formally, we can define this optimization problem as follows:

Definition 5 (Optimal anonymization with utility requirement). *For a given dataset T, an optimal anonymization solution can be achieved if it satisfies the privacy requirement $(UD(T) \geq UD_{threshold})$ and also achieves the highest AD.*

where $UD_{threshold}$ represents the threshold value of the data utility.

Based on the above optimization objectives, we can further define the multi-objective anonymization problem according to Pareto dominance [28], in which the values of AD and UD are optimized at the same time.

Definition 6 (Pareto Dominance). *Let $\mathcal{S}_i$ and $\mathcal{S}_j$ be decision vectors, we say that $\mathcal{S}_i$ has Pareto dominance over $\mathcal{S}_j$, denoted by $\mathcal{S}_i \succ \mathcal{S}_j$, if and only if:*

$$\begin{cases} \forall m = 1,2 \; f_m(\mathcal{S}_i) \geq f_m(\mathcal{S}_j) \\ \exists m = 1,2 \; f_m(\mathcal{S}_i) > f_m(\mathcal{S}_j). \end{cases} \tag{1}$$

where f_1 indicates AD, and f_2 indicates UD.

According to the above definition, we can see that the non-dominated anonymization solutions are the optimal solution to the multi-objective anonymization problem.

4   Conclusion

In this article, we review the existing methods of privacy protection, including their advantages and limitations. Also, we analyze the privacy protection of a publicly available medical dataset based on the existing privacy models. Our experiment evaluates the trade-off between privacy and utility, considering the balance between information loss and privacy protection. Furthermore, we define three optimization problems regarding privacy and utility issues. In the future, medical datasets can have an additional layer of privacy protection by integrating DP with k-anonymity and l-diversity. This framework can help healthcare institutions publish data more securely while preserving individual privacy.

References

1. Alnemari, A., Romanowski, C.J., Raj, R.K.: An adaptive differential privacy algorithm for range queries over healthcare data. In: 2017 IEEE International Conference on Healthcare Informatics (ICHI), pp. 397–402. IEEE (2017)
2. Anjum, A., et al.: An efficient privacy mechanism for electronic health records. Comput. Secur. **72**, 196–211 (2018)
3. Anjum, A., Raschia, G.: BangA: an efficient and flexible generalization-based algorithm for privacy preserving data publication. Computers **6**(1), 1 (2017)
4. Begum, S.H., Nausheen, F.: A comparative analysis of differential privacy vs other privacy mechanisms for big data. In: 2018 2nd International Conference on Inventive Systems and Control (ICISC), pp. 512–516. IEEE (2018)
5. Belsis, P., Pantziou, G.: Protecting anonymity in wireless medical monitoring environments. In: Proceedings of the 4th International Conference on PErvasive Technologies Related to Assistive Environments, pp. 1–6 (2011)
6. Belsis, P., Pantziou, G.: A k-anonymity privacy-preserving approach in wireless medical monitoring environments. Pers. Ubiquit. Comput. **18**, 61–74 (2014)
7. Bhuiyan, M.Z.A., Wang, G., Choo, K.K.R.: Secured data collection for a cloud-enabled structural health monitoring system. In: 2016 IEEE 18th International Conference on High Performance Computing and Communications; IEEE 14th International Conference on Smart City; IEEE 2nd International Conference on Data Science and Systems (HPCC/SmartCity/DSS), pp. 1226–1231. IEEE (2016)
8. Carvalho, T., Moniz, N., Faria, P., Antunes, L.: Survey on privacy-preserving techniques for data publishing. arXiv preprint arXiv:2201.08120 (2022)
9. Chong, K.M.: Privacy-preserving healthcare informatics: a review. In: ITM Web of Conferences, vol. 36, p. 04005. EDP Sciences (2021)
10. Domingo-Ferrer, J., Martínez, S., Sánchez, D.: Decentralized k-anonymization of trajectories via privacy-preserving tit-for-tat. Comput. Commun. **190**, 57–68 (2022)
11. Dwork, C.: Differential privacy: a survey of results. In: Agrawal, M., Du, D., Duan, Z., Li, A. (eds.) TAMC 2008. LNCS, vol. 4978, pp. 1–19. Springer, Heidelberg (2008). https://doi.org/10.1007/978-3-540-79228-4_1

12. Ebadi, H., Sands, D., Schneider, G.: Differential privacy: now it's getting personal. Acm Sigplan Not. **50**(1), 69–81 (2015)
13. El Emam, K., Dankar, F.K.: Protecting privacy using k-anonymity. J. Am. Med. Inform. Assoc. **15**(5), 627–637 (2008)
14. Fatima, M., Rehman, O., Rahman, I.M.: Impact of features reduction on machine learning based intrusion detection systems. EAI Endors. Trans. Scalable Inf. Syst. **9**(6), e9–e9 (2022)
15. Ficek, J., Wang, W., Chen, H., Dagne, G., Daley, E.: Differential privacy in health research: a scoping review. J. Am. Med. Inform. Assoc. **28**(10), 2269–2276 (2021)
16. Fung, B.C.M., Wang, K., Chen, R., Yu, P.S.: Privacy-preserving data publishing: a survey of recent developments. ACM Comput. Surv. **42**(4) (2010). https://doi.org/10.1145/1749603.1749605
17. Ge, Y.F., Bertino, E., Wang, H., Cao, J., Zhang, Y.: Distributed cooperative coevolution of data publishing privacy and transparency. ACM Trans. Knowl. Discov. Data (2023). https://doi.org/10.1145/3613962
18. Ge, Y.F., Orlowska, M., Cao, J., Wang, H., Zhang, Y.: MDDE: multitasking distributed differential evolution for privacy-preserving database fragmentation. VLDB J. **31**(5), 957–975 (2022)
19. Ge, Y.F., et al.: Evolutionary dynamic database partitioning optimization for privacy and utility. IEEE Trans. Dependable Secure Comput. (2023). https://doi.org/10.1109/tdsc.2023.3302284
20. Ge, Y.F., Wang, H., Cao, J., Zhang, Y.: An information-driven genetic algorithm for privacy-preserving data publishing. In: Chbeir, R., Huang, H., Silvestri, F., Manolopoulos, Y., Zhang, Y. (eds.) WISE 2022. LNCS, vol. 13724, pp. 340–354. Springer, Cham (2022). https://doi.org/10.1007/978-3-031-20891-1_24
21. Ge, Y.F., et al.: DSGA: a distributed segment-based genetic algorithm for multi-objective outsourced database partitioning. Inf. Sci. **612**, 864–886 (2022). https://doi.org/10.1016/j.ins.2022.09.003
22. Hu, J., Sun, K., Zhang, H.: Helmholtz machine with differential privacy. Inf. Sci. **613**, 888–903 (2022)
23. Jain, P., Gyanchandani, M., Khare, N.: Big data privacy: a technological perspective and review. J. Big Data **3**(1), 1–25 (2016). https://doi.org/10.1186/s40537-016-0059-y
24. Kabir, M.E., Mahmood, A.N., Wang, H., Mustafa, A.K.: Microaggregation sorting framework for k-anonymity statistical disclosure control in cloud computing. IEEE Trans. Cloud Comput. **8**(2), 408–417 (2020). https://doi.org/10.1109/tcc.2015.2469649
25. Kong, L., Wang, L., Gong, W., Yan, C., Duan, Y., Qi, L.: LSH-aware multitype health data prediction with privacy preservation in edge environment. World Wide Web **25**, 1793–1808 (2022)
26. Li, N., Li, T., Venkatasubramanian, S.: t-closeness: privacy beyond k-anonymity and l-diversity. In: 2007 IEEE 23rd International Conference on Data Engineering, pp. 106–115. IEEE (2006)
27. Machanavajjhala, A., Kifer, D., Gehrke, J., Venkitasubramaniam, M.: l-diversity: privacy beyond k-anonymity. ACM Trans. Knowl. Discov. Data (TKDD) **1**(1), 3-es (2007)
28. Ngatchou, P., Zarei, A., El-Sharkawi, A.: Pareto multi objective optimization. In: Proceedings of the 13th International Conference on, Intelligent Systems Application to Power Systems, pp. 84–91. IEEE (2005)
29. Rajendran, K., Jayabalan, M., Rana, M.E.: A study on k-anonymity, l-diversity, and t-closeness techniques. IJCSNS **17**(12), 172 (2017)

30. Samarati, P.: Protecting respondents identities in microdata release. IEEE Trans. Knowl. Data Eng. **13**(6), 1010–1027 (2001)
31. Sarki, R., Ahmed, K., Wang, H., Zhang, Y., Wang, K.: Convolutional neural network for multi-class classification of diabetic eye disease. EAI Endors. Trans. Scalable Inf. Syst. **9**(4), e5–e5 (2022)
32. Soria-Comas, J., Domingo-Ferrer, J., Sánchez, D., Martínez, S.: Enhancing data utility in differential privacy via microaggregation-based k-anonymity. VLDB J. **23**(5), 771–794 (2014)
33. Sowmiyaa, P., Tamilarasu, P., Kavitha, S., Rekha, A., Krishna, G.: Privacy preservation for microdata by using k-anonymity Algorithm. Int. J. Adv. Res. Comput. Commun. Eng. **4**(4), 373–5 (2015)
34. Sun, X., Li, M., Wang, H.: A family of enhanced (l, α)-diversity models for privacy preserving data publishing. Futur. Gener. Comput. Syst. **27**(3), 348–356 (2011). https://doi.org/10.1016/j.future.2010.07.007
35. Sun, X., Wang, H., Li, J., Zhang, Y.: Satisfying privacy requirements before data anonymization. Comput. J. **55**(4), 422–437 (2012)
36. Sweeney, L.: k-anonymity: a model for protecting privacy. Int. J. Uncertain. Fuzziness Knowl.-Based Syst. **10**(05), 557–570 (2002)
37. Vadavalli, A., Subhashini, R.: An improved differential privacy-preserving truth discovery approach in healthcare. In: 2019 IEEE 10th Annual Information Technology, Electronics and Mobile Communication Conference (IEMCON), pp. 1031–1037. IEEE (2019)
38. Vasa, J., Thakkar, A.: Deep learning: differential privacy preservation in the era of big data. J. Comput. Inf. Syst. **63**, 1–24 (2022)
39. Venkateswaran, N., Prabaharan, S.P.: An efficient neuro deep learning intrusion detection system for mobile adhoc networks. EAI Endors. Trans. Scalable Inf. Syst. **9**(6), e7–e7 (2022)
40. Vimalachandran, P., Liu, H., Lin, Y., Ji, K., Wang, H., Zhang, Y.: Improving accessibility of the Australian my health records while preserving privacy and security of the system. Health Inf. Sci. Syst. **8**, 1–9 (2020)
41. Wang, H., Yi, X., Bertino, E., Sun, L.: Protecting outsourced data in cloud computing through access management. Concurr. Comput.: Pract. Exp. **28**(3), 600–615 (2016)
42. Yin, J., Tang, M., Cao, J., Wang, H., You, M., Lin, Y.: Vulnerability exploitation time prediction: an integrated framework for dynamic imbalanced learning. World Wide Web **25**, 401–423 (2022)
43. You, M., et al.: A knowledge graph empowered online learning framework for access control decision-making. World Wide Web **26**(2), 827–848 (2023)

Enhancing Health Information Systems Security: An Ontology Model Approach

Raza Nowrozy[✉] and Khandakar Ahmed

Victoria University, 295 Queen Street, Melbourne, VIC 3000, Australia
raza.nowrozy@live.vu.edu.au, Khandakar.Ahmed@vu.edu.au

Abstract. This study explores the implications of integrating Health Information System (HIS) on the security and privacy of sensitive patient information. It identifies existing gaps in research and proposes a novel security ontology model aimed at strengthening the defence of health information systems. The model revolves around the Ontology Conceptual Security Model, which comprehensively captures the intricate relationships between different components of HIS security. By incorporating elements such as Health Information, HIS Security Conditions, and Semantic Web Rule Language (SWRL) rules, the model promotes the establishment of rule-based access policies. It effectively combines various access control strategies, including Role-Based Access Control (RBAC), Attribute-Based Access Control (ABAC), and Mandatory Access Control (MAC). This integration ensures both flexibility and compliance with regulatory requirements. While the model represents a significant advancement in the field, it recognizes the need for further validation and addresses future challenges. Specifically, it highlights the importance of exploring advanced access control mechanisms and seamless integration with existing systems. In essence, this study presents a comprehensive framework for a robust security ontology model designed to enhance the protection of patient data within HIS systems.

Keywords: Health Information Systems (HIS) · Security · Privacy · Access Control · Ontology

1 Introduction

HIS are essential for ensuring management of sensitive patient data, but are at risk of cyber attacks. Security Ontology Model for HIS addresses this concern, facilitating standardized security and aiding organisations to identify and address potential risks [16, 25, 34]. HIS information security is critical for patient data protection, but the rise in data breaches is concerning. Standardized, adaptable ontology models can help overcome fragmentation and inconsistency in current security approaches, managing risks in the complex, dynamic environment of health information systems [20]. Comprehensive models should encompass components like authentication, authorisation, encryption, and regulations like

© The Author(s), under exclusive license to Springer Nature Singapore Pte Ltd. 2023
Y. Li et al. (Eds.): HIS 2023, LNCS 14305, pp. 91–100, 2023.
https://doi.org/10.1007/978-981-99-7108-4_8

HIPAA and NIST Cybersecurity Framework, ensuring adaptability across different HIS environments. Research on HIS security is expanding but lacks a comprehensive approach, often focusing on specific aspects, leaving other components vulnerable. Security standards like HIPAA and the NIST Cybersecurity Framework need integration in HIS studies for effective measures in actual HIS systems [3]. Continuous updates addressing emerging security challenges and empirical research for assessing security measure effectiveness are crucial.

This study introduces a novel security ontology model uniquely designed for Health Information Systems (HIS). It enhances comprehension of security concepts, contributes to HIS security standard definition, and promotes better communication among diverse stakeholders. Specifically, the ontology model combines the Ontology Conceptual Security Model, which outlines the connections between various HIS security components. It includes essential elements such as Health Information, HIS Security Conditions, and Semantic Web Rule Language (SWRL) rules. These elements are crucial in creating rule-based access policies and implementing access control strategies like Role-Based Access Control (RBAC), Attribute-Based Access Control (ABAC), and Mandatory Access Control (MAC) [37,40,41]. The integration of these strategies allows system adaptability, ensures regulatory compliance, and safeguards sensitive patient information. Furthermore, the paper deeply explores the challenges associated with creating a robust security ontology model for HIS, given its inherent complexity and the lack of universal security frameworks [3,35]. It identifies deficiencies in the present security standards and emphasises the need for user-friendly interfaces that can seamlessly integrate with other systems.

The remainder of this paper is organized as follows: Sect. 2 offers a review of existing literature, spotlighting the gaps that this research aims to fill. Section 3 presents the motivation behind the study. Section 4 discusses the Ontology Security Policy. In Sect. 5, we discuss the potential implications of the model, its limitations, and suggest potential avenues for further research. Section 6 discusses the security philosophy model for Health Information Systems, along with further discussion. Lastly, Sect. 7 concludes by summarizing the paper's key contributions to enhancing HIS security.

2   Background and Related Work

This section delves into the present status of research and development surrounding the security and scalability of health information systems (HIS). It mainly centres on security ontology models, designed with tools like Web Ontology Language (OWL) and Security Content Automation Protocol (SCAP) to safeguard patients' medical records [4,17]. However, these models often overlook key features like scalability and user acceptance, limiting their capacity to handle large data volumes and users.

The study introduces a novel security ontology model for HIS, which accounts for these shortcomings by including security concepts such as availability, confidentiality, integrity, and user acceptance factors like usability and efficiency

[2,23]. This ensures that security measures do not impede system use or efficacy. The proposed model also addresses the constraint on data access through role-based access control, aligning with the latest security standards [19,27].

In comparison to existing models, the new approach offers enhanced scalability and versatility, addressing issues such as restricted data access and the complexity of HIS [24]. Unlike previous works that lacked a comprehensive understanding of user acceptance and data volume handling, this model adapts to changing threat scenarios, thereby enhancing data security.

The surge in the use of HIS necessitates robust access control policies to guard against threats such as identity theft and insurance fraud [26]. The conceptual ontology security model serves as an organised strategy for forming and implementing these policies, identifying stakeholders and ensuring that only authorised personnel can access HIS. This comprehensive approach contributes significantly to HIS security and scalability, setting it apart from existing models that failed to address these critical aspects.

3   Research Motivations

Patient health information security is critical in healthcare, and traditional Role-Based Access Control (RBAC) systems help manage resource access [33,38,39]. However, these systems lack context-awareness, leading to potentially unnecessary access grants. Context-Aware RBAC (CA-RBAC) improves upon RBAC by considering context, such as location, time, and the accessing device. This approach ensures that access is granted only when necessary, for example, granting a doctor access to a patient's medical records only when they are in the hospital and preventing access from a public Wi-Fi network. By doing so, it provides a finer level of access control and enhances privacy and security in healthcare settings [1].

Implementing CA-RBAC involves identifying relevant contextual information, creating decision trees based on this context, and integrating these trees with the RBAC model [10]. CA-RBAC can also be implemented using ontologies, which model the relationships between various contextual factors. However, implementing CA-RBAC poses several challenges including the complexity of modeling contextual information and the potential for conflicts between RBAC and CA-RBAC models [9]. CA-RBAC has been successfully utilized in different healthcare environments like emergency rooms and home healthcare, providing access based on patient's condition, urgency, healthcare provider's role, location, time, and task [13]. Despite its advantages, implementing CA-RBAC comes with challenges, including the complexity of modeling contextual information, maintaining up-to-date context, resolving conflicts between RBAC and CA-RBAC models, and potential changes to existing healthcare infrastructure [12].

Health Information Systems (HIS) play a crucial role in contemporary healthcare, enabling the accessibility of patient data and communication between providers [28,30]. Despite stringent security measures [7,32,42], data breaches have occurred due to deficient access control policies, thus inspiring the necessity for an innovative security ontology for HIS. Particularly for multi-provider patient care, current policies can be overly restrictive, impeding necessary data access and compromising patient care. Patients frequently receive care from several providers, potentially causing inefficiency and fragmentation [5,11,44]. A novel security model that facilitates seamless provider collaboration, while ensuring authorised access to patient information, is therefore essential. This model should allow access to a patient's HIS only to their care providers, safeguarding privacy, and supporting efficient, coordinated care. The highlighted scenario emphasises the importance of robust access control policies and security models to prevent unauthorised patient data access and protect against threats such as identity theft, insurance fraud, and blackmail due to data breaches. It underscores the necessity for staff training, clear security incident response policies, and improved access control policies, emphasising the need for an advanced security model or ontology to address the risks associated with unauthorised patient data access in healthcare systems.

4   Ontology Security Policy

The increasing use of Health Information Systems (HIS) necessitates robust access control policies to protect patient privacy and prevent unauthorized access to sensitive health data. In response to this need, a security ontology is introduced, defining specific entity types, attributes, and operations within the HIS context.

Entities (E) represent the actors in the system, such as patients, healthcare providers, insurers, and regulators, each with distinct roles and responsibilities. Attributes (A) define characteristics like roles, permissions, and locations, which are critical in determining the permitted operations on HIS. Operations (O) detail actions like reading or writing medical records, prescribing medications, or accessing patient histories, varying based on the stakeholder's role and responsibilities. Together, these components form a formal policy model (E, A, O) that structures access control policies, ensuring confidentiality, integrity, and accessibility of healthcare information. This ontology model is designed to enhance the protection of patient data within HIS systems, providing a comprehensive framework for a robust security ontology.

The ontology also employs Semantic Web Rule Language (SWRL) rules to ensure healthcare providers and insurers have access to only necessary records. These rules, created based on the ontology's security conditions, define who can perform specific operations on certain attributes, assisting in regulatory compliance and data security when integrated into HIS [14,43]. By defining and implementing this ontology, the study aims to present a comprehensive framework for a robust security ontology model that not only addresses the current challenges in HIS security but also provides a scalable and adaptable solution for future advancements in healthcare technology.

Building upon a previously created privacy ontology, the security ontology model defines specific security conditions for different types of health information. For example, a healthcare provider may have read-only access to a patient's medical history, while an insurer may have restricted access to billing information. This approach regulates access to health records, protecting patients' privacy [29].

Semantic Web Rule Language (SWRL) rules complement the ontology by defining who can perform specific operations on certain attributes. Created based on the ontology's security conditions, SWRL rules assist in regulatory compliance and data security when integrated into HIS. For instance, a rule might specify that only primary care physicians can write prescriptions for a particular patient [21,36](Table 1).

Table 1. Overview of Ontology Components in HIS Security

Component	Description	Examples
Entities (E)	Actors in the system requiring protection	Patients, Healthcare Providers, Insurers, Regulators
Attributes (A)	Characteristics defining roles, permissions, and locations	Role: Doctor, Nurse; Permissions: Read, Write; Location: Hospital, Clinic
Operations (O)	Actions performed on entities based on roles	Read Medical Record, Write Prescription
Security Conditions	Part of the ontology to maintain privacy	RBAC, ABAC policies, Encryption
SWRL Rules	Specify access control policies	Rule: If Role=Doctor Then Access=Read

5   SWRL Rule-Bases

SWRL (Semantic Web Rule Language) is a rules-based language designed for rule-based reasoning, differencing, and data representation in the Semantic Web. In the context of Health Information Systems (HIS), SWRL can be used to define access control policies for sensitive patient data. In order to construct a Semantic Web Rule Language (SWRL) rule-base for Health Information Systems (HIS), it is essential to define domain vocabulary, ontology, and access rules. The vocabulary includes terms such as "patient," "provider," and "insurer." The ontology represents relationships between these entities, while the rules regulate access to sensitive patient data [22]. For example, a rule could be defined that allows a patient's primary care provider to access their medical records if the patient consents. Such rules can be represented using SWRL, a tool adept at establishing rule-based systems, especially in health information systems. The Web Ontology Language (OWL) is useful for defining entities, their relationships, and constraints, such as defining a "MedicalRecord" class and its properties like "patient" and "accessControlPolicy" [15]. Following ontology definition, SWRL can model access control policies, specifying conditions under which stakeholders can access patient data. For instance, a rule may allow access to a patient's medical history if the provider is their primary care physician or a treating specialist(Table 2). Defining access control strategies is crucial in creating a SWRL rule-base for HIS, enabling robust and flexible access control policies that regulate who has access to sensitive patient data. After defining these policies, security conditions specifying when to apply them need to be established, considering factors like user identity, type of data accessed, and access purpose [6,18,31]. These conditions can also consider the user's trust level, data sensitivity, and access context. For instance, providers with specialised authorisation may have access to sensitive data like HIV status. These conditions are vital in forming a comprehensive SWRL rule-base for HIS. Combining access control policies and security conditions allows the creation of SWRL rules that dictate the circumstances under which sensitive patient data can be accessed or denied. An example rule might allow a doctor to access a patient's medical record while they are in their care. The resulting SWRL rule-base is a collection of rules defining access control policies for all health-related stakeholders [8]. The SWRL rule-base can be incorporated into the HIS to enforce access control policies, queried to determine the permissibility of a specific access request based on the user's rights, data sensitivity, and access purpose, thus ensuring the confidentiality, integrity, and availability of sensitive patient data (Fig. 1).

Table 2. SWRL rule-base

Rule ID	Rule Description
Rule 1	$Patient(?p) \wedge Provider(?pr) \wedge (PrimaryCarePhysician(?pr, ?p) \vee TreatingSpecialist(?pr, ?p)) \rightarrow MedicalHistoryAccess(?pr, ?p)$
Rule 2	$Patient(?p) \wedge Provider(?pr) \wedge PrimaryCarePhysician(?pr, ?p) \wedge Consent(?pr, ?p) \rightarrow MedicalRecordAccess(?pr, ?p)$
Rule 3	$Patient(?p) \wedge Provider(?pr) \wedge MedicalRecordAccess(?pr, ?p) \wedge MedicalTreatment(?t) \wedge PurposeOfAccess(?pr, ?t) \rightarrow Access(?pr, ?p, ?t)$
Rule 4	$Doctor(?d) \wedge Patient(?p) \wedge MedicalRecordAccess(?d, ?p) \wedge PurposeOfAccess(?d, "Medical\ Treatment") \rightarrow Access(?d, ?p, "Medical\ Record")$

6 Discussion

Different access control models offer unique strategies for securing healthcare data. Traditional Role-Based Access Control (RBAC) manages resource access but lacks context-awareness, leading to potential unnecessary access. Context-Aware RBAC (CA-RBAC) enhances this by integrating context, such as location and time, into access decisions, offering better privacy and security. Yet, its implementation can be challenging due to the complexity of contextual modeling. The Semantic Web Rule Language (SWRL) rule-base for Health Information

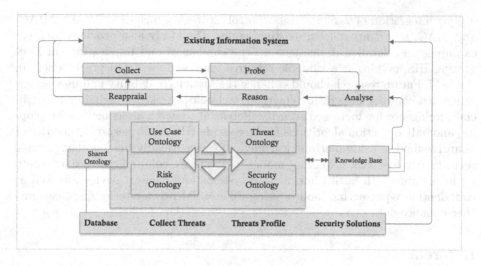

Fig. 1. Creating an SWRL rule-base for HIS

Systems (HIS) provides another approach, defining policies through ontology languages, but its effectiveness depends on the reasoning engine. Attribute-Based Access Control (ABAC) uses user attributes for more granular control, but maintaining updated user attributes can be demanding. Mandatory Access Control (MAC) ensures high-level security based on user clearance, but its inflexibility can pose management challenges. The choice of model should be based on the healthcare setting's specific needs, and a thorough evaluation and ongoing monitoring are crucial for effective security management.

The security philosophy model for Health Information Systems (HIS) has limitations and faces challenges. Despite its adaptability, the model is context-specific and doesn't cover all security aspects, focusing primarily on access control policies while overlooking network security and data encryption. It presumes equal user access across the HIS, neglecting the need for role-based controls, and requires regular updates to counter evolving threats, including those from AI and IoT. The creation of this model is complicated by the complexity of HIS, non-standardized healthcare security terms, and outdated security standards. Further difficulties include user acceptance, limited access to security data, integration issues, and scalability needs. Overcoming these challenges is vital for creating a comprehensive model ensuring patient data safety.

7 Conclusions and Future Research

This paper contributes to the field by proposing a novel ontology model for incorporating security concepts and rules in Health Information Systems (HIS). By reusing well-established ontologies and expressing security rules in SWRL, it ensures flexibility and compliance with regulatory requirements. The model's unique integration of various access control strategies, including RBAC, ABAC, and MAC, sets it apart from existing works. The study also provides concrete examples and detailed discussions on the challenges and implications of integrating HIS, making it a valuable resource for researchers and practitioners in the field. Future research should enhance the model's scalability and user acceptance and consider integrating emerging technologies like blockchain and artificial intelligence for increased security. Potential research areas include developing anomaly-detection algorithms for large-scale HIS databases, real-time threat adaptive models using machine learning, and user-friendly models that provide security risk feedback Exploring models that ensure comprehensive data safety by integrating with health information systems and medical devices, as well as confidentiality-preserving models using differential privacy techniques, can further enhance data privacy.

References

1. Alvarez-Rodríguez, J.M., Mendieta, R., Cibrián, E., Llorens, J.: Towards a method to quantitatively measure toolchain interoperability in the engineering lifecycle: a case study of digital hardware design. Comput. Stand. Interfaces **86**, 103744 (2023)
2. Bai, T., et al.: Integrating knowledge from case report: a medical-ontology based multimodal information system with structured summary (2022)
3. Blanco, J., Miguel, B., Rossi, T.: A comparative study of energy domain ontologies. In: Marchiori, M., Dominguez Mayo, F.J., Filipe, J. (eds.) WEBIST WEBIST 2020 2021. LNCS, vol. 2020, pp. 43–58. Springer, Cham (2020). https://doi.org/10.1007/978-3-031-24197-0_3
4. Cerqueira, J.: An ontology for context-aware middleware for dependable medical systems. In: Proceedings of the 11th Latin-American Symposium on Dependable Computing, pp. 79–83 (2022)
5. Ge, Y.F., Orlowska, M., Cao, J., Wang, H., Zhang, Y.: MDDE: multitasking distributed differential evolution for privacy-preserving database fragmentation. VLDB J. **31**, 1–19 (2022). https://doi.org/10.1007/s00778-021-00718-w
6. Huang, T., Gong, Y.J., Kwong, S., Wang, H., Zhang, J.: A niching memetic algorithm for multi-solution traveling salesman problem. IEEE Trans. Evol. Comput. **24**(3), 508–522 (2019)
7. Kabir, E., Mahmood, A., Wang, H., Mustafa, A.: Microaggregation sorting framework for k-anonymity statistical disclosure control in cloud computing. IEEE Trans. Cloud Comput. **8**(2), 408–417 (2015). https://doi.org/10.1109/TCC.2015.2469649
8. Kernstock, P., Przybilla, L., Thatcher, J., Krcmar, H.: Can't Get No Satisfaction?"-The Case for Broadening Information Systems Research on E-Commerce (2023)
9. Khalyasmaa, A.I., Stepanova, A.I., Stanislav, A., Eroshenko, P.V.: Matrenin: review of the digital twin technology applications for electrical equipment lifecycle management. Mathematics **11**(6), 1315–1315 (2023)
10. Lambrix, P.: Database and Web Information Systems Group: Publications (2023)
11. Lee, J.: The use of telehealth during the coronavirus (COVID-19) pandemic in oral and maxillofacial surgery - a qualitative analysis. ICST Trans. Scalable Inf. Syst. (2021). https://doi.org/10.4108/eai.2-12-2021.172361

12. Lwin, H.N.N., Punnakitikashem, P., Thananusak, T.: E-Health research in Southeast Asia: a bibliometric review. Sustainability **15**(3), 2559–2559 (2023)
13. Matos, D., Everton, E., Viegas, R., Hessel, F.: Context-aware security in the internet of things: a review. In: Barolli, L. (ed.) AINA 2023. LNCS, vol. 3, pp. 518–531. Springer, Cham (2023). https://doi.org/10.1007/978-3-031-28694-0_49
14. Mcgagh, D., et al.: A novel ontological approach to track social determinants of health in primary care. In: Polovina, R., Polovina, S., Kemp, N. (eds.) MOVE 2020. Communications in Computer and Information Science, vol. 1694, pp. 227–240. Springer, Cham (2020). https://doi.org/10.1007/978-3-031-22228-3_10
15. Minardi, R., Villani, M.L., De Nicola, A.: Semantic reasoning for geolocalized assessment of crime risk in smart cities. Smart Cities **6**(1), 179–195 (2023)
16. Nowrozy, R., Ahmed, K., Wang, H., Mcintosh, T.: Towards a universal privacy model for electronic health record systems: an ontology and machine learning approach. In: Informatics, vol. 10, p. 60. MDPI (2023)
17. Ojino, R., Mich, L., Mvungi, N.: Hotel room personalization via ontology and rule-based reasoning. Int. J. Web Inf. Syst. **18**(5/6), 369–387 (2022)
18. Ovono, G.: Sihlemoyo: conceptual linked data model for south African municipalities public services domain. In: Silhavy, R., Silhavy, P., Prokopova, Z. (eds.) CoMeSySo 2022. LNCS, vol. 2, pp. 197–208. Springer, Cham (2023). https://doi.org/10.1007/978-3-031-21438-7_17
19. Pereira, T.F., et al.: A web-based voice interaction framework proposal for enhancing information systems user experience. Procedia Comput. Sci. **196**, 235–244 (2022)
20. Pileggi, S.F.: Ontology in Hybrid Intelligence: a concise literature review (2023)
21. Prawira, K.T., Hindarto, D., Indrajit, E.: Application of enterprise architecture in digital transformation of insurance companies, 856–865 (2023)
22. Qian, J., Liu, Y.: Quantitative scenario construction of typical disasters driven by ontology data. J. Safety Sci. Resilience **4**(2), 159–166 (2023)
23. Ren, Z., Shi, J., Imran, M.: Data evolution governance for ontology-based digital twin product lifecycle management. IEEE Trans. Ind. Inf. **19**(2), 1791–1802 (2022)
24. Rezaei, Z., Vahidnia, M.H.: Effective medical center finding during COVID-19 pandemic using a spatial DSS centered on ontology engineering. GeoJournal **88**, 1–15 (2022)
25. Rousseau, J.F., Oliveira, E., Tierney, W.M., Khurshid, A.: Methods for development and application of data standards in an ontology-driven information model for measuring, managing, and computing social determinants of health for individuals, households, and communities evaluated through an example of asthma. J. Biomed. Inf. **136**, 104241 (2022)
26. Sánchez-Zas, C., Villagrá, V.A., Vega-Barbas, M., Larriva-Novo, X., Moreno, J.I., Berrocal, J.: Ontology-based approach to real-time risk management and cyber-situational awareness. Future Gener. Comput. Syst. **141**, 462–472 (2023)
27. Sansone, C., Sperlí, G.: Legal information retrieval systems: state-of-the-art and open issues. Inf. Syst. **106**, 101967–101967 (2022)
28. Sarki, R., Ahmed, K., Wang, H., Zhang, Y.: Automated detection of mild and multi-class diabetic eye diseases using deep learning. Health Inf. Sci. Syst. **8**(1), 1–9 (2020). https://doi.org/10.1007/s13755-020-00125-5
29. Sharma, A., Kumar, S.: Ontology-based semantic retrieval of documents using Word2vec model. Data Knowl. Eng. **144**, 102110–102110 (2023)
30. Singh, R., et al.: Antisocial behavior identification from Twitter feeds using traditional machine learning algorithms and deep learning. ICST Trans. Scalable Inf. Syst. **10**, e17 (2023). https://doi.org/10.4108/eetsis.v10i3.3184

31. Sun, X., Li, M., Wang, H., Plank, A.: An efficient hash-based algorithm for minimal k-anonymity. In: Conferences in Research and Practice in Information Technology (CRPIT), vol. 74, pp. 101–107 (2008)

32. Sun, X., Wang, H., Li, J.: Injecting purpose and trust into data anonymisation. In: Proceedings of the 18th ACM Conference on Information and Knowledge Management, pp. 1541–1544 (2009)

33. Sun, X., Wang, H., Li, J., Zhang, Y.: Satisfying privacy requirements before data anonymization. Comput. J. **55**(4), 422–437 (2012)

34. Tagde, P., et al.: Blockchain and artificial intelligence technology in e-health. Environ. Sci. Pollut. Res. **28**, 52810–52831 (2021)

35. Tahar, K., Martin, T., Mou, Y., Verbuecheln, R., Graessner, H., Krefting, D.: Rare diseases in hospital information systems-an interoperable methodology for distributed data quality assessments. Methods Inf. Med. AAM (2023)

36. Thuan, N.H., Dang-Pham, D., Le, H.S., Bhattacharya, P., Phan, T.Q: Introduction to Information Systems Research in Vietnam: A Shared Vision. In: Hoang Thuan, N., Dang-Pham, D., Le, H.S., Phan, T.Q. (eds.) Information Systems Research in Vietnam, pp. 1–16. Springer, Cham (2023). https://doi.org/10.1007/978-981-19-3804-7_1

37. Wang, H., Cao, J., Zhang, Y.: A flexible payment scheme and its role-based access control. IEEE Trans. Knowl. Data Eng. **17**, 425–436 (2005). https://doi.org/10.1109/TKDE.2005.35

38. Wang, H., Sun, L.: Trust-involved access control in collaborative open social networks. In: 2010 Fourth International Conference on Network and System Security, pp. 239–246. IEEE (2010)

39. Wang, H., Wang, Y., Taleb, T., Jiang, X.: Special issue on security and privacy in network computing. World Wide Web **23**, 951–957 (2020)

40. Wang, H., Yi, X., Bertino, E., Sun, L.: Protecting outsourced data in cloud computing through access management. Concurrency Comput.: Pract. Exp. **28**(3), 600–615 (2016)

41. Wang, H., Zhang, Y., Cao, J.: Effective collaboration with information sharing in virtual universities. IEEE Trans. Knowl. Data Eng. **21**, 840–853 (2009). https://doi.org/10.1109/TKDE.2008.132

42. Wang, Y., Shen, Y., Wang, H., Cao, J., Jiang, X.: MtMR: ensuring MapReduce computation integrity with Merkle tree-based verifications. IEEE Trans. Big Data **4**(3), 418–431 (2016)

43. Wawrzik, F., Rafique, K.A., Rahman, F., Grimm, C.: Ontology learning applications of knowledge base construction for microelectronic systems. Information **14**, 176–176 (2023)

44. Zhang, F., Wang, Y., Liu, S., Wang, H.: Decision-based evasion attacks on tree ensemble classifiers. World Wide Web **23**(5), 2957–2977 (2020). https://doi.org/10.1007/s11280-020-00813-y

Developing a Comprehensive Risk Management Framework for E-Health Care Delivery

Avisen Moonsamy[1,2]([✉]) [iD] and Mohiuddin Ahmed[1]

[1] Edith Cowan University, Perth, Western Australia, Australia
{a.moonsamy,mohiuddin.ahmed}@ecu.edu.au
[2] Deloitte, Risk Advisory, Perth, Western Australia, Australia

Abstract. The COVID-19 pandemic has accelerated the transformation of healthcare delivery towards E-health and telemedicine, enabling more accessible and efficient patient care. However, it introduces several additional risks, like data breaches, cyberattacks, software malfunctions, and patient privacy violations. Current risk management frameworks often fail to adequately address these specific risks in E-health, highlighting the urgent need for a more specialised approach. This paper addresses this gap by proposing a comprehensive risk management framework tailored to e-health care delivery. Our approach includes a systematic process for risk identification, assessment, mitigation, and continuous review. We explore the potential of artificial intelligence (AI) in enhancing this framework, particularly in anomaly detection and predictive modelling for risk anticipation. Furthermore, the paper discusses the legal, ethical, and societal implications of managing risks in E-health care delivery, underscoring the need for stringent data privacy measures and adherence to ethical guidelines. This research contributes to the evolving field of e-health by offering a strategic framework for mitigating its unique risks, thus ensuring safer and more secure healthcare delivery in the digital age.

Keywords: E-health · telemedicine · cyber security · risk management · data breaches · data privacy

1 Introduction

1.1 Overview of E-Health and Telemedicine

E-health and telemedicine have become increasingly central to modern healthcare systems. Eysenbach (2001) defines e-health as an emerging field in the intersection of medical informatics, public health, and business, referring to health services and information delivered or enhanced through the internet and related technologies. It represents not only a technical development but also a state of mind, a way of thinking, an attitude, and a commitment to networked, global thinking, to improve healthcare locally, regionally, and worldwide [4]. Telemedicine is a critical component of e-health, specifically dealing with the provision of healthcare services from a distance. It involves using information and communication technologies (ICT) to overcome geographical barriers, enhancing

Y. Li et al. (Eds.): HIS 2023, LNCS 14305, pp. 101–111, 2023.
https://doi.org/10.1007/978-981-99-7108-4_9

access to medical services that would often not be consistently available in distant rural communities [5]. The global COVID-19 pandemic has expedited the adoption of e-health and telemedicine, as healthcare providers sought solutions for delivering medical services remotely to adhere to social distancing regulations and ensure patient safety [7, 8]. Despite the significant benefits, the rapid digital transformation also introduces an array of new risks, including data breaches, cyberattacks, software malfunctions, and patient privacy violations [3]. Therefore, developing robust risk management strategies is crucial to address these unique challenges, particularly in e-health and telemedicine, which operate at the forefront of technological advances and are characterised by high data sensitivity [6, 9–11].

1.2 The Impact of COVID-19 on the Surge of E-Health and Telemedicine

The COVID-19 pandemic has been a transformative force for many sectors of society, and healthcare is no exception. As in-person interactions became risky due to the highly transmissible nature of the virus, e-health and telemedicine rapidly gained importance in the healthcare delivery landscape [7]. Before the pandemic, the uptake of e-health and telemedicine had been steady but relatively slow, with barriers such as a lack of technological infrastructure, digital literacy, and regulations concerning data privacy and security [11]. However, the pandemic forced a rapid reassessment of these barriers as healthcare providers scrambled to deliver services in a radically altered environment. One of the main drivers of this transformation was the need to manage patients with mild to moderate symptoms of COVID-19 remotely, reducing the strain on healthcare facilities and lowering the risk of transmission to healthcare workers and other patients. E-health applications became pivotal in this pandemic management, enabling remote patient monitoring, disseminating up-to-date information, and facilitating virtual consultations [7]. In addition, the pandemic also underscored the importance of a robust e-health readiness framework. While the rapid transition to e-health and telemedicine brought many advantages, it also exposed healthcare systems to new types of risks. Cybersecurity has become a growing concern, with the increased use of digital health technologies opening up potential vulnerabilities for data breaches and cyberattacks [3, 6, 9, 10].

1.3 The Need for a Comprehensive Risk Management Framework for E-Health and Telemedicine

The rapid advancement and adoption of e-health and telemedicine, particularly in response to the COVID-19 pandemic, has underscored the importance of robust risk management strategies in healthcare systems. The evolution of technology-driven health-care systems brings forth a new array of potential risks, including security and privacy breaches, data corruption, or system failures [3, 6]. Firstly, the security of e-health services is a primary concern. The paper by Boonyarattaphan, Bai, & Chung (2009) proposed a security framework for e-health service authentication and e-health data transmission, demonstrating the importance of securing patient data and communication during online consultations and medical services [2].

Next, privacy is another key risk factor that must be carefully managed. The advent of e-health and telemedicine involves storing and transmitting sensitive health data, making it a prime target for unauthorised access and data breaches. Hence, ensuring privacy in e-health records is critical [10]. Shrestha et al. (2016) illustrates how an enhanced e-health framework can help protect privacy in the healthcare system [9]. Their work exemplifies how innovative approaches can enhance the security and privacy of e-health and telemedicine services. Further, Ksibi, Jaidi, & Bouhoula (2021) discuss cybersecurity risks in the context of the Internet of Medical Things (IoMT) with a context-aware agent-based framework for managing cyber risks in IoMT, further indicating the need for specialised frameworks to handle the unique risks associated with e-health [6]. Croll and Croll (2007) also emphasised the need to investigate risk exposure in e-health systems. Their research shows how understanding these risks can lead to better preparedness and mitigation strategies [3]. Finally, the e-health preparedness assessment framework presented by Wickramasinghe et al. (2005) reminds us of the importance of assessing the readiness of the system to handle potential risks and challenges [11]. These studies clearly demonstrate the need for a comprehensive risk management framework for e-health and telemedicine. Such a framework would aim to identify potential risks, develop strategies to mitigate these risks and ensure the security, privacy, and reliability of e-health services.

2 Literature Review

2.1 Current Risk Management Approaches in E-Health and Telemedicine

The advent of e-health and telemedicine has brought a significant shift in the healthcare sector. However, this has also brought forth an array of new risks and challenges that need to be carefully managed. The literature presents several different approaches to addressing these risks, which can be analysed from different perspectives. Boonyarattaphan, Bai, and Chung (2009) advocate for a security framework that focuses on e-Health service authentication and e-Health data transmission. They believe that risk management in e-health must be a proactive process, and the first line of defence should be to ensure that data is accessed and transmitted securely [2]. Their security framework represents an approach that values and prioritises protecting sensitive healthcare information, thereby recognising the damage that security breaches and data loss can inflict. Complementing the security-centric approach, Croll and Croll (2007) focus on investigating risk exposure in e-health systems, which serves as a pre-emptive strategy [3]. Their work's premise is identifying risks before they become security incidents. By understanding where risk exposure is most significant, efforts can be directed to fortify these areas and reduce the likelihood of a breach. Ksibi, Jaidi, and Bouhoula (2021) address the risk management of a new generation of e-health systems with the IoMT at the core [6]. Their approach is an agent-based framework that is context-aware, effectively leveraging the capabilities of the IoMT. This framework, embedded within an environment teeming with interconnected devices and systems, demonstrates a forward-thinking perspective on risk management, in which the digital and physical realms merge to form an integrated e-health landscape. Wickramasinghe, Fadlalla, Geisler, and Schaffer (2005), on the other hand, proposed a comprehensive approach to assessing the readiness of e-health systems, which they believe to be an integral part of risk management [11].

Their framework is structured to evaluate various aspects of preparedness, such as technology readiness, organisational readiness, and the readiness of the user community. It represents a more holistic view of risk management that extends beyond the technological aspect also to include organisational and user aspects, thereby underscoring the importance of these elements in the successful implementation and use of e-health systems. These varying approaches reflect the dynamic and multi-faceted nature of risk management in e-health. They show that effective risk management requires not only robust and secure technological infrastructure but also comprehensive preparedness and risk exposure assessments.

2.2   The Role of AI in Healthcare Risk Management

Artificial Intelligence (AI) has emerged as a powerful tool in healthcare, offering capabilities that can significantly contribute to risk management. These capabilities can be seen in various aspects, such as improved diagnosis, treatment planning, patient monitoring, and even in the administrative sectors of healthcare. AI can be deployed to analyse large volumes of data quickly and accurately, helping healthcare providers to identify potential risks before they become significant issues. In e-health and telemedicine, AI could play an essential role in securing data transmission and authentication [2]. This is particularly important given the increasing prevalence of cyber threats in the healthcare sector. AI can also contribute significantly to risk management within the IoMT. Ksibi, Jaidi, & Bouhoula (2021) propose a context-aware agent-based framework for managing cyber-risks within IoMT, arguing that such a system could lead to more reliable e-health systems [6]. AI can analyse the vast amounts of data IoMT devices produce and identify potential security threats or vulnerabilities, which can then be addressed proactively. Moreover, AI can potentially improve risk management in pandemics, aiding in preparedness and response. Li & Ray (2010) discuss e-health applications for pandemic management, highlighting the potential for AI to analyse data and predict disease spread, which can help policymakers make more informed decisions [7]. Finally, AI can contribute to legal and ethical risk management in e-health. By ensuring that systems comply with regulatory requirements and ethical standards, AI can minimise the risk of breaches that could result in legal action or damage to an organisation's reputation. This includes ensuring patient data privacy and security, detecting fraudulent activities, and helping healthcare providers maintain compliance with evolving regulations.

2.3   Legal, Ethical, and Societal Implications of E-Health and Telemedicine

As e-health and telemedicine continue to evolve and permeate the healthcare landscape, they bring with them significant legal, ethical, and societal implications. It's essential that these aspects are fully considered to ensure the safe, effective, and responsible deployment and use of these technologies.

Legal Implications: The legal implications of e-health primarily revolve around issues of privacy, security, and data ownership. As Vora et al. (2018) argue, ensuring privacy and security in e-health records is paramount [10]. In many jurisdictions, legislation has been enacted to protect patient data, and healthcare providers must comply with these regulations. Legal implications also extend to issues of licensure and malpractice as healthcare delivery becomes more globalised and virtual.

Ethical Implications: Ethical issues in e-health are complex and multifaceted. One of the key concerns is the equitable distribution of these technologies. As Eysenbach (2001) asks, "What is e-health?" and perhaps more importantly, who has access to it [4]. While e-health has the potential to improve healthcare delivery, there is a risk that it could exacerbate existing health disparities if access to these technologies is not universally available. There are also ethical considerations around patient confidentiality, informed consent, and the professional-patient relationship in a digital context.

Societal Implications: The societal implications of e-health are vast and varied. On the positive side, e-health has the potential to increase access to healthcare, improve the quality of care, and reduce costs. However, these benefits must be balanced against potential downsides. For instance, the shift to e-health could potentially lead to a loss of personal interaction between healthcare providers and patients or even contribute to the digital divide if certain population segments lack access to the necessary technology. It is also important to consider how these technologies shape our perceptions of health and illness and our expectations of healthcare.

3   The Proposed Risk Management Framework

3.1   Detailed Description of the Proposed Risk Management Framework

This proposed risk management framework for e-health and telemedicine addresses the unique challenges of healthcare digitisation. It is structured around four key pillars - Data Security, Regulatory Compliance, Patient Safety, and Risk Prevention - each aimed at ensuring robust and secure e-health systems.

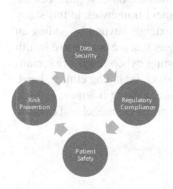

Data Security: This pillar ensures patient data's confidentiality, integrity, and availability. Recognising the growing cyber threat landscape, the framework emphasises implementing strong encryption mechanisms to protect patient data during transmission and storage. Secure authentication and authorisation protocols would be established to control access to e-health systems. In addition, a real-time monitoring system aided by AI can be instituted to identify anomalous activities indicative of a security breach, enabling swift response and mitigations [2, 9, 10].

Regulatory Compliance: The need for strict adherence to regulatory requirements like the Health Insurance Portability and Accountability Act (HIPAA), the General Data Protection Regulation (GDPR), and other country-specific laws is a critical concern. This pillar focuses on creating a framework that is designed to meet these regulatory requirements from the outset. Regular audits should be performed to ensure ongoing compliance, and any changes in legislation should be promptly incorporated into the system. Automated compliance tracking systems could also be implemented, leveraging AI to streamline the complex process of regulatory adherence [8, 9].

Patient Safety: As healthcare providers rely increasingly on e-health and telemedicine services, ensuring patient safety is paramount. This pillar of the framework focuses on the reliability and accuracy of e-health systems. High system availability should be maintained to ensure that healthcare providers can access the necessary data when required. Also, robust error-checking and fail-safe mechanisms should be incorporated to prevent misinformation and malfunctions that could harm patients. Using AI in this realm can assist in detecting potential health risks in patient data, enabling early interventions [5, 11].

Risk Prevention: The final pillar, risk prevention, advocates a proactive stance towards risk management. It involves continuously identifying and assessing risks, underpinned by a risk prediction model that leverages AI to forecast potential threats based on existing patterns and trends. Regular vulnerability assessments and threat modelling should be conducted, with mitigation plans established to address identified risks promptly. This pillar ensures that the e-health system can adapt to emerging threats and vulnerabilities, providing a resilient defence [2, 5].

The proposed risk management framework offers significant advancements compared to existing cybersecurity industry risk management frameworks while also acknowledging the value of these established systems. Existing cybersecurity risk management frameworks typically focus on data protection by identifying potential threats and vulnerabilities, implementing appropriate security controls, and managing the response to security incidents. They are comprehensive and designed to protect data confidentiality, integrity, and availability. Popular frameworks, such as the NIST Cybersecurity Framework and ISO 27000 series, offer guidance on best practices for managing cybersecurity risks. The proposed risk management framework in this study acknowledges the value of these existing approaches but extends beyond by adding an additional layer of risk assessment and management strategies that are unique to e-health and telemedicine. The proposed model enhances the existing cybersecurity risk management frameworks by incorporating a broader range of risks, including ethical, legal, and societal risks associated with e-health and telemedicine, making it a more holistic approach. Table 1 below shows a comparison between the proposed model and existing frameworks.

Table 1. Comparison between existing frameworks and the proposed model.

Frameworks	NIST Cybersecurity Framework	ISO 27001/27002	CIS Controls	COBIT	Essential 8	Proposed Risk Management Framework
Purpose	To provide a policy framework of computer security guidance for organisations to assess and improve their ability to prevent, detect, and respond to cyber-attacks.	To provide best practice recommendations on information security management, risks, and controls within the context of an overall Information Security Management System (ISMS).	To provide a prioritised set of actions to protect organisations and their data from known cyber-attack vectors.	To provide an IT governance framework that helps organisations meet objectives for the governance and management of enterprise IT.	To provide a prioritised list of practical actions to improve cyber security.	To provide a holistic risk management framework tailored for e-health and telemedicine services, focusing on not just cybersecurity but also ethical, legal, and societal implications.
Core Elements	Identify, Protect, Detect, Respond, and Recover.	Establishing the ISMS, Implementing, and operating the ISMS, Monitoring and reviewing the ISMS, and Maintaining and improving the ISMS.	Inventory and Control of Hardware Assets, Continuous Vulnerability Management, Controlled Use of Administrative Privileges, etc.	Align, Plan, Build, Run, Monitor.	Application Whitelisting, Patching Applications, Configuring Microsoft Office Macro Settings, etc.	Identify, Protect, Detect, Respond, Recover, Legal & Ethical Considerations, Societal Impact, AI Integration
AI Integration	Not inherently present.	Not inherently present.	Not inherently present.	Not inherently present.	Not inherently present.	AI is integrated into all elements, leveraging predictive analytics and pattern recognition to identify potential risks and vulnerabilities before they can be exploited.
Scope	Primarily focuses on cybersecurity risks	Primarily focuses on information security risks	Primarily focuses on cybersecurity risks	Primarily focuses on IT governance	Primarily focuses on cybersecurity risks	Covers a broader range of risks, including cybersecurity, ethical, legal, and societal implications of e-health and telemedicine.
Focus on E-health and Telemedicine	Not specifically tailored to e-health and telemedicine	Not specifically tailored to e-health and telemedicine	Not specifically tailored to e-health and telemedicine	Not specifically tailored to e-health and telemedicine	Not specifically tailored to e-health and telemedicine	Specifically designed with e-health and telemedicine in mind, considering the unique challenges of these sectors.

By building on the strengths of existing cybersecurity risk management frameworks, the proposed framework is not designed to replace these existing models but rather to extend them, incorporating sector-specific challenges associated with e-health and telemedicine. The aim is to create a more comprehensive and robust risk management strategy for healthcare providers, patients, and stakeholders involved in e-health and telemedicine. The diagram below (see Fig. 1) shows how we align each pillar with the relevant aspects of existing frameworks.

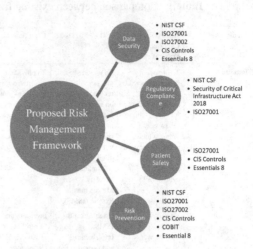

Fig. 1. Proposed Risk Management Framework

3.2 Role of AI in the Proposed Framework

Artificial Intelligence (AI) plays a significant role in the proposed risk management framework, providing powerful tools to enhance efficiency, security, and quality in the e-health and telemedicine domain. The proposed model leverages AI technology to augment traditional risk management measures, bringing about proactive and predictive capabilities. While traditional frameworks focus more on mitigation and response, the AI-driven approach in the proposed framework can proactively identify and manage risks before they materialise. For instance, machine learning algorithms can detect unusual behaviour patterns, flagging potential security breaches before they occur.

In the Data Security pillar, AI can enhance the detection of potential security threats. It can be used in conjunction with machine learning algorithms to monitor system activity and detect unusual patterns that might signify a security breach, such as abnormal login activity or unexpected data transfers [2, 9, 10]. With the growth in scale and complexity of e-health systems, AI can handle and analyse vast amounts of data at a speed and accuracy that is beyond human capability. Within the Regulatory Compliance pillar, AI can help automate and streamline the process of ensuring adherence to multiple complex regulatory standards. AI algorithms can be programmed to understand the requirements of regulations such as HIPAA and GDPR and continually audit system data and processes to ensure they remain compliant. Any deviations from compliance can be flagged for immediate correction, significantly reducing non-compliance risk [9, 10]. Regarding Patient Safety, AI plays an instrumental role in improving the reliability and accuracy of e-health systems. By leveraging predictive analysis, AI can help identify potential health risks in patient data, enabling early interventions and improving patient outcomes [5, 11]. Furthermore, AI can be utilised to ensure system availability, promptly identifying and addressing system issues that could prevent access to critical health data. In the Risk Prevention pillar, AI is a critical tool for proactive risk management. AI can analyse past security incidents and use that information to predict potential future threats. This predictive capability can inform the development of proactive measures, ensuring that e-health systems are prepared and resilient in the face of emerging threats and vulnerabilities [3, 6]. AI offers substantial benefits in addressing the unique risk management challenges of e-health and telemedicine. Its capabilities to manage vast amounts of data, identify patterns, and predict future scenarios are instrumental in enhancing these digital health systems' security, compliance, patient safety, and risk prevention capabilities.

3.3 Explanation of How the Framework Addresses the Unique Challenges of E-Health and Telemedicine

The proposed risk management framework is specifically designed to address the unique challenges of e-health and telemedicine. These challenges are diverse and complex, encompassing issues related to data security, regulatory compliance, patient safety, and proactive risk prevention. The framework's four pillars tackle these areas and are specially tailored to the digital environment of e-health and telemedicine.

Data Security: One of the biggest challenges of e-health and telemedicine is the need to secure sensitive patient data while still enabling convenient access for authorised users [2, 9, 10]. The data security pillar of the framework uses AI technology to enhance cybersecurity measures and actively monitor for potential threats. This provides robust protection against both external cyberattacks and internal misuse, ensuring patient data remains confidential and secure.

Regulatory Compliance: E-health and telemedicine systems are subject to a complex web of regulatory standards, including laws related to data privacy, health information, and telemedicine practice [4, 9]. The compliance pillar of the framework uses AI technology to continuously monitor system operations and ensure they remain in line with all relevant regulations. This not only reduces the risk of non-compliance but also helps to build trust with users, who can be confident their information is being handled in a legally compliant manner.

Patient Safety: The safety of patients is of utmost importance in e-health and telemedicine. Errors in data handling or system function can seriously affect patient health [5, 11]. The patient safety pillar of the framework focuses on using AI to improve the reliability and accuracy of the system. This includes identifying potential health risks, ensuring system availability, and flagging any unusual patterns in patient data that could signify a problem.

Risk Prevention: Given the rapid evolution of technology and cyber threats, it is crucial for e-health and telemedicine systems to be proactive in identifying and managing risks [3, 6]. The risk prevention pillar of the framework uses AI technology to analyse past incidents and predict potential future threats. This enables the development of proactive measures to enhance system resilience and ensure the system remains secure and effective even as technology and threats evolve. By addressing these unique challenges, the proposed risk management framework provides a comprehensive and tailored solution for managing risk in e-health and telemedicine. Its strategic use of AI technology further enhances its effectiveness, enabling it to adapt and respond to the dynamic and rapidly changing digital health environment.

4 Conclusion

E-health and telemedicine are rapidly transforming the healthcare sector, bringing unprecedented convenience, accessibility, and efficiency to patient care. However, the digital nature of these services presents unique risks and challenges, encompassing data security, regulatory compliance, patient safety, and risk prevention. These challenges necessitate robust and comprehensive risk management strategies specifically tailored for e-health and telemedicine. This paper has outlined and detailed such a risk management framework, drawing upon current approaches while integrating innovative AI-powered solutions. The framework's four pillars - data security, regulatory compliance, patient safety, and risk prevention - ensure a holistic approach to risk management that can be customised according to an organisation's specific needs and challenges. The role of AI in this proposed framework is significant and transformative. AI's predictive capabilities, real-time monitoring, and powerful analytics can significantly enhance traditional risk management strategies, allowing for proactive rather than reactive measures. Furthermore, AI can automate several aspects of risk management, freeing up valuable resources and further improving efficiency. In conclusion, effective risk management is essential for the sustainable growth and success of e-health and telemedicine. Further research and application of the framework across various healthcare contexts would be beneficial for refining and validating the approach.

References

1. Biancone, P., Secinaro, S., Marseglia, R., Calandra, D.: E-health for the future. Managerial perspectives using a multiple case study approach. Technovation **120**, 102406 (2023). https://doi.org/10.1016/J.TECHNOVATION.2021.102406
2. Boonyarattaphan, A., Bai, Y., Chung, S.: A security framework for e-Health service authentication and e-Health data transmission. In: 2009 9th International Symposium on Communications and Information Technology, ISCIT 2009, pp. 1213–1218 (2009). https://doi.org/10.1109/ISCIT.2009.5341116
3. Croll, P.R., Croll, J.: Investigating risk exposure in e-health systems. Int. J. Med. Inform. **76**(5–6), 460–465 (2007). https://doi.org/10.1016/J.IJMEDINF.2006.09.013
4. Eysenbach, G.: What is e-health? J. Med. Internet Res. **3**(2), 1–5 (2001). https://doi.org/10.2196/JMIR.3.2.E20
5. González, M.E., Quesada, G., Urrutia, I., Gavidia, J.V.: Conceptual design of an e-health strategy for the Spanish health care system. Int. J. Health Care Qual. Assur. **19**(2), 146–157 (2006). https://doi.org/10.1108/09526860610651681/FULL/PDF
6. Ksibi, S., Jaidi, F., Bouhoula, A.: Cyber-risk management within IoMT: a context-aware agent-based framework for a reliable e-health system. ACM Int. Conf. Proc. Ser. 547–552 (2021). https://doi.org/10.1145/3487664.3487805
7. Li, J.H., Ray, P.: Applications of e-health for pandemic management. In: 12th IEEE International Conference on E-Health Networking, Application and Services, Healthcom 2010, pp. 391–398 (2010). https://doi.org/10.1109/HEALTH.2010.5556536
8. Li, J.H., Ray, P., Seale, H., MacIntyre, R.: An e-health readiness assessment framework for public health services - pandemic perspective. In: Proceedings of the Annual Hawaii International Conference on System Sciences, pp. 2800–2809 (2012). https://doi.org/10.1109/HICSS.2012.95

9. Shrestha, N.M., Alsadoon, A., Prasad, P.W.C., Hourany, L., Elchouemi, A.: Enhanced e-health framework for security and privacy in the healthcare system. In: 2016 6th International Conference on Digital Information Processing and Communications, ICDIPC 2016, pp. 75–79 (2016). https://doi.org/10.1109/ICDIPC.2016.7470795
10. Vora, J., et al.: Ensuring privacy and security in E-health records. In: CITS 2018 - 2018 International Conference on Computer, Information and Telecommunication Systems (2018). https://doi.org/10.1109/CITS.2018.8440164
11. Wickramasinghe, N.S., Fadlalla, A.M.A., Geisler, E., Schaffer, J.L.: A framework for assessing e-health preparedness. Int. J. Electron. Healthcare 1(3), 316–334 (2005). https://doi.org/10.1504/IJEH.2005.006478

Neurological and Cognitive Disease Studies

Knowledge-Based Nonlinear to Linear Dataset Transformation for Chronic Illness Classification

Markian Jaworsky[1]($\boxtimes$), Xiaohui Tao[1], Jianming Yong[2], Lei Pan[3], Ji Zhang[1], and Shiva Raj Pokhrel[3]

[1] School of Mathematics, Physics, and Computing, University of Southern Queensland, Toowoomba, Australia
{Markian.Jaworsky,Xiaohui.Tao,Ji.Zhang}@usq.edu.au
[2] School of Business, University of Southern Queensland, Springfield, Australia
Jianming.Yong@usq.edu.au
[3] School of Information Technology, Deakin University, Waurn Ponds, Geelong, Australia
{l.pan,shiva.pokhrel}@deakin.edu.au

Abstract. Nonlinear patterns are challenging to interpret, validate, and are resource-intensive for deep learning (DL) and machine learning (ML) algorithms to predict chronic illness. Transformation of nonlinear features to a linear representation enables the human understanding of AI results and traditional and proven ML algorithms. We propose the counts of terms cross-checked against the chapters of the International Classification of Disease (ICD) to replace the raw representation of key nonlinear variables in health surveys to improve the chronic illness classification performance. The specific selection of nonlinear keywords viz. Male, Female, Diabetes, Cancer, Obese, Overweight, Smoked, Cigarettes, and Sugar from a health survey, transformed into a purely linear and scaled set of features propels the Multinomial Naive Bayes (MNB) algorithm to outperform standard dataset preparation and feature selection methods.

Keywords: Risk Factors · Linear Models · Nonlinear Models · Chronic Illness · Knowledge Graphs

1 Introduction

In countries where healthcare systems rely on first-line triage by General Practitioners, it is estimated that up to 85% of all cancers are diagnosed via patient signs and symptoms [30]. Consequently, diagnostic delays are a major factor in cancer deaths where diagnosis assisting tools and identifying risk factors can save lives [9]. The study of Rehman *et al.* [24] highlights that not only do large population growths contribute to the high cost of medical center costs, but aging populations also require a near-constant medical diagnosis.

Existing screening procedures for cancers include computed tomography (CT scan), which can detect early malignancy and improve the chances of successful

Y. Li et al. (Eds.): HIS 2023, LNCS 14305, pp. 115–126, 2023.
https://doi.org/10.1007/978-981-99-7108-4_10

treatment as most of those diagnosed will have already progressed to an advanced stage [14]. However, such screening remains a novel procedure and is not commonly available as a public screening service for breast, colorectal, and cervical cancers. Therefore, greater awareness and recognition of cancer symptoms and risk factors can increase the likelihood of patient survival.

The screening and diagnosis of cancers rely on medical practitioner expertise, the open research area in cancer detection to aid human judgment with precise technology-based methodology, to improve patient outcomes. A holistic and non-intrusive method for the classification of chronic illness and its risk factors is challenged by a number of dataset issues. High dimensionality, nonlinearity, imbalanced classes [12], and missing and erroneous values are common problems in healthcare research [4]. We propose to overcome these challenges by constructing a fully new set of linear and consistently scaled variables based on knowledge of all human diseases.

Neural network models depend on large-scale volumes of training data, require many trials of parameter tuning, and most likely do not achieve high performance on small datasets [18]. Nor is one likely to obtain transparency of the inner workings of a Neural network, given the many possible feature transformations that can occur, so identifying the causation of risk factors is doubtful. Furthermore, neural networks are challenged by spurious correlations [10], and incidental objects in image backgrounds have become unintended factors in classifying target labels. While deep learning performs feature engineering independently of human engineers, prior knowledge is usually mandatory before developing a deep model [17].

The contributions of this paper are:

– A novel method for converting nonlinear health survey responses into consistent linear variables. We create an entirely new dataset for training and classification, providing a standardized unit of measurement for nonlinear variables and enabling the prediction of chronic illnesses based on linear patterns easily understood by human beings.
– Our framework allows the evaluation of new risk factors for enhanced predictive power in cancer and diabetes classification, leveraging their correlated nature, and producing explainable results without overfitting or spurious correlation by incorporating internationally recognized knowledge of human diseases.

The rest of this paper is organized as follows: In Sect. 2, we discuss related works; in Sect. 3, we explain our methodology; in Sect. 4, we present our results; and finally Sect. 5 discusses future works and conclude this paper.

2   Related Work

The research of Chen et al. [3] focused on the classification of rare diseases, highlighting the value of including the demographic factors of patient age and gender in their datasets, and presented a novel nonlinear function methodology.

While a patient's age is a linear variable with predictive power, gender is a nonlinear variable that can evenly split a dataset in a binary fashion.

Random Forest and Multinomial Logistic Regression ML algorithms were chosen to classify lung cancer causes of death by the study of Deng *et al.* [5]. It was noted that Random Forests had outperformed Support Vector Machines and artificial neural networks in a prior study of breast cancer. Akram *et al.* [1] proposed a novel feature fusion method for reducing the dimensions of a dataset on skin lesion classification. The detection of the target label improved against the baseline with a transformed dataset that was a portion of its original size. A novel and automated 3-stage classification method of breast lesion images is proposed by Pandey *et al.* [19], the study performs a transformation of datasets by removing noisy image segments.

Automated image analysis is typically aided by deep learning algorithms, Convolutional Neural Networks (CNN) are used by Sarki *et al.* [26] in their study to diagnose diabetic eye disease, achieving suitable results in the multi-class classification of publicly available patient images. Multiple artificial neural networks were trained by Fan *et al.* [7] to classify nonlinear datasets by optimizing the number of input and output layers for fault detection. When choosing layers for a neural network, there are trade-offs. If too few layers are selected, the classification performance suffers. On the other hand, if many layers are chosen, the computational cost increases, and overfitting becomes a problem. Using nonlinear datasets often results in training overfitted models as their patterns are distinct and not often reproducible in unseen data. This observation is highlighted by Létinier *et al.* [15] in their study of text classification for medical records of drug reactions.

The Washington *et al.* [31] study focused on the trending research into computer vision across many industry sectors, including healthcare. Their insights highlighted that neglecting the elimination of redundant features from a dataset ultimately results in overfitted predictive models. This statement can broadly be interpreted to assume that all features existing in a dataset need to have an explainable existence; otherwise, if they are influential in predicting a target label, then the predictive model is not explainable.

Many studies opt for feature selection and extraction methods to reduce a dataset's complexity and improve classification performance. The search for optimal features, however, can be exhaustive and inconclusive, the Dokeroglu *et al.* [6] survey on this type of methodology concludes that no method is assured of finding an optimal feature subset, partly because each feature subset needs to be tested individually in classification performance against a target label. Similarly, Seo *et al.* [27] claims that the exhaustive optimal feature subset search is impractical, using their proposed method, only the top 2% to top 5% of features were the most useful for predictions.

In addition to having nonlinear characteristics, Twitter messages can be erroneously formed and are categorized as unstructured data. When fundamental values are often missing, Khan *et al.* [13] performed a feature construction process to ensure each Twitter message could be identified with geospatial coordinates.

The study also introduced new numerical values representing the message length and other linear features to indicate a message's sentiment value.

In the healthcare domain, Tao *et al.* [29] proposed recreating the responses of a Health Survey as a knowledge graph to improve the ability of the dataset to enhance data mining of chronic illnesses and the relations between patients and diseases. An automated ICD and BRFSS-based knowledge graph were presented by Jaworsky *et al.* [11], which uses term frequencies to determine the most significantly interrelated features in order to perform dimension reduction of a health survey dataset. Pham *et al.* [21,22] demonstrated that a knowledge-based approach to health status classification produced improved results compared to the baseline models, and was also able to demonstrate that a multi-label predictive model performed best when leveraging a medical domain-based knowledge graph (Fig. 1).

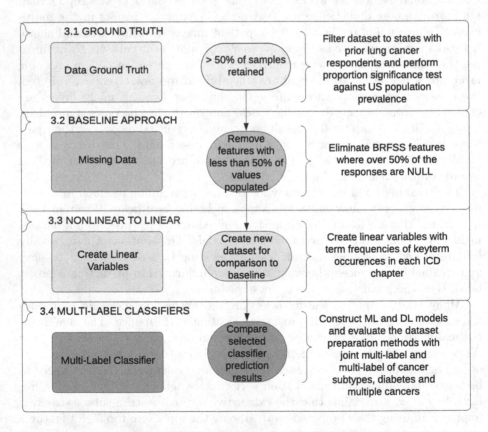

Fig. 1. Research Design—Our Methodology

3   Methodology

3.1   Data Sources and Ground Truth

In this study, we re-use the data sources identified for constructing an automated knowledge graph for the healthcare domain [11]. ICD aggregates international human disease knowledge[1] with a structure by listing each known disease relevant to each human organ system. Each disease is described with specific circumstance details, symptoms, and causes. We can determine a meaningful correlation between survey responses and our target label from this knowledge base.

The United States CDC Behavioral Risk Factor Surveillance System (BRFSS) is a publicly available annual health survey with many questions and responses about chronic illness prevalence. Personal and sensitive health information is hidden in the health survey. Nominal variable response values are described in the codebook example[2] to interpret each answer's meaning.

We prepare the health survey for all of our trials to ensure that the proportion of survey respondents with chronic illness represents the ground truth. The filters applied are the geographical state of the respondent, deselecting states without lung cancer candidates, and then comparing the prevalence of lung cancer health survey respondents to that of the wider USA population to ensure no significant difference in proportions. The prevalence of lung cancer in 2018 was 582,631 living people[3] given that the U.S. Census Bureau[4] declared the USA population at 326.8 million.

3.2   Preparation of Baseline Datasets

In our trials, we will eliminate the features where over 50%

We will then demonstrate the superior performance of the proposed methodology by comparing the classification performance of various ML and DL algorithms used in prior health survey studies against the 2 prepared baseline datasets and then against a newly transformed dataset of linear variables using our proposed methodology in this paper.

---

[1] https://www.who.int/standards/classifications/classification-of-diseases.
[2] https://www.cdc.gov/brfss/annual_data/annual_2020.html.
[3] https://seer.cancer.gov/statfacts/html/lungb.html.
[4] https://www.census.gov.

Algorithm 1. Nonlinear to Linear Transformation

    Input: Original Health Survey Dataset
    Output: New Dataset of Linear Variables
1: **procedure** COUNT KEYWORD ICD CHAPTER TERM FREQUENCY
2:     **for** Each Survey Demographic Keyword:
3:       **for** Each ICD Chapter:
4:          $ChapterICD \leftarrow Stop\ Words\ Filter$
5:          **if** $Keyword\ Exists\ in\ Chapter\ ICD$ **then**
6:             $TermFrequency \leftarrow CountKeywordFrequency$
7:             $KeywordICDChapterScore \leftarrow TermFrequency$
8:             $LinearVariableSet \leftarrow KeywordICDChapterScore$
9:          **end if**
10:       **end for do**
11:     **end for do**
12: **end procedure**
13: **procedure** CREATE NEW DATASET
14:     **for** Each Health Survey Record:
15:       **if** $Health\ Survey\ Record\ Answers\ True\ to\ Keyword$ **then**
16:          **for** Each ICD Chapter Linear Variable:
17:             $NewDatasetAppend \leftarrow LinearVariable$
18:          **end for do**
19:       **end if**
20:     **end for do**
21: **end procedure**

3.3 Nonlinear to Linear Transformation

Our knowledge-based linear variable transformation is derived using a corpus of key terms associated with cancer and diabetes and cross-referencing each term against the 26 WHO ICD chapters.

Algorithm 1 provides the step-by-step coding requirements for transforming a health survey response dataset with nonlinear responses to a new dataset that only contains consistently scaled linear variables. Nonlinear survey respondents' demographically-based keywords can be identified and selected for usage in this transformation procedure. Our selection of nonlinear keywords is listed as column names in Table 1 viz. Male, Female, Diabetes, Cancer, Obese, Overweight, Smoked, Cigarettes, and Sugar correspond to items that a response to a health survey can identify, which also correspond to the descriptions of known human diseases in the ICD.

At step 2 of Algorithm 1, for each of our survey demographic keywords, we count the frequency of these keywords appearing in each of the ICD chapters, and we repeat the construction of the set of linear variables for each ICD chapter at step 3, and for each keyword and append all the linear variables to our newly created dataset, at step 13. Our study has tested this methodology of the BRFSS survey for the years 2017–2021[5]. This methodology can be applied to the BRFSS health survey of other years or other health surveys.

---

[5] https://github.com/mjaworsky/LinearVarTransformation.

Table 1. Chronic Illness (Cancer & Diabetes) Corpus ICD Chapter Term Frequencies

ICD Chapter	male	female	diabetes	cancer	obese	overweight	smoked	cigarettes	sugar
1	0	3	2	3	0	0	0	0	0
2	17	21	0	39	0	0	0	0	0
3	0	0	0	2	0	0	0	0	0
4	1	1	0	2	0	0	0	0	0
5	4	4	89	6	0	25	0	0	3
6	0	0	1	3	0	0	3	2	0
7	0	0	2	0	0	0	0	0	0
8	1	0	9	10	0	1	0	0	0
9	0	0	10	3	1	0	0	0	1
10	0	0	1	0	0	0	0	0	0
11	1	0	2	1	0	0	0	0	0
12	0	0	2	0	0	0	0	0	1
13	0	2	0	2	0	0	0	0	0
14	11	6	10	5	2	0	0	0	0
15	0	1	2	2	0	0	0	0	0
16	26	86	7	7	0	0	0	0	0
17	30	13	0	0	0	0	0	0	0
18	0	5	10	0	0	0	0	0	0
19	0	0	20	0	0	1	0	0	0
20	17	13	1	3	0	0	0	0	0
21	28	29	4	36	1	0	0	0	1
22	1	4	0	0	0	0	0	0	0
23	0	0	0	0	0	0	0	0	0
24	1	3	2	1	0	0	0	0	0
25	0	0	0	0	0	0	0	0	0
26	2	7	0	0	0	0	0	0	0

Table 1 lists each key term in our corpus and their respective ICD chapter term frequencies. The key terms were determined by filtering out stop words from the BRFSS health survey questions and cross-referencing their existence in the ICD. The simplification of the corpus term selection allows us to find a corresponding BRFSS health survey question to determine if a patient record is a positive occurrence of that key term.

The response to the question determines a positive value to the terms male or female 'Are you male or female', 'What type of cancer was it for cancer', 'Ever told you had diabetes' for a positive response to diabetes, 'Four-categories of Body Mass Index (BMI)' for obese or overweight, 'Do you now smoke cigarettes every day, some days, or not at all' for smoked or cigarettes, and finally 'Have you had a test for high blood sugar or diabetes within the past three years' for sugar.

3.4 Classifier Performance Evaluation

There are prior ML and DL-based studies that classify chronic illness in the healthcare domain. Our selection of ML and DL classifiers is based on prior performances recorded and proposed by Bitew *et al.* [2], Prashanth & Roy [23], Ricciardi *et al.* [25], Georgakopoulos *et al.* [8].

Our TensorFlow CNN uses 3 layers, 100 back-propagation epochs, 0.01 learning rates, and a ReLU activation function. Trials of configuration were performed until the CNN model could distinguish a benign patient from a malignancy.

To detect possible chronic illness from a dataset representing the ground truth, an imbalance of benign and malignant classes [16,20,32] is expected. For this reason, we use the macro averages of the precision, the recall, and the F1-Scores to ensure that our performance is not biased toward one class at the expense of the other.

4 Results

The results listed in Table 2 are comparisons of macro precision, macro recall, and macro F1-score of baseline, feature selection, and linear variable transformation datasets. Our results represent the macro averaged 5-fold cross-validated performance of classifying a multi-label binary combination of diabetes or cancer. All metric values are rounded to 2 decimal places. The classifier names are as follows:

- AB = AdaBoost
- CNN = Convolutional Neural Network
- KNN = K-Nearest Neighbours
- LDA = Linear Discriminant Analysis
- LR = Logistic Regression
- MNB = Multinomial Naive Bayes
- RB = RUSBoost
- RF = Random Forest
- SVM = Support Vector Machine

The feature-selected datasets for 2017–2021 represent the optimum classification for selecting a subset of interrelated features with 5%, 10%, 25%, 50%, and 75% of features from the original baseline. They can be considered an exhaustive and robust feature selection.

The comparison between the baseline and feature-selected results indicates that the RB classifier improves its ability to classify our target label with a dimension-reduced dataset. We also observe that the LDA and LR classifiers can improve their performance. By selecting interrelated features, the 2nd dataset has removed outlier features.

The 3rd dataset is the product of the methodology described in Sect. 3. In this scenario, the MNB classifier significantly improves its performance by eliminating nonlinear variables and using data values that are normally distributed.

Table 2. Baseline, Feature Selected, Linear Var 5-Fold CV, Macro Precision, Macro Recall, Macro F1-Score 2017–2021 Average

Dataset	Classifier	Baseline			Feature Selection			Linear Variable		
		Precision	Recall	F1	Precision	Recall	F1	Precision	Recall	F1
2017–2021	AB	0.51	0.50	0.48	0.67	0.51	0.52	0.43	0.50	0.46
	CNN	0.26	0.52	0.20	0.41	0.50	0.40	0.37	0.50	0.37
	KNN	0.47	0.50	0.47	0.50	0.50	0.48	0.43	0.50	0.46
	LDA	0.49	0.50	0.48	**0.81**	0.61	0.58	0.43	0.48	0.45
	LR	0.48	0.50	0.47	0.66	0.50	0.47	0.43	0.50	0.46
	MNB	0.48	0.51	0.44	0.47	0.51	0.47	**0.81**	**0.77**	**0.74**
	RB	0.50	0.50	0.49	0.73	0.68	0.67	0.46	0.49	0.46
	RF	0.46	0.50	0.48	0.56	0.50	0.47	0.46	0.50	0.46
	SVM	0.46	0.50	0.48	0.46	0.50	0.48	0.46	0.50	0.46

Full result year-on-year details available via Google Sheets online[6]. When the average for the 5 years is aggregated in Table 2, we observe that the linear variable transformation performs equally as well as the optimum feature selection dataset for precision, and outperforms the baseline, and outperforms both the baseline and feature selection datasets for recall and F1-Scores.

4.1   Ablation Study

Table 2 demonstrates the distinct performance gains made by the MNB classifier when seeing the linear transformation, against the baseline datasets, including the baseline with dimension reduction. The study of Yager [33] observes that the MNB classifier has a probabilistic approach prediction and is described by Soria *et al.* [28] as being simple and linear run-time.

The data transformation from nonlinear to linear term frequency variables of health survey risk factors against each ICD chapter has optimal performance when the set of 26 linear variables is associated with each health survey keyword, as opposed to an aggregate of term frequencies of each keyword. This preserves a distinguishable scale of risk factors for each term, both from a human interpretation and for MNB-based classification. Furthermore, no improvement in classification performance is observed in combining the newly transformed linear variables with features from the original dataset, and the MNB classifier achieves its optimum performance on a pure linear format dataset.

5   Future Work and Conclusion

We have discussed the value of using a knowledge-based system to identify key terms which are correlated with signs and symptoms of chronic illness and known

---

[6] https://docs.google.com/spreadsheets/d/1QJLlhiMgUEo8EL4kXfb0khfjIHmO7X8j MTy0O9_XeZ0/edit?usp=sharing.

causes associated with health survey questions. The transformation of nonlinear responses to health survey questions enables the traditional machine learning algorithm MNB to outperform resource-intensive nonlinear algorithms prone to overfitting models. It also creates a dataset of linear features to be evaluated in a consistent unit of measure, enables the transformation of a dataset with classification results explainable to human beings, and achieves superior results in baseline dataset preparation steps and feature selection-based dimension reduction.

The transformation of nonlinear health survey keywords to a linear format via the knowledge-based ICD is limited only by the international knowledge of human diseases. Suppose a newly identified risk factor, such as a virus variant or smoking product, is not yet listed in the most recent version of the ICD. In that case, its impact on the prediction of chronic illness is not accountable. The counter-argument for introducing a knowledge constraint is the avoidance of spurious correlation, which is critical when deciding to proceed with intrusive medical procedures that can be life-saving or negatively become lifestyle-impeding. This study aims to aid medical practitioners' decision-making instead of replacing them.

Further improvement of our contribution is identifying new terms in health survey questions and the ICD that can improve the classification performance of chronic illness. The terms selected in our survey are known risk factors for diabetes and cancers. They are used to demonstrate the advantage of nonlinear to linear feature transformation. Our case study demonstrates that health survey questions that can target identifying patient demographics and risk factors are very useful in predicting chronic illness.

Declarations. –The work is conducted with approval from the Human Research Ethics Committee of the University of Southern Queensland, Australia (Approval ID: H21REA222)

References

1. Akram, T., et al.: A multilevel features selection framework for skin lesion classification. Hum.-Centric Comput. Inf. Sci. **10**, 1–26 (2020)
2. Bitew, F.H., Nyarko, S.H., Potter, L., Sparks, C.S.: Machine learning approach for predicting under-five mortality determinants in Ethiopia: evidence from the 2016 Ethiopian demographic and health survey. Genus **76**(1), 1–16 (2020)
3. Chen, I.Y., Agrawal, M., Horng, S., Sontag, D.: Robustly extracting medical knowledge from EHRs: a case study of learning a health knowledge graph. In: Proceedings of the 2020 Pacific Symposium on BioComputing, pp. 19–30. World Scientific (2019)
4. De Meulder, B., et al.: A computational framework for complex disease stratification from multiple large-scale datasets. BMC Syst. Biol. **12**(1), 1–23 (2018). https://doi.org/10.1186/s12918-018-0556-z
5. Deng, F., et al.: Predict multicategory causes of death in lung cancer patients using clinicopathologic factors. Comput. Biol. Med. **129**, 104161 (2021). https://doi.org/10.1016/j.compbiomed.2020.104161

6. Dokeroglu, T., Deniz, A., Kiziloz, H.E.: A comprehensive survey on recent meta-heuristics for feature selection. Neurocomputing (2022)
7. Fan, S.K.S., Hsu, C.Y., Jen, C.H., Chen, K.L., Juan, L.T.: Defective wafer detection using a denoising autoencoder for semiconductor manufacturing processes. Adv. Eng. Inf. **46**, 101166 (2020). https://doi.org/10.1016/j.aei.2020.101166
8. Georgakopoulos, S.V., Tasoulis, S.K., Vrahatis, A.G., Plagianakos, V.P.: Convolutional neural networks for toxic comment classification. In: Proceedings of the 10th Hellenic Conference on Artificial Intelligence, pp. 1–6 (2018)
9. Hamilton, W., Green, T., Martins, T., Elliott, K., Rubin, G., Macleod, U.: Evaluation of risk assessment tools for suspected cancer in general practice: a cohort study. Br. J. Gener. Pract. **63**(606), e30–e36 (2013)
10. Izmailov, P., Kirichenko, P., Gruver, N., Wilson, A.G.: On feature learning in the presence of spurious correlations. Adv. Neural. Inf. Process. Syst. **35**, 38516–38532 (2022)
11. Jaworsky, M., Tao, X., Yong, J., Pan, L., Zhang, J., Pokhrel, S.: Automated knowledge graph construction for healthcare domain. In: Traina, A., Wang, H., Zhang, Y., Siuly, S., Zhou, R., Chen, L. (eds.) HIS 2022. LNCS, pp. 258–265. Springer, Cham (2022). https://doi.org/10.1007/978-3-031-20627-6_24
12. Jing, X.Y., et al.: Multiset feature learning for highly imbalanced data classification. IEEE Trans. Pattern Anal. Mach. Intell. **43**(1), 139–156 (2019)
13. Khan, S.M., Chowdhury, M., Ngo, L.B., Apon, A.: Multi-class twitter data categorization and geocoding with a novel computing framework. Cities **96**, 102410 (2020). https://doi.org/10.1016/j.cities.2019.102410
14. de Koning, H.J., et al.: Reduced lung-cancer mortality with volume CT screening in a randomized trial. New England J. Med. **382**(6), 503–513 (2020)
15. Létinier, L., et al.: Artificial intelligence for unstructured healthcare data: application to coding of patient reporting of adverse drug reactions. Clin. Pharmacol. Ther. **110**(2), 392–400 (2021)
16. Liu, M., Xu, C., Luo, Y., Xu, C., Wen, Y., Tao, D.: Cost-sensitive feature selection via f-measure optimization reduction. In: Proceedings of the AAAI Conference on Artificial Intelligence, vol. 31 (2017)
17. Mosqueira-Rey, E., Hernández-Pereira, E., Alonso-Ríos, D., Bobes-Bascarán, J., Fernández-Leal, Á.: Human-in-the-loop machine learning: a state of the art. Artif. Intell. Rev., 1–50 (2022)
18. Nakano, F.K., Pliakos, K., Vens, C.: Deep tree-ensembles for multi-output prediction. Pattern Recognit. **121**, 108211 (2022). https://doi.org/10.1016/j.patcog.2021.108211
19. Pandey, D., Wang, H., Yin, X., Wang, K., Zhang, Y., Shen, J.: Automatic breast lesion segmentation in phase preserved DCE-MRIs. Health Inf. Sci. Syst. **10**(1), 9 (2022)
20. Pes, B.: Learning from high-dimensional and class-imbalanced datasets using random forests. Information **12**(8), 286 (2021)
21. Pham, T., Tao, X., Zhang, J., Yong, J.: Constructing a knowledge-based heterogeneous information graph for medical health status classification. Health Inf. Sci. Syst. **8**, 1–14 (2020)
22. Pham, T., Tao, X., Zhang, J., Yong, J., Li, Y., Xie, H.: Graph-based multi-label disease prediction model learning from medical data and domain knowledge. Knowl.-Based Syst. **235**, 107662 (2022)
23. Prashanth, R., Roy, S.D.: Novel and improved stage estimation in Parkinson's disease using clinical scales and machine learning. Neurocomputing **305**, 78–103 (2018)

24. Rehman, O., Al-Busaidi, A.M., Ahmed, S., Ahsan, K.: Ubiquitous healthcare system: architecture, prototype design and experimental evaluations. EAI Endorsed Trans. Scalable Inf. Syst. **9**(4), e6–e6 (2022)

25. Ricciardi, C., et al.: Linear discriminant analysis and principal component analysis to predict coronary artery disease. Health Inf. J. **26**(3), 2181–2192 (2020)

26. Sarki, R., Ahmed, K., Wang, H., Zhang, Y., Wang, K.: Convolutional neural network for multi-class classification of diabetic eye disease. EAI Endorsed Trans. Scalable Inf. Syst. **9**(4), e5–e5 (2022)

27. Seo, W., Park, M., Kim, D.W., Lee, J.: Effective memetic algorithm for multilabel feature selection using hybridization-based communication. Expert Syst. Appl. **201**, 117064 (2022)

28. Soria, D., Garibaldi, J.M., Ambrogi, F., Biganzoli, E.M., Ellis, I.O.: A 'nonparametric' version of the Naive Bayes classifier. Knowl.-Based Syst. **24**(6), 775–784 (2011)

29. Tao, X., Pham, T., Zhang, J., Yong, J., Goh, W.P., Zhang, W., Cai, Y.: Mining health knowledge graph for health risk prediction. World Wide Web **23**(4), 2341–2362 (2020)

30. Vedsted, P., Olesen, F.: A differentiated approach to referrals from general practice to support early cancer diagnosis-the Danish three-legged strategy. Br. J. Cancer **112**(1), S65–S69 (2015)

31. Washington, P., et al.: Challenges and opportunities for machine learning classification of behavior and mental state from images. arXiv preprint arXiv:2201.11197 (2022)

32. Xu, D., Shi, Y., Tsang, I.W., Ong, Y.S., Gong, C., Shen, X.: Survey on multioutput learning. IEEE Trans. Neural Netw. Learn. Syst. **31**(7), 2409–2429 (2019). https://doi.org/10.1109/TNNLS.2019.2945133

33. Yager, R.R.: An extension of the Naive Bayesian classifier. Inf. Sci. **176**(5), 577–588 (2006)

A Robust Approach for Parkinson Disease Detection from Voice Signal

Sarmad K. D. Alkhafaji[(✉)] and Sarab Jalal

College of Education for Pure Sciences, Computer Science Department, University Thi-Qar, Nasiriyah, Iraq
{Dr.sarmad,msc21co13}@utq.edu.iq

Abstract. Parkinson's disease (PD) is a common brain disorder that is associated with slow speech and difficulty with articulation. Mainly, clinical experts analyse patient's voice to detect PD. In this paper, we proposed a robust model using empirical mode decomposition (EMD) and machine learning algorithms. Firstly, the acquired voice signals are pre-processed and segmented into small intervals. Then, each segment is sent to EMD model. A set of entropy features are extracted and then they are fed into a K-nearest neighbor (KNN), least squares support vector machine (LS-SVM), bagged tree, SVM (support vector machine), and K-means. The proposed model is evaluated using a publicly available. Our findings showed that the proposed framework can classify voice signals with a 97% accuracy.

Keywords: Parkinson's disease · EMD · KNN · entropy features

1 Introduction

Parkinson's disease (PD) is a neurological disorder that weakens a patient's capacity to maintain normal motor function [1]. Based on global health origination, around 7–10 million people are diagnosed with PD. In addition, the number of people diagnosed with Parkinson's disorder will double in 2030. Detection Parkinson's disease in early stage can slow its development. Currently, there is no accurate test to diagnose PD. Mainly experts diagnose PD based on neurological exam, medical history, blood, voice, and brain assessments. Clinical studies proved that most patients with PD develop voice disorders by the time they are diagnosed with PD symptoms.

In recent years many researchers have explored the correlation between vocal changes and Parkinson's. Compared with other patients' information, the acquisition of voice data is simpler and more convenient. As a result, many techniques based on the analysis of speech and vocal patterns have been developed to diagnose Parkinson's disease. Designing machine learning models for analyzing voice signals to diagnose PD is considered critical to identify Parkinson's disease as early as possible. For example, studying voice patterns have become a great topic in PD diagnosis. Naranjo et al. [2] designed a PD-diagnosed model from sound signals. Haq et al., [1] suggested a PD prediction system based on machine learning. A SVM-based feature extraction model was applied to classify the input signals into health and PD. Lahmiri et al. [2] investigated

© The Author(s), under exclusive license to Springer Nature Singapore Pte Ltd. 2023
Y. Li et al. (Eds.): HIS 2023, LNCS 14305, pp. 127–134, 2023.
https://doi.org/10.1007/978-981-99-7108-4_11

changes in voice patterns to diagnose PD. Statistical metrics including Mann-Whitney-Wilcoxon, a genetic algorithm are employed to select the most powerful features from voice signals. Mostafa et al. [3] suggested a multiple feature evaluation model to diagnose PD. Sabeena et al. [4] made a comparison study of various machine learning methods for the diagnosis PD disease. Tai et al., [5] proposed a supervised learning-based model to detect PD. Jeancolas et al., [6] used machine learning models to classify voice data. They acquired data from 256 French speakers. They achieved an accuracy of 89%. Xu, Xu et al., [7] used a deep convolutional generative adversarial network. Onur Karaman et al. [8] employed a convolution neural network to classify the time-frequency characteristics of sound data. Shalin et al. [9] applied Long-term and short-term memory networks to predict Parkinson's disease. Based on the related works, although different methods of research have achieved good results on different datasets, it still lacks a robust method that is suitable for different datasets. This paper proposes a method that could be applied to most Parkinson's sound datasets.

2 Data Description

A public dataset is used to assess the proposed model. It was collected From https:// archive.ics.uci.edu/ml/datasets/Parkinson+Speech+Dataset+with++Mul tiple+Types+of+Sound+Recordings# [10]. The dataset are recorded from 20 Persons with Parkinson's (6 females and 14 males) and 20 healthy persons (10 females and 10 males).

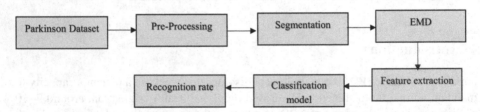

Fig. 1. Proposed Parkinson's disease detection framework

3 Materials and Methods

3.1 Proposed Parkinson's Disease Detection Framework

In this paper, PD detection model is suggested using empirical mode decomposition (EMD) and machine learning approaches. Entropy features are adopted to detect PD. Figure 1 depicts the suggested Parkinson's disease detection framework. The following section explain each step of the proposed model.

3.2 Pre-processing and Segmentation Phase

The collected voice signals are passed through a high pass filter and low pass filter of 0.5 Hz cut off 70 Hz cut off respectively. Then, the filtered signal is segmented into windows of 250 s length. The length of the window is set based on studies in [11–14].

3.3 Empirical Mode Decomposition

In this section, each segment is passed through EMD to separate the input signal into different frequency components [15, 16]. It is decomposed into a set of IMFs. IMFs are functions that have the following two properties:

1. The absolute differences between the total number of zero crossing points and a total number of function extrema are less than or equal to one.
2. The area under the curve created by the function's average lower and upper envelopes within any two consecutive extrema (one local maximum and one local minimum) is zero.

3.4 Features Extraction

In this section, we explain the features used to detect PD. From each segment, a set of entropy features are extracted to form the final features vector. In this paper, we extracted three entropy features from each segment. The three features are dispersion entropy, approximate entropy, and Shannon entropy.

3.4.1 Shannon Entropy (ShEn)

Entropy is calculated by multiplying the power level at each frequency by the logarithm of the power level's inverse. Finally, the spectral entropy of the time series is calculated using the method below [12].

$$ShEn = \sum_f p_f \log(\frac{1}{p_f})\tag{1}$$

the Shannon entropy, which calculates the mean value of the signal's information, suppose a voice signal $x = [x_1, x_2, x_3, \ldots, x_n]$ with a probability distribution function $p(x_i)$, the Shannon entropy is computed as:

$$Shanon_{entropy} = -\sum_{i=1}^{m} p_i^2 \log_2\left(p_i^2\right)\tag{2}$$

$$Shanon_{entropy} = \sum_{i=1}^{m} p_i^2 log_2\tag{3}$$

3.4.2 Approximate Entropy (ApEn)

That measures a regularity of a time series [12]. ApEn (approximate entropy) is a time series complexity metric. It is widely employed in a wide range of biological signal processing applications, including EEG epileptic activity analysis, background activity, coronary artery disease (CAD) heart rate signal analysis, and so on. It assesses a time series' randomness or regularity in various dimensions.

approximate entropy (ApEn) that measures a regularity of a time series. The ApEN is calculated using the following formula.

$$ApEn\ (z, r,\ L) = \phi^z(r) - \phi^{z+1}(r)\tag{4}$$

where $\phi^z(\mathrm{r})$ is calculated using the following formula:

$$\phi^z(\mathrm{r}) = \frac{1}{L-z+1} \sum_i \ln\left(C_i^z(r)\right) \tag{5}$$

and C_i^z is the correlation integral given by

$$C_i^z(\mathrm{r}) = \frac{1}{L-z+1} L_i^r \quad i = 1, 2, \ldots, L-z+1 \tag{6}$$

3.4.3 Dispersion Entropy (DisEn)

DisEn is a technique for characterizing time series irregularity derived from Shannon Entropy and symbolic dynamics for constructing a fast and robust algorithm to quantify the degree of irregularity of a signal segment under investigation. The approach entails representing the dynamics of a signal segment using a dispersion pattern distribution. Dispersion patterns are symbol sequences formed by the relative amplitude of samples from a whole signal segment quantized with a particular mapping function. As a result, when a signal segment can be represented with a small proportion of dispersion patterns, it has a low DisEn value compared to one that needs all conceivable dispersion patterns to be present in equal probability [12].

The following parameters are set during the implementation of a DisEn algorithm:

- **Embedding dimension:** the number of samples of each dispersion pattern utilized to represent the signal segment.
- **The number of classes:** the number of possible values for each sample in the dispersion pattern.
- **Mapping approach (logarithm sigmoid function):** which distributes the values of the dispersion pattern classes along the amplitude range of the investigated signal.
- **Time delay:** This can be used to add a lag in the algorithm's analysis of samples.

3.5 Classifiers

We used the most common classification models including SVM, LS-SVM, Bagged tree, k-means, k-nearest (KNN).

3.5.1 Least Square Support Vector Machine (LS-SVM)

The LS-SVM approach solves classification and regression problems []. It looks for the best hyperplane in the higher dimension input space to build a decision boundary between two separate sets of patterns. This technique was originally designed as a linear classifier.

3.5.2 Support Vector Machine (SVM)

Vapnik introduced SVM in 1980' [17]. SVM splits data into class labels, then it builds hyperplanes. It is commonly used for binary classification [17].

3.5.3 Bagged Trees

Ensemble approaches (methods that aggregate the predictions of many models) first appeared in the 1990s. Leo Breiman invented bagging, short for bootstrap aggregation, as one of the earliest ensemble techniques. [18]. Bagging is a broad way to construct an ensemble that combines bootstrapping with any regression (or classification) model. The structure of the approach is quite straightforward, consisting of the stages in Algorithm (1). Following that, the ensemble models are used to forecast the new sample, and the k estimates are averaged to predict the bagging model.

3.5.4 K-Nearest-Neighbour (KNN) Classifiers

K-NN is a supervised classification technique, and KNN is a non-parametric approach for solving both regression and classification problems. This technique is one of the simplest and oldest for pattern recognition. It is used in machine learning, text categorization, data mining, Etc. It frequently produces efficient performance and, in certain situations, exceeds state-of-the-art classifiers in accuracy [15]. Using the K-closest samples from the training set, the technique predicts a new sample (similar to Fig. 4) [12]. Each observation in a learning set is represented as a point in an n-dimensional space, where n is the number of predictor variables. We seek the K points that are closest to this pattern to predict the class of an observation. The target variable's class has the most representation among the K's closest neighbors. The performance of a KNN classifier is also determined by the "d" distances between the tested and training data. Manhattan, Euclidian, and Chebyshev distances are the most commonly used examples.

3.5.5 K Means Clustering

K-Means method is based on dividing and is a type of cluster algorithm. It is referred as unsupervised approach. The primary concept behind these methods is this algorithm's basis is the square error and error criterion, which seeks to reduce the cluster performance index. To attain the best possible outcome, this strategy aims to locate K divisions that meet a specified condition. Firstly, choose several dots to represent the first cluster focus points. (Typically, the first K sample dots with revenue are chosen to represent the first cluster focus point.); Secondly, we will use the minimum distance criterion to gather the remainder of the dots to their focal points, and then we will get the initial classification; if the classification is unreasonable, we will modify it (calculate each cluster focal point again), and we will iterate until we get a satisfactory classification. The division-based K-Means technique is a sort of cluster algorithm that has the advantages of being concise, efficient, and quick [37].

3.6 Performance Metrics

The five-performance metrics accuracy (Acc), specificity (Spec), sensitivity (Sen), positive predictive value (PPV), and Fscore are used to evaluate the performance of the classifiers. The formulas to calculate the aforementioned performance metrics are provided in Table 1:

Table 1. Performance metrics for the classifier.

Parameter	Expression
Accuracy	$\text{Acc } (\%) = \frac{TP+TN}{TP+FP+TN+FN} * 100\%$
Sensitivity	
Specificity	$\text{Sen } (\%) = \frac{TP}{TP+FN} * 100\%$
Precision	
F-score	$\text{Spec } (\%) = \frac{TN}{TN+FP} * 100\%$
	$\text{Pre } (\%) = \frac{TP}{TP+FP} * 100\%$
	$\text{F-score } (\%) = 2 * \frac{* \text{ Precision} * \text{Sensitivity}}{\text{Precision} + \text{Sensitivity}} * 100\%$

4 Experimental Results and Discussion

In this paper, an PD disease detection model is suggested. The proposed model was implemented in MATLAB 2022A. A publicly available UCI dataset was used to evaluate the proposed model. EMD based classification models were used to classify the dataset into healthy and unhealthy subjects. Firstly, the recorded voice signals were filtered to reduce noise. The filtered signals were then passed through the EMD to decompose the input signals into IMFs. Finally, entropy features were extracted to detect PD.

4.1 Classifiers Results Based on Different Classifiers

In this experiment, three Entropy features from each IMFS of EMD were used to form the PD model. The voice recording signals were randomly partitioned into 80% for training and 20% for testing. The extracted features were sent to the K-nearest, LS-SVM, SVM, Bagged tree, and Kmeans. Table 2 reports the classification results. It can be noticed that the KNN and Bagged tree recorded the highest accuracy compared with other classifiers.

Table 2. Classification results based on EMD and different classification models

Classifier	Accuracy	Sensitivity	Specificity	precision	F-score
KNN	0.97	1	1	0.95	0.97
Bagged tree	0.97	1	1	0.94	0.97
LS-SVM	0.93	0.95	0.94	0.90	0.92
SVM	0.93	0.95	0.94	0.90	0.92
K-means	0.86	0.75	0.68	1	0.84

4.2 Cross-Fold Validation

In this experiment, 10-cross validation metric was adopted to assess the proposed model. The voice data was divided into 10 sets. One set was used for testing, while the others for training. Table 3 reports the classification results based on 10-cross validation.

Table 3. Classification results based on EMD

Classifier	Fold 1	Fold 2	Fold 3	Fold 4	Fold 5	Fold 6	Fold 7	Fold 8	Fold 9	Fold 10
KNN	1	1	1	1	1	1	1	1	0.95	0.95
Bagged tree	1	1	1	0.90	1	1	1	1	1	1
LS-SVM	1	0.90	1	1	1	1	0.95	1	1	1
SVM	1	1	0.90	1	1	1	1	1	1	1
K-means	1	1	1	1	1	1	1	1	0.95	0.95

4.3 Complexity Time of the Proposed Model

We examined the complexity time of the proposed model to detect the Parkinson's disease detection. The dataset was divided into several samples' sizes. Each experiment, the complexity time of classifiers were recorded. We noticed that the LS-SVM recorded the highest time while the SVM was recorded the lowest time (Fig. 2).

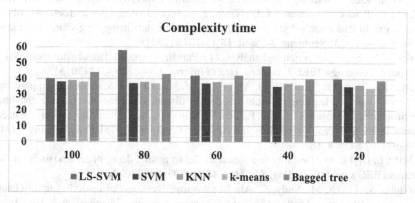

Fig. 2. The proposed method's time complexity. Time (seconds)

5 Conclusion

Based on EMD feature extraction methods, this paper has presented a framework for the detection of Parkinson's disease. The PD dataset from the UCI database is used for testing. we compute the entropy, Shannon and approximation-based features for ML classification after extracting the IMFs using the EMD approach. A ten-fold cross validation method is used to reduce the overfitting problem in ML algorithms. And the confusion matrix has been used to assess the performance of the four classifier models, SVM, KNN, bagged tree and k _means. The experimental results demonstrate the potential of the suggested framework employing the KNN technique a suitable classification accuracy of 97% was achieved. The suggested method can be used in future research to classify other complex diseases across a larger dataset.

References

1. Haq, A.U., et al.: Feature selection based on L1-norm support vector machine and effective recognition system for Parkinson's disease using voice recordings. IEEE Access **7**, 37718–37734 (2019)
2. Lahmiri, S., Shmuel, A.: Detection of Parkinson's disease based on voice patterns ranking and optimized support vector machine. Biomed. Sig. Process. Control **49**, 427–433 (2019)
3. Mostafa, S.A., et al.: Examining multiple feature evaluation and classification methods for improving the diagnosis of Parkinson's disease. Cogn. Syst. Res. **54**, 90–99 (2019)
4. Sabeena, B., Sivakumari, S., Amudha, P.: A technical survey on various machine learning approaches for Parkinson's disease classification. Mater. Today Proc **10**, 1–5 (2020)
5. Tai, Y.C., Bryan, P.G., Loayza, F., Peláez, E.: A voice analysis approach for recognizing Parkinson's disease patterns. IFAC-PapersOnLine **54**(15), 382–387 (2021)
6. Jeancolas, L., et al.: Voice characteristics from isolated rapid eye movement sleep behavior disorder to early Parkinson's disease. Parkinsonism Relat. Disord. **95**, 86–91 (2022)
7. Xu, Z.J., Wang, R.F., Wang, J., Yu, D.H.: Parkinson's disease detection based on spectrogram-deep convolutional generative adversarial network sample augmentation. IEEE Access **8**, 206888–206900 (2020)
8. Karaman, O., Çakın, H., Alhudhaif, A., Polat, K.: Robust automated Parkinson disease detection based on voice signals with transfer learning. Expert Syst. Appl. **178**, 115013 (2021)
9. Shalin, G., Pardoel, S., Lemaire, E.D., Nantel, J., Kofman, J.: Prediction and detection of freezing of gait in Parkinson's disease from plantar pressure data using long short-term memory neural-networks. J. Neuroeng. Rehabil. **18**(1), 1–15 (2021)
10. Sakar, B.E., et al.: Collection and analysis of a Parkinson speech dataset with multiple types of sound recordings. IEEE J. Biomed. Health Inform. **17**(4), 828–834 (2013)
11. Lafta, R., Zhang, Ji., Tao, X., Li, Y., Diykh, M., Lin, J.-W.: A structural graph-coupled advanced machine learning ensemble model for disease risk prediction in a telehealthcare environment. In: Roy, S.S., Samui, P., Deo, R., Ntalampiras, S. (eds.) Big data in engineering applications. SBD, vol. 44, pp. 363–384. Springer, Singapore (2018). https://doi.org/10.1007/978-981-10-8476-8_18
12. Alsafy, I., Diykh, M.: Developing a robust model to predict depth of anesthesia from single channel EEG signal. Phys. Eng. Sci. Med. **45**(3), 793–808 (2022)
13. Abdulla, S., Diykh, M., Siuly, S., Ali, M.: An intelligent model involving multi-channels spectrum patterns based features for automatic sleep stage classification. Int. J. Med. Inform. **171**, 105001 (2023)
14. Diykh, M., Abdulla, S., Deo, R.C., Siuly, S., Ali, M.: Developing a novel hybrid method based on dispersion entropy and adaptive boosting algorithm for human activity recognition. Comput. Methods Programs Biomed. **229**, 107305 (2023)
15. Zhang, T., Zhang, Y., Sun, H., Shan, H.: Parkinson disease detection using energy direction features based on EMD from voice signal. Biocybern. Biomed. Eng. **41**(1), 127–141 (2021)
16. Diykh, M., Miften, F.S., Abdulla, S., Saleh, K., Green, J.H.: Robust approach to depth of anaesthesia assessment based on hybrid transform and statistical features. IET Sci. Meas. Technol. **14**(1), 128–136 (2020)
17. Diykh, M., et al.: Texture analysis based graph approach for automatic detection of neonatal seizure from multi-channel EEG signals. Measurement **190**, 110731 (2022)
18. Diykh, M., Abdulla, S., Oudah, A.Y., Marhoon, H.A., Siuly, S.: A novel alcoholic EEG signals classification approach based on adaboost k-means coupled with statistical model. In: Siuly, S., Wang, H., Chen, Lu., Guo, Y., Xing, C. (eds.) HIS 2021. LNCS, vol. 13079, pp. 82–92. Springer, Cham (2021). https://doi.org/10.1007/978-3-030-90885-0_8

Analysis on Association Between Vascular Risk Factors and Lifestyle Factors with the Risk of Dementia/Alzheimer's Disease Using Medical Ontologies

Wenjuan Hong, Can Wang, Chenping Hu, Yanhua Chen, Xiyan Zhang, Zhisheng Huang, and Hongyun Qin[✉]

Department of Psychiatry, Shanghai Pudong New Area Mental Health Center, Tongji University School of Medicine, Pudong, Shanghai 200124, China
qinhongyun07@163.com

Abstract. Purpose: This Study Aims to Investigate How Lifestyle Factors Play a Role in the Connection Between Vascular Risk Factors (VRFs) and Dementia/Alzheimer's Disease (AD), As Well As the Underlying Associations Between These Variables, Within a Community Located in Pudong New Area, Shanghai, China.

Methods: We Utilized the Internationally Recognized Medical Ontology, SNOMED CT, to Identify Relevant Concepts Concerning Lifestyle and Vascular Risk Factors. These Metrics Served As the Foundation for Analyzing Our Collected Patient Data. We Conducted a Population-Based Cohort Study of Individuals Aged 60 Or Above; Participants Underwent Repeated in-Person Neuropsychological Assessments Between June 2011 and 2012. Additionally, We Conducted a Systematic Review to Monitor the Onset of Dementia/AD From July to December 2017 As a Follow-Up.

Results: The hierarchical structure of SNOMED CT identified 3466 sub-concepts relevant to VRFs and lifestyle. Our analysis particularly emphasized: 1) hypertension, 2) diabetes mellitus (DM), 3) dyslipidemia, 4) obesity, 5) tobacco smoking, and 6) alcohol consumption, with the inclusion of regular physical exercise (RPE) as an influential lifestyle factor. The incidence rate for dementia/AD was found to be 13.6%

Conclusions: Adopting a healthy lifestyle appears to alleviate the adverse impacts of VRFs on the onset of dementia/AD. Using standardized medical concepts enables us to further understand the relationship between VRFs and healthy lifestyles in diminishing the prevalence of dementia/AD.

Keywords: Alzheimer's Disease · dementia · Risk analysis · Medical Ontologies · Terminologies

Abbreviation

VRFs Vascular risk factors
AD Alzheimer's disease

Y. Li et al. (Eds.): HIS 2023, LNCS 14305, pp. 135–145, 2023.
https://doi.org/10.1007/978-981-99-7108-4_12

MMSE Mini-Mental State Examination
MoCA Montreal Cognitive Assessment Scale
CDR   Clinical Dementia Rating
DM   diabetes mellitus
RPE   regular physical exercise

1 Introduction

Dementia is characterized by a deterioration in cognitive function, impacting an individual's ability to perform daily tasks. It is not a specific disease, but rather a syndrome (a collection of symptoms) that can be caused by several different conditions, such as Alzheimer's disease (AD), vascular dementia (VaD), or Lewy body dementia. AD is the predominating form of dementia, accounting for 60–80% of all cases. It is a progressive neurodegenerative disorder that affects memory, cognition, and behavior, marked by the accumulation of neuropathological proteins such as beta-amyloid and tau, leading to neuronal death and cerebral atrophy.

Lifestyle encompasses an individual's daily habits, behaviors, and decisions. This includes dietary choices, physical activity, sleep patterns, work-life balance, social interactions, and recreational pursuits. Additionally, one's chosen lifestyle can reflect the core values, beliefs, and health orientations that guide their actions. For instance, an individual who prioritizes their health will likely engage in regular exercise, maintain a balanced diet, and follow an optimal sleep routine.

Lifestyle exerts a profound influence on health and well-being. A healthy lifestyle can alleviate risks of chronic illnesses like cardiovascular disease, diabetes, and cancer, improving both physical and mental health. In contrast, detrimental habits such as smoking, alcohol consumption, and physical inactivity can increase the risk of disease and negatively impact one's health.

Empirical evidence indicates that specific lifestyle determinants can reduce the risk for AD or slowing its progression. Noteworthy factors include:

1. Regular physical exercise (RPE): Empirical data suggests physical engagement can help reduce the risk for AD and improve cognitive abilities among those already diagnosed individuals. Additionally, it elevates mood, sleep quality, and overall physiological health.
2. Dietary pattern: A diet abundant in fruits, vegetables, whole grains, and lean proteins, while limited in saturated and trans fats, appears protective against AD. Mediterranean dietary patterns, rich in monounsaturated fats like olive oil, emerge as especially advantageous.
3. Cognitive stimulation: Pursuits that challenge the mind, such as reading, puzzle solving, or acquiring new skills, appear to diminish AD risks while improving cognitive function.

4. Social engagement: Robust social networks and familial ties can potentially lower the risk of developing AD while elevating overall well-being.
5. Chronic health condition management: Effective control of chronic diseases, such as hypertension, diabetes, and depression, may minimize the risk for developing AD while improving overall health status.

It is important to understand that while lifestyle modifications may decrease the risk of AD, they do not guarantee absolute prevention or cure. Certain lifestyles can exacerbate the risk of vascular diseases, such as strokes, myocardial infarctions, and peripheral artery diseases. For instance:

1. Tobacco consumption: Smoking significantly increases the risk for vascular disease, instigating vascular damage and thrombotic events; smoking cessation can reduce such risks.
2. Physical inactivity: Sedentary lifestyle elevates the chance of vascular disease, whereas regular physical engagement benefits vascular health, reduces inflammation, and improves blood circulation.
3. Unhealthy diet: Diets high in saturated fats, trans fats, cholesterol, salt, and added sugars can escalate vascular disease risk. Conversely, a balanced diet consisting of fruits, vegetables, grains, lean proteins, and healthy fats proves protective of vascular diseases.
4. Obesity: Excess weight burdens the cardiovascular system. Maintaining a healthy weight via balanced nutrition and physical activity is vital for vascular health.
5. High blood pressure: Hypertension can damage blood vessels and increase the risk of developing vascular disease. A healthy lifestyle inclusive of regular physical engagement, nutritious dietary patterns, and stress relief can help regulate blood pressure.

This study aims to investigate the relationship between vascular risk factors (VRFs) and lifestyle factors with dementia/AD risk. We utilize the renowned medical ontology/terminology, SNOMED CT, to find relevant concepts regarding lifestyle and VRF to gain more insights into this topic.

2 Methods

2.1 Medical Ontology and Terminology

Medical ontology [1] and terminology are two related but distinctive concepts integral to the medical domain.

Medical ontology refers to the formal categorization of concepts and their interrelations within a specific medical field. It utilizes standardized language to facilitate effective communication and logical deduction. By providing a unified understanding of domain-specific concepts and their interdependencies, an ontology enables automated reasoning and informed decision-making processes.

In contrast, medical terminology is characterized by a collection of standardized terms and definitions within the field of medicine; they are used to describe diseases, conditions, procedures, and additional medical notions. This ensures concise and unequivocal discourse concerning medical concepts, thereby enabling precise documentation, accurate coding, and systematic billing for medical services.

Commonly used medical terminologies include the International Classification of Diseases (ICD), Current Procedural Terminology (CPT), and Systematized Nomenclature of Medicine (SNOMED). These terminologies undergo periodic updates to accommodate new advances in the medical field and shifts in clinical practice.

In recent years, there has been an increasing emphasis on the development and application of medical ontologies and terminologies to support research, data sharing and clinical decision-making in the field of medicine. By offering a unified linguistic framework, these tools have the potential to increase the efficacy and quality of healthcare provision and research.

SNOMED CT (Systematized Nomenclature of Medicine - Clinical Terms) is a comprehensive and standardized medical terminology system. It is often used to encode clinical data in electronic health records (EHRs). It consists of more than 350,000 concepts and over 1 million terms for diseases, symptoms, procedures, drugs, devices, and other clinical concepts. SNOMED CT standardizes the representation and structuring of clinical data, facilitating an easier and more efficient communication among different healthcare systems and environments.

SNOMED CT operates in conjunction with other medical terminologies, such as ICD and CPT, to improve the precision of patient data documentation and support clinical decision-making.

The International Health Terminology Standards Development Organization (IHTSDO), a non-profit organization, oversees the ongoing development and maintenance of SNOMED CT. There is an increased utilization of SNOMED CT globally, with many countries adopting it as their standard terminology for EHRs and clinical data exchange.

To explore all the sub-concept related to the top concept of "Health-related behavior finding" (SNOMED CT Concept ID: 365949003), employ the following semantic query (i.e., SPARQL query) on the ontology SNOMED CT:

```
PREFIX ...
select distinct ?id ?label
where {
?id rdfs:subClassOf snomed:365949003.
?id sct:hasEnglishLabel ?label.
}
```

2.2 For the Perspective of Clinical Experience

Various vascular risk factors (VRFs), including midlife obesity [2–4], hypertension [5–7], diabetes mellitus (DM) [8, 9], tobacco smoking [10, 11], hypercholesterolemia [12, 13], and markers such as the APOE genotype [14], play pivotal roles in the pathogenesis and etiology of Alzheimer's disease (AD) [5, 10, 15–18]. Research suggests that midlife VRFs correlate with amyloid accumulation in the brain during later years, as shown by positron emission tomography using florbetapir [15]. These VRFs may either exacerbate AD-associated impairments or directly result in AD [15].

A linear relationship has been established between overall scores for a healthy lifestyle (weight, height, tobacco smoking, physical activity, and alcohol consumption) and the number of years lived without diseases such as type-2 diabetes mellitus (T2DM), coronary heart disease, stroke, cancer, asthma, chronic obstructive pulmonary disease, and dementia [8, 18, 19]. The Lifestyle for Brain Health Index has been shown to assist in preventing dementia in individuals below 80 years of age, according to a comprehensive study across multiple European centers [8, 20].

Our previous epidemiological studies indicated that individuals aged 60 and above (June 2011–2012) with new-onset hypertension displayed an increased risk for dementia, particularly AD [21]. A 6-year follow-up study (from July to December 2017) revealed that about 17.5% (77 out of 441) of subjects with mild cognitive impairment (MCI) progressed to AD. Interestingly, this rate is less than the 28% reported in a meta-analysis [22] and also lower than that observed in the group with new-onset hypertension. These observations encouraged us to further explore the connection between healthy lifestyle scores and VRFs.

2.3 The Hypothesis

Our hypothesis proposed that exposure to VRFs is associated with a higher prevalence of dementia/AD. Additionally, we believed that lifestyle factors could potentially mediate and intensify this relationship. To test this hypothesis, we utilized a well-characterized, population-based cohort with spatially detailed data on long-term exposure to various lifestyle factors, accompanied by clinical evaluations of dementia/AD.

This study centered on a cohort comprising individuals aged 60 and above at baseline. These participants underwent multiple in-person neuropsychological evaluations between June 2011 and 2012 and were then systematically screened for emerging dementia/AD from July to December 2017. Our cohort analysis encompassed a total of 1,231 participants over the 6-year follow-up period. All participants gave their written consent, and the study was approved by the ethical committee of the School of Medicine, Tongji University.

3   Results

3.1   The Sub-concepts in SNOMED CT of VRFs and Life Style

Using the top concept titled "Health-related behavior finding" (SNOMED CT Concept ID: 365949003), we extracted 1012 sub-concept labels/355 sub-concepts from the SNOMED CT, as depicted in Fig. 1:

1	http://www.ihtsdo.org/SCT_65568007	Cigarette smoker	SNOMEDCT2018
2	http://www.ihtsdo.org/SCT_65568007	Cigarette smoker (finding)	
3	http://www.ihtsdo.org/SCT_65568007	Cigarette smoker (life style)	
4	http://www.ihtsdo.org/SCT_70545002	Narcotic drug user	
5	http://www.ihtsdo.org/SCT_70545002	Narcotic drug user (finding)	
6	http://www.ihtsdo.org/SCT_70545002	Narcotic drug user (life style)	
7	http://www.ihtsdo.org/SCT_373613000	Cleans own needles (finding)	
8	http://www.ihtsdo.org/SCT_373613000	Cleans own needles	
9	http://www.ihtsdo.org/SCT_373870008	Cleans needles with bleach (finding)	
10	http://www.ihtsdo.org/SCT_373870008	Cleans needles with bleach	
11	http://www.ihtsdo.org/SCT_228273003	Finding relating to alcohol drinking behaviour	
12	http://www.ihtsdo.org/SCT_228273003	Alcohol drinking behaviour	
13	http://www.ihtsdo.org/SCT_228273003	Alcohol drinking behavior	
14	http://www.ihtsdo.org/SCT_228273003	Finding relating to alcohol drinking behavior	
15	http://www.ihtsdo.org/SCT_228273003	Finding relating to alcohol drinking behavior (finding)	
16	http://www.ihtsdo.org/SCT_228366006	Finding relating to drug misuse behaviour	
17	http://www.ihtsdo.org/SCT_228366006	Drug misuse behaviour	
18	http://www.ihtsdo.org/SCT_228366006	Drug misuse behavior	

Fig. 1. Screenshot of the semantic query result; examples of sub-concept labels of Health-related behavior finding in SNOMED CT

In contrast, using the top concept "life style" (SNOMED CT Concept ID: 60134006) yielded narrower results primarily associated with criminal behavior, illustrated in Fig. 2.

From the top concept "Eating/feeding/drinking finding" (SNOMED CT Concept ID: 116336009), we obtained 1099 sub-concept labels and 455 sub-concepts. Using the top concept "Motor behavior (observable entity)" (SNOMED CT Concept ID: 68130003), we found 24 sub-concept labels/1 sub-concept. Thus, the total number of "life style" related sub-concepts discovered in the SNOMED CT is 811 (calculated as 355 + 455 + 1).

For the top concept "Vascular disorder" (SNOMED CT Concept ID: 27550009), we found 6460 sub-concept labels/2534 sub-concepts in SNOMED CT. The top concept "Disorder of glucose metabolism (disorder)" (SNOMED CT Concept ID: 73211009) produced 394 sub-concept labels/120 sub-concepts (Fig. 3).

We noted that "dyslipidemia", crucial to our study, is not classified as a vascular disorder but is instead viewed as a metabolic disorder. Consequently, we included "dyslipidemia" as one of the top concepts. Using the top concept "dyslipidemia" (SNOMED CT Concept ID: 109041000119107), we identified 5 sub-concepts in SNOMED CT. These relevant concepts form the foundational framework for our investigation (Table 1).

	id	⬍	la
1	http://www.ihtsdo.org/SCT_105551000		Criminal life style
2	http://www.ihtsdo.org/SCT_105551000		Criminal life style (life style)
3	http://www.ihtsdo.org/SCT_105552007		Sexual offender
4	http://www.ihtsdo.org/SCT_105552007		Sexual offender (life style)
5	http://www.ihtsdo.org/SCT_105553002		Child molester
6	http://www.ihtsdo.org/SCT_105553002		Child molester (life style)
7	http://www.ihtsdo.org/SCT_105554008		Rapist
8	http://www.ihtsdo.org/SCT_105554008		Rapist (life style)
9	http://www.ihtsdo.org/SCT_105555009		Stalker
10	http://www.ihtsdo.org/SCT_105555009		Stalker (life style)
11	http://www.ihtsdo.org/SCT_105556005		Peeping Tom
12	http://www.ihtsdo.org/SCT_105556005		Peeping Tom (life style)
13	http://www.ihtsdo.org/SCT_105557001		Thief
14	http://www.ihtsdo.org/SCT_105557001		Thief (life style)
15	http://www.ihtsdo.org/SCT_105558006		Burglar
16	http://www.ihtsdo.org/SCT_105558006		Burglar (life style)
17	http://www.ihtsdo.org/SCT_105559003		Shoplifter
18	http://www.ihtsdo.org/SCT_105559003		Shoplifter (life style)

Fig. 2. Screenshot of the semantic query result; examples of sub-concept labels of life style in SNOMED CT

	id	⬍	
1	http://www.ihtsdo.org/SCT_5969009		Diabetes mellitus associated with genetic syndrome
2	http://www.ihtsdo.org/SCT_5969009		Genetic syndromes of diabetes mellitus
3	http://www.ihtsdo.org/SCT_5969009		Diabetes mellitus associated with genetic syndrome (disorder)
4	http://www.ihtsdo.org/SCT_70694009		Diabetes mellitus AND insipidus with optic atrophy AND deafness
5	http://www.ihtsdo.org/SCT_70694009		Marquardt-Loriaux syndrome
6	http://www.ihtsdo.org/SCT_70694009		DIDMOAD syndrome
7	http://www.ihtsdo.org/SCT_70694009		DIDMOAD - Diabetes insipidus,diabetes mellitus, optic atrophy and deafness
8	http://www.ihtsdo.org/SCT_70694009		Diabetes insipidus,diabetes mellitus, optic atrophy and deafness
9	http://www.ihtsdo.org/SCT_70694009		Wolfram syndrome

Fig. 3. Screenshot of the semantic query result; examples of sub-concept labels of Vascular disorder in SNOMED CT

In this preliminary analysis, we focused on a selected subset of concepts from the concept hierarchy of SNOMED CT. Based on clinical experience and ease of data collection, concepts such as tobacco smoking, alcohol consumption, physical activity, high blood pressure (HBP), diabetes mellitus, and dyslipidemia were chosen for this research. We intend to explore other concepts in subsequent studies.

Table 1. The top concepts and the sub-concepts of VRFs and life style

Top concept	SNOMED CT Concept ID	Sub-concept labels/sub-concepts
Health related behavior finding	365949003	1012/355
Eating/feeding/drinking finding	116336009	1099/455
Motor behavior	6813003	24/1
Vascular disorder	27550009	6460/2534
Disorder of glucose metabolism (disorder)	73211009	394/120
Dyslipidemia	109041000119107	5/1
Total		8994/3466

3.2 The Incident of AD in the Cohort

The study involved 1231 participants with a mean age of 66.94 ($\pm$7.18) years. Of these, 811 individuals (or 66.0%) were female. Participants aged 65 and above recorded a lower mean Mini-Mental State Examination (MMSE) score with a difference of 1.2 (95% confidence interval, 0.9–1.5). A dose-response relationship was observed between the number of Vascular Risk Factors (VRFs) and the incidence of dementia/AD, particularly when the VRF count was 2 or fewer. Upon inclusion, 30.8%, 44.7%, 20.6%, 3.5%, and 0.5% of the participants had 4, 3, 2, 1, and 0 metrics at the optimal lifestyle level, respectively.

During the follow-up period, 13.6% of the participants were diagnosed with dementia/AD. The Spearman correlation analysis revealed a positive association between the number of VRFs and the adoption of healthy lifestyles, with a correlation coefficient (r) of 0.192 (P = 0.000). The bivariate logistic regression analysis identified advanced age (with an odds ratio OR = 1.088, P = 0.000), a lower education background (OR = 0.601, P = 0.023), and the absence of Regular Physical Activity (RPA) (OR = 1.473, P = 0.034) as potential risk factors for dementia/AD.

4 Discussion

In our study, we identified 8,994 sub-concept labels/sub-concepts related to lifestyle and 3,466 for VRFs. Within SNOMED CT, factors such as hypertension, DM, dyslipidemia, obesity, tobacco smoking, alcohol consumption, and RPA fall under different top concepts.

Dyslipidemia is characterized by abnormal levels of lipids—such as triglycerides, cholesterol, and fat phospholipids—in the blood. While often linked to diet and lifestyle, dyslipidemia is a recognized risk factor for atherosclerotic cardiovascular disease (ASCVD). Yet, maintaining optimal lipid levels is more pertinent to ASCVD prevention than to dementia/AD prevention. This is because lipids, being water-insoluble, must combine with apolipoprotein (Apo) to become soluble lipoproteins in the blood, thereby ensuring they don't pose direct threats to the brain.

Obesity refers to excessive body fat accumulation. Hypertension denotes elevated arterial blood pressure, while DM describes a disorder of carbohydrate metabolism. Given their distinct pathologies, dyslipidemia, obesity, hypertension, and DM are classified under separate top concepts.

However, Canadian study showed a correlation between increases in systolic blood pressure (SBP) and BMI [23]. This implies that dyslipidemia, obesity, and other metabolic irregularities might function as intermediary phenotypes for primary hypertension [23]. Hypertension and DM are leading causes of cardiovascular disease (CVD), due to their collective impact on both large and small blood vessels [23, 24]. Therefore, despite their initial pathologies varying, their harmful effects on vascular health are consistent, leading to conditions such as CVD and AD. This differentiation might explain why dyslipidemia and obesity are classified as metabolic disorders, while hypertension is seen as a vascular disorder, even though all are considered VRFs in medical classifications.

Throughout our study's follow-up, only 13.6% of participants were diagnosed with dementia/AD. Diseases linked with VRFs, like hypertension, type 2 diabetes, obesity, and dyslipidemia, elevate the risk of dementia/AD. Potential mechanisms include altered cerebral structure, cerebral microcirculation disturbances, reduced amyloid protein clearance, and increased Aβ deposition in nerve cells [25]. The exact mechanism of Aβ-related pathology, however, remains unclear [26].

Nearly a third of participants exhibited healthy lifestyles—abstaining from smoking and alcohol, actively engaging in RPA, and maintaining a normal BMI—and showed no signs of VRFs such as hypertension, diabetes mellitus, dyslipidemia, or obesity. This observation suggests that Pudong's elderly population generally leads a healthy life with preserved cognitive abilities. As the number of VRFs increased, participants seemed to adopt healthier lifestyles, perhaps to counteract these risk factors and mitigate other health risks. Our findings reinforce the idea that embracing a healthy lifestyle, especially activities like RPA, can potentially offset and diminish dementia/AD risk.

5 Conclusions

A healthy lifestyle, characterized by regular physical exercise, abstaining from smoking, and moderate alcohol consumption, can potentially reduce the impact of VRFs on dementia/AD onset. This study offers a structured approach to comprehend the interaction between healthy living and VRFs concerning dementia/AD incidence, laying the groundwork for future clinical and research endeavors.

6 Strengths and Limitations

One of the primary strengths of our study is the utilization of artificial intelligence technology, which enables us to gain a comprehensive understanding of dementia/AD-related diseases and lifestyle information. This knowledge was then applied to investigate the cohort in the Pudong New Area.

However, our investigation does have certain limitations. Firstly, based on literature reviews and clinical experiences, we only selected 7 metrics from the 3,466 sub-concepts in SNOMED CT. This selection process inevitably overlooked some important factors, such as the frequency of RPE and the complications associated with DM and hypertension. Secondly, our cohort survey is retrospective, which might impact the validity of the results.

Acknowledgements. We would like to acknowledge Zhengai Lin (University College London), for hard working on the editor of the manuscript.

Authors' Contributions. HY Qin guided the implementation of the research, the other authors collated and analyzed the data. ZS Huang gave essential points for the analysis of data. All authors have read and approved the manuscript and ensure that this is the case. HY Qin is the corresponding authors.

Fundings. This research was funded by Shanghai Pudong Municipal Health Commission (No. PWZbr 2022-09 and PKJ2022-Y77), and Shanghai Municipal Health Commission (No. 202240093).

Declarations.

Competing Interests. None.

Ethics Approval and Consent to Participate. The research project was examined and approved by the ethics committee of the School of Medicine within Tongji University (Shanghai, China).

Consent to Publish. Not applicable.

Code Availability. Not applicable.

Availability of Data and Materials. The datasets used and/or analyzed are available from the corresponding author upon reasonable request.

References

1. Singh, R., et al.: Antisocial behavior identification from Twitter feeds using traditional machine learning algorithms and deep learning. EAI Endorsed Trans. Scalable Inf. Syst. **10**(4), e17 (2023)
2. Fitzpatrick, A.L., et al.: Midlife and late-life obesity and the risk of dementia: cardiovascular health study. Arch. Neurol. **66**(3), 336–342 (2009)
3. Gustafson, D., et al.: An 18-year follow-up of overweight and risk of Alzheimer disease. Arch. Intern. Med. **163**(13), 1524–1528 (2003)
4. Anstey, K.J., et al.: Body mass index in midlife and late-life as a risk factor for dementia: a meta-analysis of prospective studies. Obes. Rev. **12**(5), e426–e437 (2011)
5. Gottesman, R.F., et al.: Midlife hypertension and 20-year cognitive change: the atherosclerosis risk in communities neurocognitive study. JAMA Neurol. **71**(10), 1218–1227 (2014)

6. Walker, K.A., et al.: Association of midlife to late-life blood pressure patterns with incident dementia. JAMA **322**(6), 535–545 (2019)
7. Baloyannis, S.J., Baloyannis, I.S.: The vascular factor in Alzheimer's disease: a study in Golgi technique and electron microscopy. J. Neurol. Sci. **322**(1–2), 117–121 (2012)
8. Baumgart, M., et al.: Summary of the evidence on modifiable risk factors for cognitive decline and dementia: a population-based perspective. Alzheimers Dement. **11**(6), 718–726 (2015)
9. Baglietto-Vargas, D., et al · Diabetes and Alzheimer's disease crosstalk. Neurosci. Biobehav. Rev. **64**, 272–287 (2016)
10. Chang, R.C., et al.: Neuropathology of cigarette smoking. Acta Neuropathol. **127**(1), 53–69 (2014)
11. Baron, J.A.: Beneficial effects of nicotine and cigarette smoking: the real, the possible and the spurious. Br. Med. Bull. **52**(1), 58–73 (1996)
12. Rockwood, K., et al.: Use of lipid-lowering agents, indication bias, and the risk of dementia in community-dwelling elderly people. Arch. Neurol. **59**(2), 223–227 (2002)
13. Loera-Valencia, R., et al.: Alterations in cholesterol metabolism as a risk factor for developing Alzheimer's disease: potential novel targets for treatment. J. Steroid Biochem. Mol. Biol. **190**, 104–114 (2019)
14. Huang, W., et al.: APOE genotype, family history of dementia, and Alzheimer disease risk: a 6-year follow-up study. Arch. Neurol. **61**(12), 1930–1934 (2004)
15. Gottesman, R.F., et al.: Association between midlife vascular risk factors and estimated brain amyloid deposition. JAMA **317**(14), 1443–1450 (2017)
16. Gottesman, R.F., et al.: Associations between midlife vascular risk factors and 25-year incident dementia in the Atherosclerosis Risk in Communities (ARIC) cohort. JAMA Neurol. **74**(10), 1246–1254 (2017)
17. Ng, T.P., et al.: Metabolic syndrome and the risk of mild cognitive impairment and progression to dementia: follow-up of the Singapore longitudinal ageing study cohort. JAMA Neurol. **73**(4), 456–463 (2016)
18. Samieri, C., et al.: Association of cardiovascular health level in older age with cognitive decline and incident dementia. JAMA **320**(7), 657–664 (2018)
19. Nyberg, S.T., et al.: Association of healthy lifestyle with years lived without major chronic diseases. JAMA Intern. Med. (2020)
20. Vos, S.J.B., et al.: Modifiable risk factors for prevention of dementia in midlife, late life and the oldest-old: validation of the LIBRA index. J. Alzheimers Dis. **58**(2), 537–547 (2017)
21. Qin, H., Zhu, B., Wang, L., Guo, Y., Cao, Z., Hu, C.P.: Follow-up investigation of the effect of the new-onset and untreated hypertension on the elderly patients with mild cognitive impairment in community. Chin. Gen. Pract. **23**(13), 1640–1646, 1653 (2020)
22. Hu, C., et al.: The prevalence and progression of mild cognitive impairment among clinic and community populations: a systematic review and meta-analysis. Int. Psychogeriatr. **29**(10), 1595–1608 (2017)
23. Litwin, M., Kułaga, Z.: Obesity, metabolic syndrome, and primary hypertension. Pediatr. Nephrol. **36**(4), 825–837 (2021)
24. Strain, W.D., Paldánius, P.M.: Diabetes, cardiovascular disease and the microcirculation. Cardiovasc. Diabetol. **17**(1), 57 (2018)
25. Jacobson, A.M., et al., Diabetes Control and Complications Trial/EDIC Research Group: Biomedical risk factors for decreased cognitive functioning in type 1 diabetes: an 18 year follow-up of the Diabetes Control and Complications Trial (DCCT) cohort. Diabetologia **54**(2), 245–255 (2011)
26. Dansson, H.V., et al.: Predicting progression and cognitive decline in amyloid-positive patients with Alzheimer's disease. Alzheimers Res. Ther. **13**(1), 151 (2021)

COVID-19 Impact Studies

Unveiling the Pandemic's Impact: A Dataset for Probing COVID-19's Effects on E-Learning Activities and Academic Performance

Yanjun Liu[1], Daizhong Luo[1], Kate Wang[2], and Jiao Yin[3](✉)

[1] School of Artificial Intelligence, Chongqing University of Arts and Sciences, Chongqing 402160, China
[2] School of Health and Biomedical Sciences, RMIT University, Melbourne 3064, VIC, Australia
kate.wang@rmit.edu.au
[3] Institute for Sustainable Industries and Liveable Cities, Victoria University, Melbourne, VIC 3011, Australia
jiao.yin@vu.edu.au

Abstract. During the COVID-19 pandemic, educational institutions worldwide were affected and forced to switch to online education. This paper presents an open-source dataset that examines the influence of the pandemic on students' e-learning activities and academic performance. The dataset, collected from the C Programming Language course at Chongqing University of Arts and Sciences from 2019 to 2022, includes e-learning activities and final exam grades. Correlation analysis reveals a strong association between final exam scores, online assignments, and experiment results. Regression models are then built using random forest, linear regression, and Bayesian algorithms to investigate the impact of COVID-19. These models exhibit consistent trends, showing improved performance each year after a decline in 2020 and outperforming the results from 2019. This indicates that online learning gradually became the primary factor influencing students' academic performance after the initial chaotic adaptation period in 2020. The findings of this study provide valuable insights for educators and institutions, enhancing their understanding of the effects of online education and the pandemic on students' academic performance.

Keywords: COVID-19 pandemic impact · E-learning activity · Academic performance · Regression model

The work reported in this paper was partly supported by the higher education teaching reform research project "Exploration and Practice of Digital Transformation in the Fundamentals of Programming Course", funded by the Chongqing Education Commission, China, and a project sponsored by the Natural Science Foundation of Chongqing, China (Grant No. cstc2013jcyjA40066).

Y. Li et al. (Eds.): HIS 2023, LNCS 14305, pp. 149–160, 2023.
https://doi.org/10.1007/978-981-99-7108-4_13

1   Introduction

Due to the ongoing advancements in Internet technology, e-learning has emerged as a crucial component of higher education and continues to gain popularity and widespread adoption [11,20]. However, the correlation between students' e-learning behaviors, traits, and academic performance remains largely unexplored. To delve into these associated matters, a substantial volume of data on students' e-learning activities is required, encompassing personal information, subject matter content, online learning behavior, and more. Acquiring such data is challenging, and very few open-source datasets are currently accessible.

In addition, the outbreak of the COVID-19 pandemic in 2020 compelled schools and educational institutions worldwide to transition to online education [4,13], resulting in numerous studies investigating the connection between e-learning and students' academic performance. However, existing studies primarily focus on analyzing the influence of e-learning on student performance during the pandemic, with limited research comparing the impact of e-learning activities on student academic performance before and during the pandemic.

To partially address the aforementioned issues, this paper introduces an open-source dataset that investigates the impact of COVID-19 on the relationship between e-learning activities and students' academic performance. The dataset is derived from our teaching practices of the C Programming Language at Chongqing University of Arts and Sciences, China, spanning from 2019 to 2022. This paper aims to enhance understanding and utilization of e-learning tools while providing valuable insights into studying students' e-learning behaviors.

To summarize, the contributions of this paper are threefold:

- Firstly, we construct an open-source dataset, available on GitHub[1], to provide a valuable resource for researchers interested in investigating this field.
- Secondly, the paper comprehensively analyses correlations between academic performance and various e-learning activities, shedding light on their interrelationships.
- Lastly, a comparative study of academic performance is conducted, contrasting the pre-pandemic era with the pandemic era, providing valuable insights into the effects of the pandemic on educational outcomes.

2   Literature Review

With the application of information technology in the field of education and the continuous enrichment of e-learning resources, such as video classrooms, online teaching platforms, virtual laboratories, etc., e-learning has become a necessity for higher education institutions and is being promoted in educational institutions worldwide [3,9]. E-learning not only improves the quality and efficiency of education but also provides students with a more convenient way of learning. Students can access knowledge and information through the Internet, which

---

[1] https://github.com/liuyanjun66/E-learning-Data.

enables e-learning and interaction. In addition, higher education institutions can use technologies such as data analysis and artificial intelligence to optimize education management and teaching quality.

E-learning has generated a large amount of student online learning behavior data. How to use these data and machine learning models to predict students' academic performance and provide timely teaching feedback is the core topic in the field of e-learning analytics, attracting much attention from scholars worldwide. Paper [14] proposed a self-adaptive feature fusion strategy based on learning behavior classification, aiming to mine effective e-learning behavioral features to improve the performance of learning performance prediction models. Zhang W. et al. [21] summarized 19 behavior indicators in the online learning platform and proposed a student performance prediction model covering the whole learning process. Another work [2] designed two prediction models to detect the factors that influence students' learning achievement in MOOCs.

The development of education informatization is becoming increasingly rapid, especially under the influence of the COVID-19 pandemic, which has further propelled its progress. The outbreak of COVID-19 in early 2020 has accelerated the rapid development of e-learning. COVID-19's impact on higher education has also become a hot topic for scholars worldwide. For example, paper [10] reviewed the impact of COVID-19 on educational institutions and assessed the prevalence of e-learning changes. Paper [12] revealed some existing problems, challenges, and advantages of using e-learning systems to replace traditional education. Paper [1] conducted a comparative study examining students' grades before and during the COVID-19 pandemic to understand how it has affected their academic performance.

Though significant work has been conducted on e-learning and the impact of COVID-19 on education, several areas could benefit from further improvement. Firstly, there is a need for more publicly available datasets to enable the replication of research findings and inspire further related studies. Secondly, many studies heavily rely on questionnaire surveys and primarily employ statistical analysis methods, with limited utilization of more objective auto-generated log data from e-learning platforms and machine-learning models for predicting academic performance. Lastly, most studies predominantly focus on examining the impact of COVID-19 during the pandemic era, with a lack of comparative studies between the pre-pandemic and pandemic stages. This paper provides a solution for the aforementioned problems.

3 Dataset Construction

3.1 Data Collection

The dataset includes the e-learning activity log data of the course C Programming Language, collected from online learning platforms. Spanning four consecutive years (2019–2022), the course is delivered to freshmen students as compulsory and was offered only in the fall semester during these four years. The number of students enrolled in the course was 297 in 2019, 389 in 2020, 406 in

2021, and 400 in 2022. The dataset is collected from students in two majors, i.e., Artificial Intelligence and Computer Science, at Chongqing University of Arts and Sciences, China. It contains the following four categories of information:

(1) Student personal information: including student ID, name, gender, major, and class. We replaced student names and ID numbers with fake identifiers to protect student privacy.
(2) E-learning information: recording students' learning behavior on the MOOC platform, Smart Education of Chongqing[2]. It includes the total online learning hours, the total number of logins, comments, and test scores during the video learning process. In addition, a video learning score is also recorded to represent the completion rate of the instructional videos watched by students.
(3) Assignment and experiment scores: representing the results of in-class experiments and post-class assignments. Both were conducted on another online learning platform, CourseGrading[3], which can provide students with real-time feedback and help them continually modify their codes until correctness. Among them, the in-class experiments are conducted in lab classrooms with the guidance of instructors and mainly involve programming tasks. The number of experiments varied yearly but was usually between 5 and 8 in total. In contrast, the post-class assignments are completed independently by students after classes and include different types of questions, such as programming tasks, multiple-choice questions, and fill-in-the-blanks. The programming tasks in the post-class assignments are slightly more challenging than those in the in-class experiments. The number of assignments also varied yearly, usually between 4 and 8.
(4) Final exam scores: the final end-of-semester, off-line, closed-book exam scores, with a maximum score of 100. In this paper, they are used as the indicator of students' academic performance in C Programming Language.

3.2 Statistical Analysis and Visualization

Student Personal Information. The gender distributions of enrolled students from 2019 to 2022 are shown in Fig. 1, indicating consistent trends over the four years. The number of male students remains consistently 2–3 times higher than the number of female students.

E-Learning Information. We visualize the boxplots of online hours, number of logins, number of comments, and test scores from 2019 to 2022, as shown in Fig. 2. By comparing the data from these four years, it is evident that, after the outbreak of the pandemic in 2020, the online hours, the number of logins, and the number of comments decreased compared to the pre-pandemic year of 2019. This can be attributed to most courses being conducted offline before the pandemic.

---

[2] https://www.cqooc.com/.
[3] https://course.educg.net/.

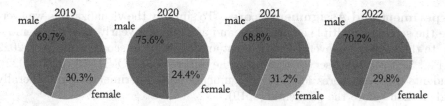

Fig. 1. Distribution of students' gender

As one of the few courses that offered an online learning platform, the course C Programming Language attracted more attention and time from students. However, following the outbreak of COVID-19, almost all courses shifted to online or hybrid teaching mode, significantly increasing students' overall online learning time. Nonetheless, the relative amount of online learning time students could allocate specifically for this course decreased.

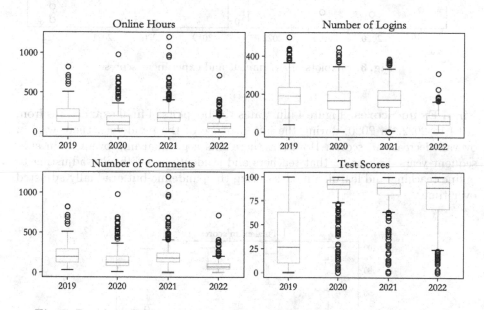

Fig. 2. Boxplots of e-learning information collected from a MOOC platform

By contrast, the average test scores significantly increased after the outbreak compared to 2019. The main reason for this is a rule change implemented in 2020. Since then, students have been allowed to take these quiz tests up to three times, and the platform recorded the highest score as the final score. However, before 2020, students only had one opportunity to take these tests.

Experiment and Assignment Scores. To simplify the visualization, we average the scores of multiple experiments and assignments yearly and only demonstrate the boxplots of average assignment and experiment scores from 2019–2022 in Fig. 3. It can be observed that after the outbreak of COVID-19 (2020–2022), students' average scores for both assignments and experiments were generally higher than before the pandemic (2019).

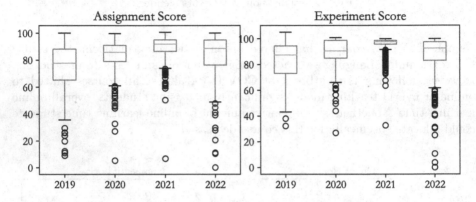

Fig. 3. Boxplots of assignment and experiment scores

Final Exam Scores. Figure 4 illustrates the boxplots of final exam scores from 2019 to 2022. In 2020, during the initial phase of the pandemic, there was an overall decrease in scores. However, there was a gradual improvement in subsequent years, indicating that teachers and students had difficulty adjusting to online teaching and learning modes during the pandemic but gradually adjusted over time.

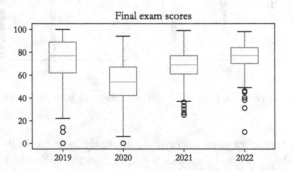

Fig. 4. Boxplots of final exam scores

3.3   Correlation Analysis

We conducted a correlation analysis between students' e-learning behaviors and their academic performance, measured in terms of final exam scores, to analyze the relationship between them. Figure 5 illustrates that final exam scores are primarily correlated with average assignment scores (0.2), average experiment scores (0.13), and online hours (0.13).

This finding aligns with our expectations, as it supports the notion that performance in the practical-oriented course C Programming Language is strongly associated with scores in practical assignments and experiments. Moreover, the positive correlation between online hours and final exam scores indicates that online learning contributes to improved academic performance. Conversely, final exam scores demonstrate relatively weak correlations with the number of logins (0.068) and the number of comments (0.0016). Furthermore, a weak negative correlation exists between final exam scores and test scores (-0.038).

In addition, strong correlations were observed between online assignment scores and online experiment scores (0.73), online hours and the number of logins (0.51), test scores and average assignment scores (0.44), test scores and the number of comments (0.41), and test scores and average experiment scores (0.4). On the other hand, weak negative correlations were observed between test scores and online hours (-0.027), as well as the number of logins (-0.025).

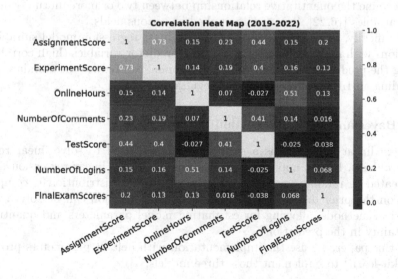

Fig. 5. Correlation matrix of e-learning data

4   Regression Analysis

In this section, we constructed regression models to predict students' final exam scores, which are continuous values ranging from 0 to 100, using the collected e-learning data. Three classic machine learning models were employed: random forest (RF), linear regression (LR), and Bayesian regression (Bayes), as described below [15, 19].

4.1   Random Forest

Random Forest is an ensemble learning method based on a combination of decision trees. It is commonly used for data classification problems and non-parametric regression problems [7, 18]. In classification, Random Forest returns the class option with the highest number of votes, while regression returns the average value of all the outputs of the decision trees.

The Random Forest regression model consists of multiple regression trees combined together. Random Forest regression can effectively analyze nonlinear data with collinearity and interaction effects without assuming a predefined model form [8]. However, Random Forest cannot make predictions beyond the range of the training dataset, which can lead to overfitting when modeling data with specific noise.

4.2   Linear Regression

Linear regression is a statistical analysis method in mathematical statistics used to determine the quantitative relationship between two or more mutually dependent variables [16, 22]. It is widely applied in various fields.

Specifically, this study adopts the Lasso linear regression model suitable for situations with multicollinearity among the predictor variables (high correlation among the predictor variables). The Lasso model can reduce the standard error by adding an L1 penalty term to the regression estimate.

4.3   Bayesian Linear Regression

Bayesian linear regression is a statistical method used to solve linear regression problems. In this approach, the parameters of the linear regression model are treated as random variables, and their posterior distribution is computed based on the prior distribution. Bayesian linear regression can be solved using numerical methods, allowing for estimating model parameters and quantifying uncertainty in the predictions.

In this paper, we use the implementation with default parameters provided by scikit-learn[4] to implement these three models.

4.4   Results of Regression Models

To assess the performance of these three models, we employed two categories of evaluation metrics. The first category measures the errors between predicted values and true values, including root mean square error (RMSE), mean absolute

---

[4] https://scikit-learn.org/stable/.

error (MAE), and mean absolute percentage error (MAPE) [6]. The second category measures the correlation between predicted values and true values, including Pearson correlation (Pear corr) and Spearman correlation (Spear corr) [5,17].

During the data preprocessing phase, we discarded samples with missing values and samples with a final exam score below 15. Additionally, we trimmed outliers in the online hours variable, capping them at a maximum value of 400. Subsequently, we consolidated the data from 2019 to 2022 into a comprehensive dataset and partitioned it into training and testing sets, employing an 8:2 ratio. Table 1 presents the results of the three models on the testing set. The RF model demonstrates the highest predictive performance among the three models, while the LR and Bayes models exhibit comparable prediction performance.

Table 1. Results of regression models on the e-learning dataset

Model	RMSE	MAE	MAPE	Pearson	Spearman
RF	15.6116	12.3007	0.2572	0.3276	0.3542
LR (Lasso)	15.9887	12.7958	0.2361	0.2031	0.1943
Bayes	15.9520	12.6928	0.2306	0.1969	0.1854

Regarding prediction error, the RMSE of the three models ranges from 15.6 to 16, the MAE ranges from 12.3 to 12.8, and the MAPE ranges from 0.23 to 0.26. As for the correlation between the predicted and true values, the Pearson coefficient ranges from 0.19 to 0.33, and the Spearman coefficient ranges from 0.18 to 0.36.

5   COVID-19 Implication

The outbreak of the COVID-19 pandemic had a profound influence on online learning worldwide. Schools were compelled to suspend in-person classes to prioritize student safety and ensure uninterrupted educational progress. Consequently, teachers and students swiftly transitioned to online education and learning platforms. This shift in the learning environment necessitated students to adapt their study methods and habits, requiring them to demonstrate greater levels of concentration and self-discipline. As a result, this transformation is anticipated to impact students' academic performance.

To investigate the impact of the COVID-19 pandemic, we further divided the dataset into four groups based on four consecutive years and then evaluated the performance of these models on each group separately. The results are presented in Table 2. Results show that the performance of all models is equivalent and follows the same trend over the four-year period. They performed poorly in 2019 but even worse in 2020. However, after the outbreak of COVID-19, there was a year-by-year improvement in their performance from 2020 to 2022. Taking the RF algorithm as an example, regarding prediction errors, RMSE decreased from

18.03 to 9.10, MAE decreased from 14.85 to 7.1, and MAPE decreased from 0.32 to 0.1. Regarding correlation, the Pearson value increased from 0.09 to 0.42, and the Spearman value increased from 0.07 to 0.39. Compared to the pre-pandemic period, all three models' prediction performance in 2020 was slightly worse than in 2019. The predictions in 2021 were better than in 2019, with lower RMSE and MAE values and higher Pearson and Spearman correlation values. The prediction performance in 2022 showed a significant improvement for all three models.

Table 2. Performance comparison of regression models between pre-pandemic and during-pandemic eras

Model	Period	Year	RMSE	MAE	MAPE	Pearson	Spearman
RF	Pre-pandemic	2019	15.60	13.37	0.19	0.17	0.16
	During-pandemic	2020	18.03	14.85	0.32	0.09	0.07
		2021	13.55	11.52	0.22	0.34	0.35
		2022	9.10	7.10	0.12	0.42	0.39
LR(Lasso)	Pre-pandemic	2019	15.12	12.64	0.19	0.19	0.19
	During-pandemic	2020	16.91	13.98	0.31	0.27	0.21
		2021	13.32	10.74	0.20	0.31	0.31
		2022	9.52	7.52	0.12	0.29	0.28
Bayes	Pre-pandemic	2019	15.01	12.48	0.18	0.21	0.19
	During-pandemic	2020	16.76	13.84	0.30	0.28	0.22
		2021	13.37	10.87	0.18	0.29	0.31
		2022	9.47	7.56	0.10	0.34	0.35

Based on our teaching practice, we believe that the reason for the poor performance in 2019 is that, before the pandemic, offline learning was still the main approach for students to acquire knowledge, and e-learning activities played a relatively weak role in determining the final exam results. However, after the outbreak of the pandemic, following a relatively chaotic adaptation period in 2020, online learning gradually became mainstream. As a result, the predictive ability of e-learning activities in determining students' academic performance has improved over time. Consequently, the performance of all models showed improvement from 2020 to 2022.

6   Conclusion

This paper constructed and released an e-learning dataset collected from the teaching practice of the course C Programming Language at Chongqing University of Arts and Sciences for four consecutive years, from 2019 to 2022. We conducted a correlation analysis to analyze the relationships between e-learning activities and students' academic performance. The results show that the final exam scores were mainly correlated with online assignment scores, online experiment scores, and online hours. To further investigate the impact of COVID-19 on education, we conducted regression analysis on the entire dataset and each year separately, using three classic machine learning algorithms. The results show that all three models achieved the worst performance in 2020, indicating that the outbreak of COVID-19 has disrupted the regular teaching and learning process. Therefore, predicting students' academic performance during that year was more challenging. However, as the impact of the pandemic diminishes over time, students' online learning behaviors can better predict their academic performance. Thus, all three models performed best in 2022, surpassing the prepandemic period in 2019. The reason is that before the pandemic, students' academic performance relied more on their offline learning activities. In contrast, online learning gradually became mainstream during the pandemic, and students' online learning behaviors can better reflect their academic performance. This research can enhance our understanding of the effectiveness and adaptability of online learning and provide valuable insights for future education during similar crisis periods.

References

1. Abdullah, M., Al-Ayyoub, M., AlRawashdeh, S., Shatnawi, F.: E-learningdjust: E-learning dataset from Jordan university of science and technology toward investigating the impact of covid-19 pandemic on education. Neural Comput. Appl., 1–15 (2021)
2. Alshabandar, R., Hussain, A., Keight, R., Khan, W.: Students performance prediction in online courses using machine learning algorithms. In: 2020 International Joint Conference on Neural Networks (IJCNN), pp. 1–7. IEEE (2020)
3. Chen, Y., Han, S., Chen, G., Yin, J., Wang, K.N., Cao, J.: A deep reinforcement learning-based wireless body area network offloading optimization strategy for healthcare services. Health Inf. Sci. Syst. **11**(1), 8 (2023)
4. Ebner, M., et al.: Covid-19 epidemic as e-learning boost? chronological development and effects at an Austrian university against the background of the concept of "e-learning readiness". Future Internet **12**(6), 94 (2020)
5. Ge, Y.F., Cao, J., Wang, H., Chen, Z., Zhang, Y.: Set-based adaptive distributed differential evolution for anonymity-driven database fragmentation. Data Sci. Eng. **6**(4), 380–391 (2021)
6. Ge, Y.F., Wang, H., Cao, J., Zhang, Y.: An information-driven genetic algorithm for privacy-preserving data publishing. In: Chbeir, R., Huang, H., Silvestri, F., Manolopoulos, Y., Zhang, Y. (eds.) WISE 2022. LNCS, vol. 13724, pp. 340–354. Springer, Cham (2022). https://doi.org/10.1007/978-3-031-20891-1_24
7. Hong, W., et al.: Graph intelligence enhanced bi-channel insider threat detection. In: Yuan, X., Bai, G., Alcaraz, C., Majumdar, S. (eds.) NSS 2022. LNCS, pp. 86–102. Springer, Cham (2022). https://doi.org/10.1007/978-3-031-23020-2_5
8. Hong, W., et al.: A graph empowered insider threat detection framework based on daily activities. ISA Transactions (2023)
9. Islam, N., Beer, M., Slack, F.: E-learning challenges faced by academics in higher education. J. Educ. Training Stud. **3**(5), 102–112 (2015)

10. Khan, M.A.: Covid-19's impact on higher education: a rapid review of early reactive literature. Educ. Sci. **11**(8), 421 (2021)
11. Kibuku, R.N., Ochieng, D.O., Wausi, A.N.: e-learning challenges faced by universities in Kenya: a literature review. Electr. J. e-Learning **18**(2), 150–161 (2020)
12. Maatuk, A.M., Elberkawi, E.K., Aljawarneh, S., Rashaideh, H., Alharbi, H.: The covid-19 pandemic and e-learning: challenges and opportunities from the perspective of students and instructors. J. Comput. High. Educ. **34**(1), 21–38 (2022)
13. Moustakas, L., Robrade, D.: The challenges and realities of e-learning during covid-19: the case of university sport and physical education. Challenges **13**(1), 9 (2022)
14. Qiu, F., et al.: E-learning performance prediction: mining the feature space of effective learning behavior. Entropy **24**(5), 722 (2022)
15. Shaodong, H., Yingqun, C., Guihong, C., Yin, J., Wang, H., Cao, J.: Multi-step reinforcement learning-based offloading for vehicle edge computing. In: 2023 15th International Conference on Advanced Computational Intelligence (ICACI), pp. 1–8. IEEE (2023)
16. Singh, R., et al.: Antisocial behavior identification from twitter feeds using traditional machine learning algorithms and deep learning. EAI Endorsed Trans. Scalable Inf. Syst. **10**(4), e17–e17 (2023)
17. Vimalachandran, P., Liu, H., Lin, Y., Ji, K., Wang, H., Zhang, Y.: Improving accessibility of the Australian my health records while preserving privacy and security of the system. Health Inf. Sci. Syst. **8**, 1–9 (2020)
18. Yin, J., Tang, M., Cao, J., You, M., Wang, H.: Cybersecurity applications in software: Data-driven software vulnerability assessment and management. In: Daimi, K., Alsadoon, A., Peoples, C., El Madhoun, N. (eds.) Emerging Trends in Cybersecurity Applications, pp. 371–389. Springer, Cham (2022). https://doi.org/10.1007/978-3-031-09640-2_17
19. Yin, J., You, M., Cao, J., Wang, H., Tang, M.J., Ge, Y.-F.: Data-driven hierarchical neural network modeling for high-pressure feedwater heater group. In: Borovica-Gajic, R., Qi, J., Wang, W. (eds.) ADC 2020. LNCS, vol. 12008, pp. 225–233. Springer, Cham (2020). https://doi.org/10.1007/978-3-030-39469-1_19
20. You, M., et al.: A knowledge graph empowered online learning framework for access control decision-making. World Wide Web **26**(2), 827–848 (2023)
21. Zhang, W., Huang, X., Wang, S., Shu, J., Liu, H., Chen, H.: Student performance prediction via online learning behavior analytics. In: 2017 International Symposium on Educational Technology (ISET), pp. 153–157. IEEE (2017)
22. Zhang, X., et al.: Radiomics under 2d regions, 3d regions, and peritumoral regions reveal tumor heterogeneity in non-small cell lung cancer: a multicenter study. La radiologia medica, 1–14 (2023)

Understanding the Influence of Multiple Factors on the Spread of Omicron Variant Strains via the Multivariate Regression Method

Zhenkai Xu[1], Shaofu Lin[1(✉)], Zhisheng Huang[2,3], and Yu Fu[1]

[1] Faculty of Information Technology, Beijing University of Technology, Beijing 100124, China
linshaofu@bjut.edu.cn
[2] Department of Computer Science, Vrije University Amsterdam, Amsterdam, Netherlands
[3] Clinical Research Center for Mental Disorders, Shanghai Pudong New Area Mental Health Center, Tongji University School of Medicine, China and Deep Blue Technology Group, Shanghai, China

Abstract. The Omicron variant of SARS-CoV-2, emerging in November 2021, has rapidly spread worldwide due to its high transmissibility and ability to evade vaccines. It is still not fully under control, and there is a need to enhance our scientific understanding of the Omicron variant. Investigating the influencing factors and the correlated characteristics of the transmission of the Omicron variant remains an important issue in COVID-19 prevention and control. This study utilized data from various sources to investigate Omicron's transmission factors. Focusing on populous countries like China, France, and the US, a multiple regression model was optimized through the Gauss-Newton method to reveal links between daily Omicron cases and variables like climate, population, healthcare, and vaccination and etc. Results showed vaccination rates, healthcare facility numbers, and population density as pivotal factors influencing transmission. Higher vaccination rates and more healthcare facilities correlated with lower Omicron transmission, while dense population areas experienced higher spread. These findings hold significance for guiding public health decisions and shaping vaccination strategies amidst the Omicron variant's ongoing impact.

Keywords: Omicron · Multiple Regression · COVID-19 Pandemic · Quantitative Analysis

1 Introduction

On November 26, 2021, the World Health Organization (WHO) named the B.1.1.529 variant of the SARS-CoV-2 as Omicron and identified it as a variant of concern (VOC). Since then, Omicron has rapidly spread among populations, posing severe challenges to global public health systems and socio-economic development. According to the latest data from the WHO, as of July 2023, the global cumulative confirmed cases have surpassed 76.8 million, with a death toll of 6.9 million. As a new variant of the COVID-19 pandemic, the Omicron variant has rapidly spread worldwide over the past year. Its high

Y. Li et al. (Eds.): HIS 2023, LNCS 14305, pp. 161–174, 2023.
https://doi.org/10.1007/978-981-99-7108-4_14

transmissibility and immune escape characteristics present new challenges in terms of transmission and control of the disease. Although the WHO has announced that COVID-19 no longer constitutes an international public health emergency, Dr. Tedros Adhanom Ghebreyesus [1] has warned that if there is a significant increase in cases or deaths in the future, he will not hesitate to convene another Emergency Committee meeting and declare a global health emergency once again. There are still many unanswered questions regarding the COVID-19 pandemic, particularly the Omicron variant, such as the factors contributing to the emergence of the Omicron variant, its unknown characteristics, and the factors influencing its spread. Therefore, this study employs multiple regression analysis to investigate the multifactorial influences on the transmission of the Omicron variant, aiming to provide scientific decision-making support for epidemic prevention and the prevention of similar respiratory infectious diseases. The remaining sections of this paper are organized as follows:

Section 2 comprehensively introduces the current understanding and research progress on the Omicron variant, analyzing the research achievements of various factors influencing the transmission of Omicron. Section 3 describes the data sources. Section 4 presents our research methodology and findings. Section 5 analyzes and discusses the experimental results and Sect. 6 provides our experimental conclusions and relevant recommendations.

2 Related Work

2.1 Understanding of Omicron

Following the outbreak of the Delta variant of SARS-CoV-2, the emergence of the Omicron variant poses a significant threat to global public health. Researchers have conducted extensive studies on the genetic characteristics, clinical symptoms, and transmissibility of the Omicron variant.

Collier et al. (2022) [2] found that Omicron exhibited enhanced resistance to neutralizing antibodies, while Khalifa et al. [3] discovered that this variant might cause milder symptoms compared to previous variants, although the mortality rate among hospitalized Omicron variant patients was slightly higher than that of the Delta variant. Zhang et al. [4] investigated the D614G mutation of the SARS-CoV-2 virus, which shared some similarities with the Omicron variant. The study revealed that this mutation made the spike protein on the virus surface more prone to binding with human cells, thereby increasing the infectivity of the virus. Osman Özüdoğru et al. [5] compared the clinical conditions of Delta and Omicron variant patients using a questionnaire survey and found a higher reinfection rate among Omicron variant patients compared to Delta variant patients. Lino et al. [6] discovered numerous mutations in regions associated with higher transmissibility, stronger viral binding affinity, antibody escape, and affinity in the Omicron variant.

The studies [2–6] mentioned above provide foundational and comprehensive information about Omicron. Overall, these studies have found that the Omicron variant possesses distinct genomic characteristics compared to other variants [7] and exhibits different symptoms and characteristics upon infecting individuals. Additionally, these studies suggest that the Omicron variant may cause milder symptoms than other variants but can pose challenges to the effectiveness of vaccines. These findings contribute to a better understanding of the features and transmission of the Omicron variant, providing a scientific basis for tackling the pandemic.

2.2 Research on Factors Influencing Omicron Transmission

In the study of the factors influencing the spread of Omicron variant, scholars have conducted research from different aspects including population, healthcare interventions, and environmental factors.

Asamoah et al. (2022) [8] used a compartmental model to study the impact of vaccine coverage, population mobility, and population density on Omicron transmission in South Africa. The study found that higher vaccine coverage and reduced population mobility were effective in controlling the spread of the virus. Dumitrescu et al. (2022) [9] employed a mathematical model to investigate the impact of various factors, including population mobility and vaccine coverage, on the dynamics of Omicron transmission in Europe. The study revealed that vaccination and reducing population mobility were effective in controlling the spread of the virus. Funk et al. (2022) [10] examined the transmission of Omicron in the United Kingdom and found that reducing social contacts and increasing vaccine coverage were effective measures to control the virus's spread. The study also indicated that early detection and contact tracing could effectively prevent outbreaks. J. Lee et al. (2021) [11] employed a qualitative analysis to investigate the frequency of utilization of telemedicine guidance within the population of individuals afflicted by COVID-19, thereby instigating a reevaluation of the COVID-19 pandemic from diverse perspectives through the application of qualitative analytical methodologies. Gao et al. (2022) [12] used statistical models to analyze the influence of population structure and environmental factors on the dynamics of Omicron transmission in China. The study identified population density, temperature, and humidity as important factors affecting the spread of the virus. Kang et al. (2022) [13] studied various intervention measures to control Omicron transmission in the United States, including vaccination, testing, and contact tracing. The study found that vaccination was the most effective intervention measure for controlling the spread of the virus. Lee et al. (2022) [14] analyzed the impact of population mobility on the dynamics of Omicron transmission in South Korea using a mathematical model. The study concluded that reducing population mobility could effectively control the spread of the virus. Liu et al. (2022) [15] investigated the dynamics of Omicron transmission in Beijing, China using a mathematical model. The study identified population density, social contacts, and vaccine coverage as important factors influencing the spread of the virus. Moghadas et al. (2022) [16] used a mathematical model to study the impact of vaccines and non-pharmaceutical interventions on the dynamics of Omicron transmission in Canada. The study found that vaccination was the most effective intervention measure for controlling the spread of the virus, followed by reducing social contacts. Ong et al. (2022) [17] studied the transmission dynamics of Omicron in Singapore and found that vaccine coverage and reducing population mobility were highly effective in controlling virus transmission. The study also highlighted that early detection and contact tracing could effectively prevent outbreaks. Wang et al. (2022) [18] used a mathematical model to analyze the impact of vaccine coverage, population density, and population mobility on the dynamics of

Omicron transmission in China. The study found that vaccine coverage and reducing population mobility were highly effective in controlling virus transmission. Fu et al. [19] constructed experimental data based on publicly available datasets of COVID-19, such as Johns Hopkins and China Meteorological Data Network. They used the Gauss-Newton iteration method to quantitatively analyze the relationship between the epidemic spread and various features, concluding that population density had the highest positive correlation with epidemic transmission.

These studies [8–19] provide insights into the factors influencing the transmission of Omicron, considering various aspects such as population dynamics, vaccination, mobility, and environmental factors. The findings contribute to a better understanding of the mechanisms behind Omicron transmission and provide valuable information for guiding effective strategies in pandemic control.

3 Data Sources

The data for this study primarily cover six aspects, including pandemic data, variant strain data, climate data, population and flight data, air quality data, and healthcare facility and vaccine data.

(1) Pandemic data: This study utilized the COVID-19 dataset provided by the Johns Hopkins University Center for Systems Science and Engineering (CSSE). This dataset has been collecting global pandemic data since January 22, 2020, and provides real-time updates on the pandemic situation during the early stages. The experimental data for this study span from January 22, 2020, to December 31, 2022, including cumulative confirmed cases, cumulative recoveries, cumulative deaths, and the daily number of new cases as the featured data elements.

(2) Variant strain data: This study used the variant strain data provided by the website Covariants (https://covariants.org/), which tracks global COVID-19 variant strains. This website, created by researchers and developers, provides detailed information on various SARS-CoV-2 variant strains, including their names, transmission trends, potential impacts, and information on the effectiveness of available vaccines and treatments. For this study, the percentage of each variant strain's occurrence from January 22, 2020, to December 31, 2022, was selected as the featured data element.

(3) Climate data: This dataset was collected from various meteorological stations worldwide through the China Meteorological Data Service Center (http://data.cma.cn/). The study selected daily climate records from different regions from January 22, 2020, to December 31, 2022. The featured data elements include daily maximum temperature, daily minimum temperature, wind speed, precipitation, dew point temperature, atmospheric pressure, gust, elevation, absolute humidity, and relative humidity.

(4) Population and flight data: The data were obtained from the United Nations Department of Economic and Social Affairs, Population Division (https://population.un.org/wpp/). The study selected population and flight data from different regions from January 22, 2020, to December 31, 2022. The featured data elements include total population, population density, total number of flights, domestic flight count, and international flight count.

(5) Air quality data: The dataset was sourced from the open-access air quality website, World Air Quality Index (WAQI) (https://aqicn.org/data-platform/covid19/). The study selected air quality data from different regions from January 22, 2020, to December 31, 2022. The featured data elements include concentrations of pollutants such as NO_2, PM_{10}, $PM_{2.5}$, PM_1, SO_2, O_3, CO, air quality index (AQI), particulate matter concentration (from NEPH), ultraviolet index (UVI), pollution (POL), and dominant wavelength (WD).

(6) Healthcare facility and vaccine administration data: The data were obtained from the Centers for Disease Control and Prevention (CDC) in the United States (https://www.cdc.gov/coronavirus/2019-ncov/). The study selected vaccine administration data and the number of healthcare facilities (including nucleic acid testing centers and medical emergency centers) from different regions from January 22, 2020, to December 31, 2022.

We collected a dataset comprising 33 different dimensions of features from 35 countries. The epidemic data, population data and flight data were obtained through publicly available datasets, while the variant strains, air quality, climate data, as well as healthcare institution and vaccine administration data were acquired by crawling the data sources using Python. Due to feasibility considerations in data collection, we selected only these 35 countries. To ensure an adequate amount of data for model training, we divided the dataset into training set and testing set in a ratio of 9:1. The training set includes data from January 22, 2020, to October 13, 2022, while the testing set comprises data from October 14, 2022, to December 31, 2022 (Table 1).

Table 1. Feature display of fusion data set

Feature Category	Feature Range
Date	2020.01.22–2022.12.31
Country	Afghanistan, Australia, Austria, Brazil, Canada, Chile, China, Colombia, Estonia, Ethiopia, Finland, France, Germany, Greece, Iceland, India, Indonesia, Iran, Iraq, Japan, Korea, Mexico, Netherlands, New Zealand, Norway, Poland, Russia, Serbia, Singapore, South Africa, Spain, Sweden, Thailand, United Kingdom, United States
Epidemic	Confirmed, Recovered, Deaths, New
Climate	Tmax, Tmin, Wind_speed, Precipitation, DP_F, Pressure, Wind_gust, Altitude, Ab_humidity, Re_humidity
Population	Pop, Density
Air quality	NO_2, PM_{10}, $PM_{2.5}$, PM_1, SO_2, O_3, CO, AQI, NEPH, UVI, POL, WD
Flight	Flight_total, Flight_domestic, Flight_international
Medical Assistance	Vaccination rates, Medical institutions

Tmax, Tmin, Wind_speed, Precipitation, DP_F, Pressure, Wind_gust, Altitude, Ab_humidity, and Re_humidity represent the daily maximum temperature, daily minimum temperature, wind speed, precipitation, dew point temperature, atmospheric pressure, instantaneous wind speed, altitude, absolute humidity, and relative humidity, respectively. Pop and Density represent the total population and population density, respectively. NO_2, PM_{10}, $PM_{2.5}$, PM_1, SO_2, O_3, CO, AQI, NEPH, UVI, POL, and WD represent the concentrations of NO_2, PM_{10}, $PM_{2.5}$, PM_1, SO_2, O_3, CO in the air, as well as the Air Quality Index (AQI), nephelometric turbidity unit (NEPH), UV index (UVI), pollution level (POL), and dominant wavelength (WD), respectively. Flight_total, Flight_domestic, and Flight_international represent the total number of flights, number of domestic flights, and number of international flights, respectively. Vaccination rates and medical institutions represent the vaccination rates and the number of medical institutions, respectively.

4 Research Method

The quantitative relationship model proposed in this paper between Omicron variant transmission and multiple feature factors consists of the following three steps:

1) Time series calculation of the increment of the daily number of new cases of Omicron variant;
2) Quantitative analysis of the relationship between multivariate regression and feature data;
3) Model optimization using the Gauss-Newton iteration method.

4.1 Calculation Method of Daily New Omicron Cases

In this study, we obtained the daily number of new cases of the Omicron variant and the daily proportion of Omicron cases among all cases. The proportion of Omicron cases, as a variable, forms a time series composed of discrete numbers that vary over time. To eliminate the issue of missing data for different proportions on each day, we have used the ARIMA method to remove the level changes in the series, i.e., to remove seasonality or trends, which helped stabilize the mean of the time series. As a result, we have obtained a stable percentage value, denoted as y_t', representing the percentage of Omicron cases among daily new cases, where y_t represents the value of new cases on a given date and y_{t-1} represents the value on the previous day.

$$y_t' = y_t - y_{t-1} \tag{1}$$

By multiplying the daily number of new cases Y by the percentage of Omicron cases y_t', we obtain the daily number of new Omicron cases y, for that day. Similarly, by this method, we can obtain the number of new deaths, the cumulative number of deaths and the cumulative number of infections per day.

$$y = Y \times y_t' \tag{2}$$

4.2 Multiple Regression Analysis of Factors Affecting the Transmission of Omicron Variant

We have utilized the Gauss-Newton iteration method to optimize multiple regression and address the quantitative analysis problem between multiple factors and the number of new Omicron cases. Multiple Regression Analysis (MRA) is a commonly used quantitative analysis method that describes the relationship between variables through a mathematical model. This relationship can be either linear or nonlinear. In multiple regression analysis, a subset of variables is considered as independent variables, and one variable is treated as the dependent variable, establishing a mathematical relationship among multiple variables.

For a given sample vector $\vec{x} = \left(x^{(1)}, x^{(2)}, \ldots, x^{(m)}\right)^T$, where m represents the number of features in the sample, in the multiple regression model, we select one feature from the sample as the dependent variable y, and the other features that influence the dependent variable are denoted as $\vec{x} = \left(x^{(1)}, x^{(2)}_- \ldots, x^{(m-1)}\right)^T$. The mathematical form of the multiple regression analysis model is expressed as follows:

$$y = W \cdot \vec{x} + b \tag{3}$$

where $W = (w^{(1)}, w^{(2)}, \ldots, w^{(m-1)})$ is the weight matrix, representing the weights provided by each feature in predicting y. It intuitively shows the importance of each feature in predicting y. b is the intercept, representing the constant impact apart from the effects of independent variables in the prediction.

4.3 Multiple Regression Analysis Model Optimization via Gauss-Newton Iteration Method

The Gauss-Newton iteration method is an iterative approach derived from the least squares method and is commonly used to estimate parameters in nonlinear regression models. The basic idea of the Gauss-Newton iteration method is to construct a Taylor series expansion to continuously fit the nonlinear relationship between variables. Through multiple iterations and adjustments of the model parameters, the method aims to minimize the sum of squared residuals between the model results and the sample data. This iterative process ultimately yields the optimal regression coefficients, providing a mathematical approximation of the nonlinear relationship between variables using the Taylor series.

$$\hat{y}_i = f(x_i, r) + \epsilon_i, \ (i = 1, 2, \ldots, n) \tag{4}$$

Based on the above equation, we employ the multiple regression model and the Gauss-Newton iteration method for quantitative analysis. The multiple regression model is suitable for cases where multiple variables influence a single variable. It can fit the relationship between variables and assess the correlation among them. The Gauss-Newton iteration method utilizes a Taylor series expansion to continuously fit the nonlinear relationship between variables. Through multiple iterations and adjustments of the model parameters, it aims to minimize the sum of squared residuals between the model results and the sample data, thereby obtaining the optimal regression coefficients.

Therefore, we have transformed the nonlinear regression problem into a multiple linear regression problem by minimizing the sum of squared residuals to estimate the relationship between the independent and dependent variables. In each iteration, this method utilizes matrix differentiation and solving normal equations to update the model parameters until it converges to a local optimal solution. Due to the faster convergence of the Newton iteration method, it is more practical than other methods such as gradient descent, especially for larger sample sizes or a higher number of independent variables. Based on the selected observed variable data, we have constructed a multiple nonlinear regression model as follows.

$$y = f(X, \beta) + \varepsilon \tag{5}$$

In this model, y represents the dependent variable, indicating the daily number of new cases in the experiment. X is the set of independent variables, representing the data for each feature factor in the experiment. β is a location parameter, and ε is the error term, an unobservable random variable with a mean of 0 and a variance $\sigma^2 > 0$. The above model can be used for predictive analysis to determine the nonlinear relationship between each independent variable and the dependent variable. The Gauss-Newton iteration method is employed to iteratively estimate the regression parameters β of the nonlinear regression model.

5 Results and Analysis

5.1 Construction and Training of Multiple Regression Model

The implementation process of the quantitative analysis model can be found in Fig. 1 and includes the following steps:

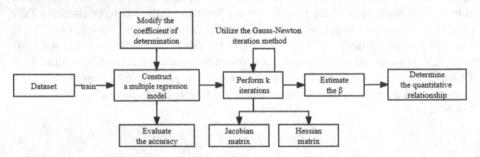

Fig. 1. Flowchart of the quantitative analysis model.

(1) Construct a multiple regression model and train it using the data.
(2) Evaluate the accuracy of the model by modifying the coefficient of determination.
(3) Use the multiple regression model to determine the quantitative relationship between multiple factors and the daily number of new cases of Omicron variant.

(4) Assign different initial values for the factors x_0.
(5) Utilize the Gauss-Newton iteration method to perform k iterations, calculate the Jacobian matrix J and Hessian matrix H, B, compute the increment Δ_x.
(6) Estimate the unknown parameter β by completing the iterations and determine the quantitative relationship between different factors and the daily number of new cases.
(7) Obtain the estimated values of β and determine the quantitative relationship between different factors and the daily number of new cases.

We have conducted a multiple regression model and training on the valid dataset of the selected 35 countries. Through the multiple regression model, we have determined the quantitative relationship between multiple factors and the daily number of new cases. We have evaluated the predictive ability of the model by adjusting the adjusted R-squared value. We have then selected initial values for the Gauss-Newton iteration method based on the model parameters. The quantitative relationship between multiple factors and the daily number of new cases is shown in the table below (Table 2):

Table 2. Regression equation parameter.

y	Confirmed	Recovered	Deaths	
	0.06	0.17	−0.28	
x_i	Wind_speed	Precipitation	DP_F	Pressure
	−16.46	84.64	−4.67	2.02
	Altitude	Ab_humidity	Re_humidity	Pop
	6.71e−7	−0.17	−0.112	5.8e9
	Density	NO_2	PM_{10}	$PM_{2.5}$
	54282.5	1.95e3	49.42	55.59
	PM_1	SO_2	O_3	CO
	45.29	−21.91	65.56	12.61
	AQI	NEPH	UVI	POL
	0.14	−8.45	−1.46	23.68
	WD	Flight_total	Flight_domestic	Fligth_international
	1.91	189.547	379.995	187.5932
	Vaccination rates	Medical institutions	Tmax	Tmin
	−78253.7	−14256.5	−4.52	−2.97
	Wind_gust			
	73.72			
Parameters	ε	Adjusted R Square		
	293.18	0.79		

The y-value contains three target factors: Confirmed, Recovered and Deaths. Meanwhile, x_i contains 29 indicator factors, which includes: Wind_speed, Precipitation, DP_F, Pressure, Altitude, Ab_humidity, Re_humidity, Pop, Density, NO_2, PM_{10}, $PM_{2.5}$, PM_1, SO_2, O_3, CO, AQI, NEPH, UVI, POL, WD, Flight_domestic, Flight_international, Vaccination rates, Medical institutions, Tmax, Tmin and Wind_gust.

This study employs quantitative analysis using the source data. The objectives are as follows:

(1) Analyze the quantitative relationship between multiple factor features (x_i) and the daily number of cases (y), and generate predictions for y.
(2) While controlling other factors, adjust the values of x_i to generate predictions for y.
(3) Utilize the source data as input and train the model using the Gauss-Newton iteration method. This process allows us to determine the coefficients between x_i and y, thereby establishing the quantitative relationship.

According to the aforementioned method, we have obtained the coefficient equations between the daily number of new cases of Omicron variant and the feature factors listed in the table for each country. Thus the quantitative relationship between the daily number of new cases and the feature factors in each country has been determined.

5.2   Calculation and Analysis of the Coefficients for Multiple Factors

After constructing the multiple regression model, we have calculated the average coefficients for the same features across all countries. Thus we have got the quantitative relationship between each feature and the daily number of new cases of Omicron variant that exhibits strong generalization performance and is applicable to the selected countries. The results are summarized in the following table:

In Table 3, the Feature column represents the different characteristic factors, the Particle column represents the units taken by the different factors for normalization, and the Influence column represents the coefficient of influence.

If the Influence value is greater than 0, it indicates a positive correlation between the factor and the daily number of new cases, meaning that an increase in the factor is associated with an increase in the daily new cases.

Based on the above Table 3 and Fig. 2, the following conclusions can be inferred.

Among the selected features, the population density per square kilometer has the highest positive correlation with the daily number of new cases, followed by the number of flights. For every 1% increase in population density per square kilometer, there is an approximate 1.141% increase in daily new cases. Similarly, for every 1% increase in population, there is an approximate 1.093% increase in daily new cases.

Table 3. Quantitative relationship between characteristic factors and the daily number of new cases of Omicron.

Features	Particle	Influence/%
Density	$+1\%/km^2$	1.0786217
Pop	$+1\%/km^2$	1.1412287
Flight_total	$+1\%$	1.0932741
Flight_domestic	$+1\%$	0.9869113
Flight_international	$+1\%$	0.9426679
UVI	$+1\ \mu g/m^3$ in the range of 100–200 $\mu g/m^3$	0.8062715
$PM_{2.5}$	$+1\ \mu g/m^3$ in the range of 100–200 $\mu g/m^3$	0.0127804
PM_{10}	$+1\ \mu g/m^3$ in the range of 0–100 $\mu g/m^3$	0.0116004
NO_2	$+0.3\ \mu g/m^3$ in the range of 0–30 $\mu g/m^3$	0.0186019
SO_2	$+0.1\ \mu g/m^3$ in the range of 0–10 $\mu g/m^3$	0.0209683
PM_1	$+1\ \mu g/m^3$ in the range of 100–200 $\mu g/m^3$	0.0145565
Wind_speed	$+1$ m/s in the range of 0–10 m/s	0.0984426
Precipitation	$+1\%$	−0.0181508
Re_humidity	$+1\%$	−0.0157905
DP_F	$+1\ °C$ in the range of 0–50 °C	−0.0150023
Tmin	$+1°C$ in the range of 0–50 °C	−0.0275235
Tmax	$+1°C$ in the range of 0–50 °C	−0.0222132
Vaccination	$+1\%$	−3.0561276
Medical_institutions	$+1\%$	−2.0943653

In the selected features, vaccination rate and the number of healthcare facilities have a negative correlation with the spread of the virus. For every 1% increase in vaccination rate, the total daily number of new cases decreases by approximately 3.056%. Similarly, for every 1% increase in the number of healthcare facilities, the total daily number of new cases decreases by approximately 2.094%.

Factors such as daily maximum temperature, daily minimum temperature, and dew point temperature have a negative correlation with the daily number of new cases. Within the range of 0–50 °C, for every 1 °C increase in temperature, the daily new cases can decrease by approximately 0.022%, 0.028%, and 0.015% respectively. Climate and air factors also have a weak impact on the spread of the virus. For example, the factor with the highest influence coefficient, SO2, within the range of 0–10 $\mu g/m^3$, for every 0.1 $\mu g/m^3$ increase, the daily new cases will increase by 0.021%. However, overall, the impact of air quality and climate factors on the spread of the virus is far less significant compared to the influence of population mobility and population density.

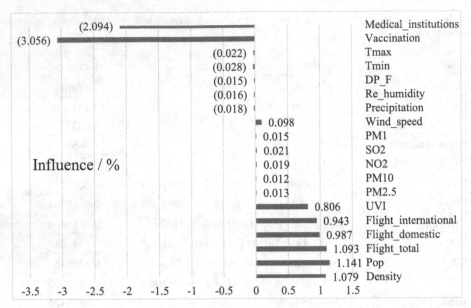

Fig. 2. Quantitative relationship between characteristic factors and the daily number of new cases of Omicron

5.3　Further Analysis

Based on the above analysis, the following implications can be drawn:

(1) In epidemic prevention and control policies, more consideration should be given to controlling population mobility and population density in order to effectively control the spread of the virus.
(2) Climate and air quality factors have a certain influence on the spread of the Omicron variant, but they cannot be relied upon to reduce the spread of the virus in areas with high population density.
(3) Increasing vaccination rates and the number of healthcare facilities can significantly mitigate the spread of the Omicron variant. It may be advisable to establish more healthcare facilities and further promote vaccination in areas with high population density and significant population mobility.

6　Conclusions and Future Work

In this study, we have conducted a quantitative analysis of the impact of multiple factors on the spread of the Omicron variant by integrating multiple datasets and using Gaussian-Newton iteration optimized multivariate regression. We have obtained quantitative relationships between various factors and the daily number of the new cases of Omicron variant.

Based on the experimental results, we have found that increasing vaccination rates and the number of healthcare facilities help to suppress the spread of the Omicron variant, while an increase in population size and population density accelerates its spread, and that weather and climate have limited effects on the spread of Omicron. Therefore, among the multiple factors influencing the spread of the Omicron variant, we need to pay close attention to controlling population density and large-scale population mobility to prevent the widespread transmission of the variant among the population. We also need to promote the rapid vaccination of the population against COVID-19 and establish healthcare facilities in areas with high population density, as this will help slow down the spread of the Omicron variant. Furthermore, it is not advisable for governments of different nations to entertain the expectation that the transmission of viruses can be completely eradicated through natural weather and climate changes.

This study has explored the quantitative analysis of multiple factors influencing the spread of the Omicron variant using the Gaussian-Newton iteration optimized multivariate regression method. However, due to differences in the level of informatization and economic development among countries, there may be errors in the daily number of confirmed cases reported by different countries. Furthermore, the study has not considered the impact of changes in epidemic prevention and control policies or measures implemented by different countries or regions on the epidemic data. Therefore, future work should address these issues and further investigate the topic.

References

1. World Health Organization: Statement on the fifteenth meeting of the International Health Regulations (2005) Emergency Committee regarding the coronavirus disease (COVID-19) pandemic, 5 May 2023. https://www.who.int/news/item/05-05-2023-statement-on-the-fifteenth-meeting-of-the-international-health-regulations-(2005)-emergency-committee-regarding-the-coronavirus-disease-(covid-19)-pandemic
2. Collier, D.A., et al.: Age-related immune response heterogeneity to SARS-CoV-2 vaccine BNT162b2. Nat. Med. **28**(3), 385–391 (2022). https://doi.org/10.1038/s41591-021-01593-w
3. Khalifa, Y.M., Zakaria, M.K., Alsowaida, Y.A., Alzamil, F.A.: The emergence of the Omicron (B.1.1.529) SARS-CoV-2 variant of concern: a systematic review. J. Infect. Public Health **15**(2), 153–160 (2022). https://doi.org/10.1016/j.jiph.2021.11.012
4. Zhang, L., et al.: The D614G mutation in the SARS-CoV-2 spike protein reduces S1 shedding and increases infectivity (2021)
5. Özüdoğru, O., Bahçe, Y.G., Acer, Ö.: SARS CoV-2 reinfection rate is higher in the Omicron variant than in the Alpha and Delta variants. Ir. J. Med. Sci. **192**, 751–756 (2023). https://doi.org/10.1007/s11845-022-03060-4
6. Lino, A., Cardoso, M.A., Martins-Lopes, P., Gonçalves, H.M.R.: Omicron – the new SARS-CoV-2 challenge? Rev. Med. Virol. **32**(4), e2358 (2022). https://doi.org/10.1002/rmv.2358
7. WHO.: Classification of Omicron (B.1.1.529): SARS-CoV-2 Variant of Concern (2021). https://www.who.int/news/item/26-11-2021-classification-of-omicron-(b.1.1.529)-sars-cov-2-variant-of-concern
8. Asamoah, O.E., Adu, B., Ampofo, W.K.: Impact of vaccination coverage, mobility patterns, and population density on the spread of Omicron in South Africa: a compartmental model analysis. Int. J. Infect. Dis. **116**, 29–35 (2022)
9. Dumitrescu, I.E., Loh, S.A., Xue, X., Koopmans, M.P.G.: Mathematical modeling of Omicron variant transmission dynamics in Europe: effect of human mobility and vaccination coverage (2022)
10. Funk, S., Flaxman, S., Volz, E.: Real-time tracking of the Omicron variant in the UK: insights from early data. Lancet. Public Health **7**(1), e26–e27 (2022)

11. Lee, J., Park, J.S., Wang, K.N., Feng, B., Tennant, M., Kruger, E.: The use of telehealth during the coronavirus (COVID-19) pandemic in oral and maxillofacial surgery – a qualitative analysis. EAI Endorsed Trans. Scalable Inf. Syst. **18**, e34 (2021)
12. Gao, L., Wu, J.T., Lin, Q., He, D., Wang, M.H.: Investigating the transmission dynamics of Omicron in China (2022)
13. Kang, E., Ki, M., Kim, J.K., Choi, B.: Effectiveness of various interventions against Omicron: an analysis of the COVID-19 outbreak in the United States. J. Infect. Chemother. **28**(3), 381–385 (2022)
14. Lee, S., Han, K., Lee, J.Y.: Impact of human mobility on the transmission dynamics of Omicron in South Korea: a modeling study (2022)
15. Liu, X., Wang, Y., Zhang, J.: Mathematical modeling and analysis of Omicron transmission dynamics in Beijing, China (2022)
16. Moghadas, S.M., Shoukat, A., Fitzpatrick, M.C.: Impact of vaccination and non-pharmaceutical interventions on Omicron variant transmission in Canada (2022)
17. Ong, S.W.X., Chiew, C.J., Ang, L.W.: Impact of vaccination and mobility on the transmission dynamics of the Omicron variant in Singapore (2022)
18. Wang, Q., Chen, C., Xu, K.: Quantifying the impact of vaccination coverage, population density, and human mobility on Omicron transmission dynamics in China (2022)
19. Fu, Y., Lin, S., Xu, Z.: Research on quantitative analysis of multiple factors affecting COVID-19 spread. Int. J. Environ. Res. Public Health **19**(6), 3187 (2022)

Analyzing the Impact of COVID-19 on Education: A Comparative Study Based on TOEFL Test Results

Puti Xu[1], Wei Hong[1], Jiao Yin[1(✉)], Kate Wang[2], and Yanchun Zhang[1]

[1] Institute for Sustainable Industries and Liveable Cities, Victoria University, Melbourne, VIC 3011, Australia
{puti.xu,wei.hong2}@live.vu.edu.au, {jiao.yin,yanchun.zhang}@vu.edu.au
[2] School of Health and Biomedical Sciences, RMIT University, Melbourne, VIC 3064, Australia
kate.wang@rmit.edu.au

Abstract. The COVID-19 pandemic and subsequent lockdown policies have significantly impacted the education sector worldwide. However, there has been a lack of analysis regarding the influence of the pandemic on academic performance from a global perspective. To fill this gap, this paper collects global TOEFL test results from 2017 to 2021, to investigate the impact of the COVID-19 pandemic on education worldwide. The test results from every two consecutive years are paired into groups to examine the performance change across different regions and test sections (reading, listening, writing, and speaking). The results reveal a consistent and significant increase in most test sections across all regions for the paired 2020-2019 group, which reflects the initial stage of the pandemic. However, for the paired group 2021-2020, there is no significant difference observed for most test sections and regions. These findings suggest that, during the outbreak of the pandemic in 2020, online learning increased the flexibility for students to access resources and maintain attendance, resulting in better results compared to 2019. However, this positive effect has diminished in 2021 with the normalization of the pandemic. In contrast, based on the data collected before the pandemic, there were no significant and consistent changes in scores across regions and test sections.

Keywords: COVID-19 impact · TOEFL test · Academic performance

1 Introduction

In response to the COVID-19 pandemic, numerous education institutions in different countries had to implement home-based teaching and tests [5]. Due to the wide adoption of online learning, researchers have begun to investigate the impact of the pandemic on academic performance. Extensive research studies

Y. Li et al. (Eds.): HIS 2023, LNCS 14305, pp. 175–184, 2023.
https://doi.org/10.1007/978-981-99-7108-4_15

have explored the impact of the pandemic on education sectors across some subjects and regions [3,12,16]. However, one significant shortcoming is that most studies focused only on one or several subjects and countries, lacking the evolving impact during different stages of the pandemic.

In order to address gaps in the previous studies, the research question in this paper is: "How does academic performance across regions change before the COVID-19 pandemic, at the peak of the COVID-19 pandemic, and after the peak of the COVID-19 pandemic?" The research question aims to explore how the educational outcomes across regions differ before and during the COVID-19 pandemic. Therefore, the paper makes contributions to future academic studies and practice from two perspectives:

- Firstly, this paper statistically shows that COVID-19 pandemic and corresponding educational modes bring benefits to the education sector through an analysis of the TOEFL test worldwide.
- Secondly, it provides brief insights into the dynamic impact of pandemics through the pandemic and possible explanations for the findings based on the analysis and previous research studies.

The rest of this paper is arranged as follows: Sect. 2 identifies the key gaps from previous studies. Section 3 presents the research method and data source. The findings from the data analysis are displayed and discussed in Sect. 4 and 5 respectively. Finally, Sect. 6 illustrates the implications while Sect. 7 concludes the paper with future directions.

2   Literature Review

Some experts researched the impact of the pandemic on the academic performance of students in primary and secondary schools. A study on fourth-grade primary school students in Germany revealed a drastic decline in mean reading achievement between 2016 and 2021 [8]. However, a study of 100 primary students in Spain indicated that more than 40% of the respondents reported no significant change in their academic performance during the pandemic [9]. Additionally, an academic study on senior secondary students revealed a significant decrease in academic performance after the COVID-19 pandemic began [10]. Some scholars also found that, compared with the pre-pandemic mathematics achievements among over 368 secondary students in Spain, there was a significant decrease after the implementation of lockdown policies [11].

Moreover, extensive research studies were conducted on the influence of the pandemic on study performance in universities. An investigation of 200 US public higher education institutions showed that GPA slightly increased after the implementation of online studies [2]. However, findings based on research at Nueva Ecjia University of Science and Technology suggested that the academic performance did not show significant changes after the widespread adoption of online education [1].

Despite the comprehensive findings, a major missing part is the comparative studies worldwide. In general, the current research is lacking in the analysis of cultural diversity and education system differences in multiple countries and regions. In addition, most studies lack a comprehensive analysis of the dynamics of pandemic effects before and during the outbreak. Therefore, it is necessary and important to conduct a comprehensive comparison along the time span and across the regions.

3   Methodology

3.1   Data Collection and Pre-processing

In this paper, a quantitative methodology is applied to explore the changes in academic performance, which is applied in multiple research studies. For example, it is applied in a research study on an E-health system during the period of pandemic [7], where statistics are presented concisely with graphs and charts. Therefore, it is appropriate to apply the quantitative methodology to conduct research with concise and direct comparisons across different periods and regions.

The data source is selected with reference to two important criteria, the availability and consistent standardization [14,15]. Generally, public databases from international institutions can be accessed through online sources and in many cases, the data is collected with consistent criteria. For example, public databases are utilized in the research of a certain classification approach of analyzing alcoholic EEG signals [4].

Therefore, the data sets of the TOEFL test are selected for data analysis. TOEFL is a globally recognized test with four sections including Reading, Listening, Speaking, and Writing, allowing for in-depth exploration of different subsections. The TOEFL data is sourced from the reports[1] of Education Testing Service (ETS)[2], a non-profit organization certified by the international institutions, which ensures the reliability of data because of consistent sampling and calculation criteria. Moreover, the reports sourced from ETS cover a substantial time span and a wide range of countries, which is appropriate for comparative studies both in time and space.

On the other hand, it is crucial to select the appropriate time periods for the research [6,17]. The outbreak of COVID-19 was in 2020 [8], and multiple education institutions gradually eased their restriction in 2021 [18]. For the pre-pandemic period, the years 2017, 2018, and 2019 are selected. In the paper, the annual results from 2017 to 2021 will be reorganized into four groups for comparison purposes, which are Group 1 (2018-2017), Group 2 (2019-2018), Group 3 (2020-2019), and Group 4 (2021-2020).

However, the consistency of comparison should be maintained. If one country is missing any years in the dataset, it will be excluded from the analysis. Additionally, the databases of COVID-19 cases and deaths are introduced to serve

---

[1] https://www.ets.org/toefl/teachers-advisors-agents/ibt/scores.html.
[2] https://www.etsglobal.org/fr/en/content/who-we-are.

as an indicator of pandemic severity. Therefore, countries that are not on the COVID-19 report[3] will also be excluded for data consistency concerns.

In addition, it is necessary to assess whether the sample size is appropriate. In total, 147 countries or regions are selected. Among them, 34 are selected out of 51 in Africa, while 25 are selected out of 47 in America. In Asia, 23 are selected out of 35, while 43 are selected in Europe out of 53. In the Middle East, all of the 19 are selected. However, only 3 countries or regions satisfy the data selection criteria in the Pacific out of 23, which is not sufficient to represent the academic performance of this grand region. As a result, Pacific countries or regions will be included in the overall worldwide analysis, while the Pacific grand region itself will be excluded from the grand region analysis.

3.2   Research Design

The paired sample t-test is applied for the comparison between two years within each group. In general, the paired sample t-test compares the means of the two measurements from the same units [13], which is appropriate to compare the differences in the mean scores between two years within each group of the same countries. Hypotheses are formulated to compare whether the results are equal or not between two consecutive years.

Therefore, the hypotheses for paired sample t-test aim to test whether the mean difference between the two years within the group is equal to zero or not [13]:

H_0: $m_1 - m_2 = 0$ (The mean difference of the populations within the group is equal to 0).

H_1: $m_1 - m_2 \neq 0$ (The mean difference of the populations within the group is not equal to 0).

4   Results

Total Scores in the World and Different Regions. As shown in Table 1, star marks are used to indicate the significance level of the results, which represent a p-value less than 5% with one star and a p-value less than 1% with two stars. As Table 1 shows, none of the p-values in Group 1 reaches the preset significance level (5%), indicating that in all regions, the average total scores do not exhibit significant changes between 2018 and 2017. However, half of the p-values in Group 2 pass the 5% significance threshold, which suggests considerable differences in total scores worldwide. Specifically, in comparison with the result in 2018, the average total scores in Asia and the Middle East were significantly higher in 2019 by 0.565 and 1 point, respectively. At the same time, the test results from Africa, America, and Europe do not show significant differences for Group 2 (2019-2018). As for Group 3 (2020-2019), the significance levels of all of the regions are less than 0.05 or 0.01, and positive mean differences are

---

[3] https://ourworldindata.org/covid-vaccinations?country=OWID-WRL.

observed, which suggests that compared with 2019, the means of the total scores were significantly higher in 2020 across all regions. In Group 4, the significance level indicates there are no significant differences in the mean scores in the five regions.

Table 1. Group mean difference across regions (total scores based)

Group	World	Africa	America	Asia	Europe	Mid East
G1 (2018-2017)	−0.075	−0.441	−0.32	0.304	−0.023	0
G2 (2019-2018)	0.395*	0.353	−0.12	0.565*	0.349	1*
G3 (2020-2019)	2.367**	2.706**	2.731**	2.087**	2.119**	2.368**
G4 (2021-2020)	−0.041	−0.735	−0.32	0.261	0.535	0

*p < 0.05, **p < 0.01

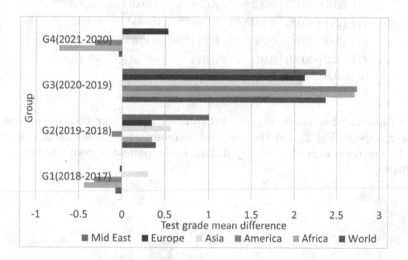

Fig. 1. Mean difference of total scores for each group across regions

We visualize the test score mean difference for all the groups and regions in Fig. 1, and it clearly shows the significant increase in total TOEFL scores worldwide between the years 2020 and 2019.

Section Scores Worldwide. The results in Table 2 reveal significant differences in the academic performance changes among different test sections worldwide in the four groups. As the first row in Table 2 shows, there exists a slight performance drop in the Reading and Writing test when comparing the result in 2018 with the result in 2017, and the significance level for this conclusion is as high as 0.01. However, in Group 2 and Group 3, the significance levels of Reading, Listening, and Speaking and the mean differences indicate significant increases in these test sections. Compared with the results in Group 2, the mean difference values are considerable higher in Group 3 (0.769 > 0.286, 0.714 > 0.259, 0.116 > 0.095), indicating a major improvement in performance in 2020. Surprisingly, in Group 4, there are no significant differences for the four test sections of TOEFL worldwide since no star is marked. Therefore, the mean differences value and significance level show that the increase in mean scores of the four test sections between 2020 and 2019 is the most significant, while no significant changes are observed between 2021 and 2020.

Table 2. Group mean difference globally (section grade based)

Group	Reading	Listening	Speaking	Writing
G1 (2018-2017)	−0.238**	0.088	0.000	−0.170**
G2 (2019-2018)	0.286**	0.259**	0.095*	−0.041
G3 (2020-2019)	0.769**	0.714**	0.116*	0.653**
G4 (2021-2020)	0.075	0.014	−0.014	−0.109

*$p < 0.05$,**$p < 0.01$

We draw the bar chart of mean difference for the four test sections across all the groups in Fig. 2, and the surge of test performance for all four sections could be clearly observed in Group 3, which compares the result between 2020 and 2019.

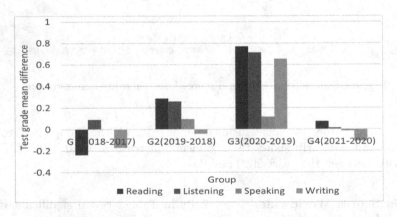

Fig. 2. Mean difference of for each group globally (section grade based)

Table 3. Group mean difference across regions (section grade based)

Region	Group	Reading	Listening	Speaking	Writing
Africa	G1 (2018-2017)	−0.412**	0.118	−0.088	−0.206
	G2 (2019-2018)	0.059	0.412*	0.176	−0.088
	G3 (2020-2019)	0.735**	0.735**	0.412**	0.588**
	G4 (2021-2020)	0.029	−0.206	−0.176	−0.206
America	G1 (2018-2017)	−0.280*	0.000	0.120	−0.160*
	G2 (2019-2018)	0.120	−0.080	0.000	0.000
	G3 (2020-2019)	0.808**	0.808**	0.115	0.769**
	G4 (2021-2020)	−0.080	0.040	−0.120	−0.200
Asia	G1 (2018-2017)	0.000	0.130	−0.130	−0.261
	G2 (2019-2018)	0.261	0.261*	0.304*	−0.130
	G3 (2020-2019)	0.739**	0.696**	0.000	0.565**
	G4 (2021-2020)	0.348*	0.261*	−0.087	0.043
Europe	G1 (2018-2017)	−0.256*	0.023	0.023	−0.070
	G2 (2019-2018)	0.442**	0.186	−0.047	−0.047
	G3 (2020-2019)	0.786**	0.714**	0.024**	0.643**
	G4 (2021-2020)	0.070	0.070	0.326**	−0.047
Mid East	G1 (2018-2017)	−0.263	0.105	0.105	−0.263
	G2 (2019-2018)	0.579**	0.526**	0.105	0.105
	G3 (2020-2019)	0.842**	0.789**	−0.105	0.737**
	G4 (2021-2020)	0.105	−0.158	−0.105	−0.053

*$p < 0.05$,**$p < 0.01$

Performance Breakdown for Sections and Regions. In order to further investigate the dynamics of how the score changes across the four sections and in all regions, we break down the results based on both regions and test sections in Table 3. Different patterns of mean differences and significance levels are observed across the regions and test sections. Specifically, the results in Group 3 (2020-2019) show the most significant increase in test scores across different regions. Within this Group, the average scores in Reading, Listening, and Writing enjoyed an overwhelming and significant increase when comparing the result of 2020 with the result of 2019. However, except for Africa, the results suggest that the scores in Speaking do not have a significant change.

In Group 1 (2018-2017), despite a few significant changes in some regions in terms of some sections, the majority of the regions did not see a significant change in most of the test sections. In detail, only the p-values and mean differences in Reading in Africa, America, and Europe and Writing in America indicate a significant decrease.

Additionally, in Group 4, there only exist significant increases in Reading and Listening scores in Asia, and Speaking score in Europe, while the test scores of other sections across the rest regions exhibit no significant changes between the year 2021 and 2020.

The results in Group 2 (2019-2018) are the most divided among the four groups. On one end, the reading score in Africa, America, and the Middle East witnessed a significant increase in 2019, while the Listening score in Asia and the Middle East saw a significant increase. On the other hand, the test score for Speaking shows a significant increase in Asia, while the score for Writing does not exhibit a significant increase in the Middle East.

Therefore, out of all the complicated change patterns across the regions and test sections, the overall increase in test scores in Group 3 (2020-2019) is the most significant and obvious.

5 Discussion

The findings from the previous part offer insights into how different stages of the COVID-19 pandemic have factored into the changes in TOEFL test results. At the initial stage of the pandemic, the increase in total scores in the world and most regions are much more significant than the improvement before the COVID-19 pandemic. Similarly, the mean differences in the four test sections are also more significant in the early stages of the pandemic. However, after reaching the peak of the COVID-19 pandemic, the results show that the upward trend of substantial increase across the test sections and regions diminished.

For this phenomenon, our best guess is, the increase in mean scores during the pandemic is very likely due to the widespread application of online learning and testing worldwide. On the one hand, online courses facilitate flexible interaction and timely revision, which enhance the daily study processes. An academic study among secondary students shows that online learning during the COVID-19 pandemic might stimulate the creativity of students [11]. On the other hand, the flexibility of the online home testing of language tests might help students achieve better results[4].

The flexibility of online learning might also help explain the diminishing of the increase in test results globally. A study in 2022 [5] claims that online learning increases the flexibility of the materials and the attendance rate in digital lectures is significantly higher than the traditional ones, thus boosting the academic performance. When transitioning from online courses to face-to-face learning after the pandemic, the attendance rate might decrease in certain institutions, which might result in a performance drop. Another academic study [18] among some Chinese international students also finds that the abrupt and substantial reduction of digital learning disrupts the 'pandemic-style' study process, which to some extent brings negative effects on daily studies due to the lack of flexibility.

---

[4] https://ischoolconnect.com/blog/coronavirus-impact-on-tests-like-gre-gmat-ielts-toefl/.

6   Implications

The study provides an overview of the academic performance changes worldwide with consistent TOEFL standards. During the pandemic, it is very common that an educational institution would set up online courses and this study has provided theoretical implications that the countermeasures such as online learning during the pandemic may present opportunities for improving study outcomes. Therefore, the adoption of a new education mode, particularly the online learning mode, may help students to achieve better academic performance on a global scale.

Another important implication of this paper is the dynamic impact of the COVID-19 pandemic on a global scale. Previously, many research studies only investigate specific periods during the COVID-19 pandemic in limited countries or regions. However, it is possible that there were similar patterns of changes in test results before the COVID-19 pandemic. Moreover, very few studies have investigated whether the impacts of the pandemic have differed along different stages. The study provides great insights into different stages of the pandemic, suggesting the directions for future studies in terms of the dynamic COVID-19 impact on education.

7   Conclusion

In conclusion, the study examines the changes in academic performance during different periods of the COVID-19 pandemic through a comprehensive analysis of TOEFL test results worldwide. The findings indicate there is a significant increase in TOEFL scores across different test sections after the COVID-19 pandemic broke out globally. However, the improvement in performance stopped after the pandemic reached its peak. The study contributes to the understanding of the similarities and differences among different learning areas globally, which provides insights into the changing impacts of the pandemic during different periods.

However, some limitations need to be addressed in future studies. Firstly, the current databases available only include integer values, which might reduce the accuracy of the studies. Secondly, the scope of this paper is limited to the results of the TOEFL test, neglecting other language proficiency tests. Thirdly, the indicator for academic performance is quite limited in this paper since only TOEFL test score is used, and other indicators, such as attendance rate and study time, could be investigated in the future. Therefore, future studies should encompass a broad range of language studies, various indicators of the study effects, and multiple time periods in order to reveal the dynamic impact of the pandemic on education.

References

1. Capinding, A.T.: Analysis of learning and academic performance of education students before and during the coronavirus disease pandemic. Eur. J. Educ. Res. **10**(4), 1953–1962 (2021)

2. Cavanaugh, J., Jacquemin, S., Junker, C.: A look at student performance during the COVID-19 pandemic. Qual. Assur. Educ. **31**(1), 33–43 (2023)
3. Chen, Y., Han, S., Chen, G., Yin, J., Wang, K.N., Cao, J.: A deep reinforcement learning-based wireless body area network offloading optimization strategy for healthcare services. Health Inf. Sci. Syst. **11**(1), 8 (2023)
4. Diykh, M., Abdulla, S., Oudah, A.Y., Marhoon, H.A., Siuly, S.: A novel alcoholic EEG signals classification approach based on AdaBoost k-means coupled with statistical model. In: Siuly, S., Wang, H., Chen, L., Guo, Y., Xing, C. (eds.) HIS 2021. LNCS, vol. 13079, pp. 82–92. Springer, Cham (2021). https://doi.org/10.1007/978-3-030-90885-0_8
5. Haugom, E.: The effect of changing from campus-based to digital teaching on student attendance: a case study of Norwegian business students. Heliyon **8**(11), e11307 (2022)
6. Hong, W., et al.: A graph empowered insider threat detection framework based on daily activities. ISA Trans. (2023). https://doi.org/10.1016/j.isatra.2023.06.030
7. Jahan, S., Ali, F.: Advancing health information system with system thinking: learning challenges of E-health in Bangladesh during COVID-19. In: Siuly, S., Wang, H., Chen, L., Guo, Y., Xing, C. (eds.) HIS 2021. LNCS, vol. 13079, pp. 15–23. Springer, Cham (2021). https://doi.org/10.1007/978-3-030-90885-0_2
8. Ludewig, U., et al.: COVID-19 pandemic and student reading achievement: findings from a school panel study. Front. Psychol. **13**, 876485 (2022)
9. Manuel Prieto, J., Salas Sánchez, J., Tierno Cordón, J., Álvarez-Kurogi, L., González-García, H., Castro López, R.: Social anxiety and academic performance during covid-19 in schoolchildren. PLoS ONE **18**(1), e0280194 (2023)
10. Nwokocha, A.C., Elijah Etukudo, U.: The effect of COVID-19 on academic achievement of senior secondary school students in English language. Int. J. Engl. Lang. Educ. **10**(1), 44 (2022). https://doi.org/10.5296/ijele.v10i1.20075
11. Patston, T.J., et al.: Secondary education in COVID lockdown: more anxious and less creative-maybe not? Front. Psychol. **12**, 391 (2021)
12. Sarki, R., Ahmed, K., Wang, H., Zhang, Y., Wang, K.: Convolutional neural network for multi-class classification of diabetic eye disease. EAI Endors. Trans. Scalable Inf. Syst. **9**(4), e5–e5 (2022)
13. University, K.S.: SPSS tutorials: paired samples T test (2023). https://libguides.library.kent.edu/spss/pairedsamplesttest
14. Vimalachandran, P., Liu, H., Lin, Y., Ji, K., Wang, H., Zhang, Y.: Improving accessibility of the Australian my health records while preserving privacy and security of the system. Health Inf. Sci. Syst. **8**, 1–9 (2020)
15. Wang, H., Yi, X., Bertino, E., Sun, L.: Protecting outsourced data in cloud computing through access management. Concurr. Comput.: Pract. Exp. **28**, 600–615 (2014). https://doi.org/10.1002/cpe.3286
16. Yin, J., You, M., Cao, J., Wang, H., Tang, M.J., Ge, Y.-F.: Data-driven hierarchical neural network modeling for high-pressure feedwater heater group. In: Borovica-Gajic, R., Qi, J., Wang, W. (eds.) ADC 2020. LNCS, vol. 12008, pp. 225–233. Springer, Cham (2020). https://doi.org/10.1007/978-3-030-39469-1_19
17. You, M., et al.: A knowledge graph empowered online learning framework for access control decision-making. World Wide Web **26**(2), 827–848 (2023)
18. Zhao, X., Xue, W.: From online to offline education in a post-pandemic era: challenges encountered by international students in UK universities. Front. Psychol. **13**, 8642 (2023)

Advanced Medical Data and AI Techniques

BiblioEngine: An AI-Empowered Platform for Disease Genetic Knowledge Mining

Mengjia Wu[1], Yi Zhang[1], Hua Lin[2], Mark Grosser[2], Guangquan Zhang[1], and Jie Lu[1]

[1] University of Technology Sydney, Ultimo, NSW, Australia
{mengjia.wu,yi.zhang,guangquan.zhang,jie.lu}@uts.edu.au
[2] 23Strands, Pyrmont, NSW, Australia
{hua.lin,mark.grosser}@23strands.com

Abstract. Recent decades have seen significant advancements in contemporary genetic research with the aid of artificial intelligence (AI) techniques. However, researchers lack a comprehensive platform for fully exploiting these AI tools and conducting customized analyses. This paper introduces BiblioEngine, a literature analysis platform that helps researchers profile the research landscape and gain genetic insights into diseases. BiblioEngine integrates multiple AI-empowered data sources and employs heterogeneous network analysis to identify and emphasize genes and other biomedical entities for further investigation. Its effectiveness is demonstrated through a case study on stroke-related genetic research. Analysis with BiblioEngine uncovers valuable research intelligence and genetic insights. It provides a profile of leading research institutions and the knowledge landscape in the field. The gene co-occurrence map reveals frequent research of NOTCH3, prothrombotic factors, inflammatory cytokines, and other potential risk factors. The heterogeneous biomedical entity network analysis highlights infrequently studied genes and biomedical entities with potential significance for future stroke studies. In conclusion, BiblioEngine is a valuable tool enabling efficient navigation and comprehension of expanding biomedical knowledge from scientific literature, empowering researchers in their pursuit of disease-specific genetic knowledge.

Keywords: Artificial intelligence · Network analytics · Disease genetics

1 Introduction

In recent decades, contemporary genetic research has witnessed notable advancements by leveraging Artificial Intelligence (AI) techniques. These techniques have enabled the analysis of large-scale, high-dimensional, and multi-modal data [5,9,10], which particularly help identify the associations between diseases and gene mutations in the disease genetic context. Nevertheless, an important challenge persists in the absence of a comprehensive platform that aids

© The Author(s), under exclusive license to Springer Nature Singapore Pte Ltd. 2023
Y. Li et al. (Eds.): HIS 2023, LNCS 14305, pp. 187–198, 2023.
https://doi.org/10.1007/978-981-99-7108-4_16

biomedical researchers in efficiently comprehending the explosive knowledge embedded within the rapidly accumulating scientific literature. To address this gap, this paper introduces BiblioEngine, a literature knowledge-mining platform that incorporates analytical techniques empowered by natural language processing (NLP) and network analytics. By harnessing multiple AI-empowered data sources, BiblioEngine equips the original research papers with research concepts and biomedical entities. Additionally, it employs a heterogeneous network analysis framework to unveil the significance and specificity of these biomedical entities, ultimately generating comprehensive rankings across four distinct categories.

This paper additionally presents a case study that investigates stroke genetic knowledge through literature analysis. First, it elucidates the research intelligence and knowledge landscape within the field, highlighting prominent institutions such as Inserm, Harvard University, and Karolinska Institutet, as well as the emerging influence of the University of Cambridge and Massachusetts General Hospital. Secondly, it unravels the genetic knowledge pertaining to stroke, identifying NOTCH3 as the most frequently studied gene. Additionally, it demonstrates that other genes tend to be studied in conjunction, forming three distinct groups: prothrombotic factors, inflammatory cytokines, and other potential risk factors. Through gene importance-specificity analysis, six genes are identified as meriting further investigation due to their current potential, albeit limited evidence. The overall rankings derived from the study highlight several biomedical entities that warrant further exploration regarding their associations with stroke.

Our major contributions are two-fold: First, it introduces a workflow that harmoniously integrates AI-empowered tools and network analytics to facilitate the efficient assimilation of disease-related genetic knowledge derived from scientific literature. Second, it presents an in-depth and comprehensive case study centered on stroke, elucidating the current research landscape in this area. Additionally, the case study highlights frequently studied genes and identifies potential genes and mutations that warrant further investigation.

The remainder of this paper is organized as follows: Sect. 2 delineates the methodology and workflow of BiblioEngine, providing a detailed explanation of its functioning. Section 3 presents the case study conducted on stroke, including the research findings and corresponding results. Finally, Sect. 4 concludes the paper by summarizing the key insights and discussing the limitations encountered during the study.

2   Platform Framework and Methodology

The framework and workflow of BiblioEngine are depicted in Fig. 1. The platform operates by receiving research paper inputs from the PubMed database. These papers are then mapped to OpenAlex[1] and Pubtator[2] to retrieve standardized

---

[1] https://openalex.org/.
[2] https://www.ncbi.nlm.nih.gov/research/pubtator/.

hierarchical research concepts and entities that are studied within the research papers. Subsequently, the platform encompasses two distinct task trajectories. The first trajectory is dedicated to the discovery of research intelligence, and the second trajectory focuses on revealing gene knowledge derived from the literature via heterogeneous biomedical entity network analysis.

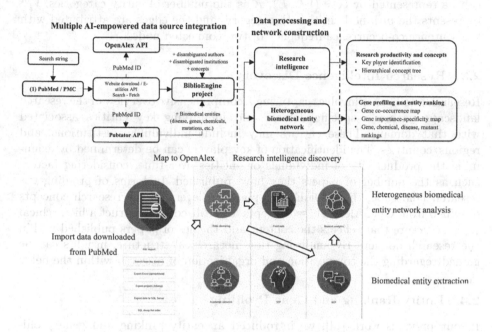

Fig. 1. Genetic knowledge mining framework

2.1   Multiple AI-Empowered Data Source Integration

The BiblioEngine platform integrates two AI-empowered data sources, namely Pubtator and OpenAlex, to maximize the utilization of curated literature metadata provided by these repositories. OpenAlex offers hierarchical research concepts that reflect the underlying research content. Those concepts are derived from Wikipedia entries and are associated with research papers through a topic modeling process. Furthermore, the BiblioEngine platform integrates the Pubtator entity extraction function, which enables the identification of diverse biomedical entities from PubMed articles. These entities include diseases, genes, chemicals, mutations, cell lines, and more. The extracted entities are subsequently mapped to biomedical thesauri, enriching their semantic context. Moreover, the platform leverages corresponding entity databases to retrieve comprehensive information regarding the identified entities, including official symbols, names, mutation sites, and other relevant details.

2.2   Data Processing and Network Construction

The Pubtator API enables the extraction of biomedical entities, encompassing four primary categories: diseases, chemicals, genes, and mutations. In order to facilitate subsequent analysis, a weighted heterogeneous network is constructed, incorporating these four biomedical entity categories. The constructed network can be represented by $G = (V^K, E)$, K is the number of entity categories, V_i^m represents the mth node in the ith category, and the edges are attributed with the sentence co-occurrence frequency of two connected nodes.

2.3   Research Intelligence Discovery

Research intelligence involves capturing a comprehensive overview of the research landscape within a specific domain and identifying key entities associated with that domain. These entities may include individuals, institutions, and regions/countries. The identification of key players can be determined by examining the productivity of individuals or entities over time, considering factors such as the number of papers they have published. In terms of profiling the research landscape, the BiblioEngine platform leverages the research concepts obtained from OpenAlex. These concepts are utilized to construct a hierarchical topic structure that reflects the content and themes of papers published within the research domain. By analyzing this hierarchical structure, insights can be gained regarding the composition and organization of research within the field.

2.4   Entity Ranking and Gene Profiling

In our previous work [14], we introduced an entity ranking and gene profiling approach that focuses on identifying key biomedical entities and uncovering gene characteristics in relation to a specific target disease. This approach utilizes centrality measures and network-based intersection ratios as proxies to assess the significance and specificity of biomedical entities within the context of the disease. Specifically, degree, closeness, and betweenness centrality measures are employed to the nodes' ability to aggregate, disseminate, and transfer information within a network. The calculations are provided below:

$$Degree(V_i^m) = \frac{\sum_{j=1}^{K} \sum_{n=1}^{|V_j|} A_{V_i^m V_j^n}}{|V_K| - 1} \tag{1}$$

$$Closeness(V_i^m) = \frac{|V_K| - 1}{\sum_{j=1}^{K} \sum_{n=1}^{|V_j|} d_{V_i^m V_j^n}} \tag{2}$$

$$Betweenness(V_i^m) = \frac{2 \sum_{x,y=1}^{K} \sum_{a=1}^{|V_x|} \sum_{b=1}^{|V_y|} \frac{\sigma(V_x^a V_y^b)_{V_i^m}}{\sigma(V_x^a V_y^b)}}{(|V_K| - 1)(|V_K| - 2)} \tag{3}$$

where $|V_K|$ denotes the number of all K categories of nodes in the network and $|V_j|$ is the number of nodes in the jth category, $d_{V_i^m V_j^n}$ is the distance from node

V_i^m to node V_j^n, $\sigma(V_x^a V_y^b)$ is all shortest path counts from node V_x^a to V_y^b and $\sigma(V_x^a V_y^b)_{V_i^m}$ is the path counts that pass through node V_i^m.

In addition to the three centrality measures mentioned earlier, we also calculate an additional indicator known as the intersection ratio. This indicator is used to assess the specificity of biomedical entities in relation to the target disease. which is defined as follows:

$$Intersection\ ratio(V_i^m) = \frac{w(V_i^m, V_{disease}^t)}{\sum_{a=1}^{|V_{disease}|} w(V_i^m, V_{disease}^a)} \tag{4}$$

where $V_{disease}^t$ represents the node(s) of the target disease, and $w(V_i^m, V_{disease}^t)$ refers to the weight of the edge connecting V_i^m and $V_{disease}^t$.

To obtain comprehensive rankings for each category of biomedical entities, we utilize a non-dominated sorting algorithm [14] that combines the three centrality measures as proxies for entity importance. This algorithm also incorporates the intersection ratio later to generate more comprehensive rankings. The non-dominated sorting algorithm ensures that entities are ranked in a non-dominated order, considering their importance as well as their specificity.

3   Case Study: Stroke Genetic Research Analysis

To showcase the effectiveness of the BiblioEngine platform, we conducted a case study centered around stroke genetic investigation. Stroke is a prevalent cardiovascular disease with detrimental implications for individuals and public health but poses a complex genetic landscape that remains incompletely understood. Using the BiblioEngine platform, we generated results that shed light on the research landscape and conveyed genetic knowledge pertinent to stroke. To enhance the visual representation of these findings, we employed Xmind[3] software and the Circos visualization web application[4].

3.1   Data Collection and Processing

Using the search strategy described below in PubMed, 4,557 original research papers were retrieved from PubMed for further analysis.

((("stroke/genetics" [MeSH Terms] OR ("Stoke" [All Fields] AND "genom*" [All Fields])) AND "humans" [MeSH Terms]) NOT ("Review" [Publication Type] OR "systematic review" [Publication Type])) AND (humans[Filter])
Search date: 31/05/2023

In accordance with the workflow of the BiblioEngine platform, the research papers obtained were mapped to the OpenAlex database, and subsequently, biomedical entities were extracted using Pubtator. The fundamental statistics

---

[3] https://xmind.app/.
[4] http://mkweb.bcgsc.ca/tableviewer/visualize/.

regarding the 4,557 research papers and the concepts/entities mined from them are presented in Table 1. Continuing with the network construction process described in Sect. 2.2, a co-occurrence network of heterogeneous biomedical entities was established. This network comprises 6,150 nodes and 42,021 edges.

Table 1. Basic statistics of the 4,557 research papers

Data source	Field	Count	Top five instances
OpenAlex	Author	13,284	Martin Dichgans, Hugh S. Markus, James F. Meschia, Bradford B. Worrall, Rainer Malik
OpenAlex	Institution	2,980	Harvard University, University of Cambridge, Inserm, Ludwig-Maximilians-Universität München, Massachusetts General Hospital
OpenAlex	Concept	110	Genotype, allele, single-nucleotide polymorphism, ischemic stroke, leukoencephalopathy
Pubtator	Disease	950	Stroke, Ischemic stroke, hypertension, atherosclerosis, leukoencephalopathy
Pubtator	Gene	1,868	NOTCH3, MTHFR, APOE, ACE, IL6
Pubtator	Chemical	495	Cholesterol, lipid, homocysteine, triglyceride, cysteine
Pubtator	Mutant	2,405	rs1801133, rs1799963, rs1799983, rs1801131, rs1800795

3.2 Key Players and Knowledge Landscape in Stroke Genetic Studies

This section delivers the first trajectory of results. In Fig. 2, the ranking changes of the top ten leading research institutions are depicted. The time period is divided into six windows, with the first window ending in 2000, followed by five 5-year gaps.

Notably, the University of Cambridge and Massachusetts General Hospital have experienced notable rises in their rankings over the past decade. Analysis of research papers originating from these institutions indicates that their improved rankings can be attributed to the high productivity of research teams led by Hugh S. Markus and Jonathan Rosand, respectively. Harvard University, Karolinska Institutet, and Ludwig-Maximilians-Universität München consistently maintain high rankings throughout the entire time span, demonstrating their enduring research leadership and contributions within the field. The rankings of other institutions exhibit fluctuating trends, which may be influenced by factors such as the migration of key research teams or time gaps between research progress and publication.

Subsequently, we proceeded to extract the hierarchical relationships among all concepts and present the visualization of the hierarchical concept tree in Fig. 3. This hierarchical concept tree provides a visual representation of the

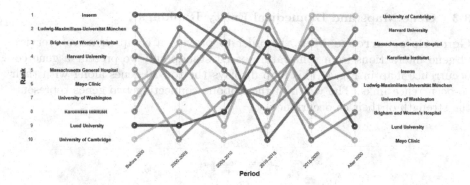

Fig. 2. Research institution ranking change in consecutive time windows

knowledge landscape pertaining to genetic studies of stroke. The numbers accompanying each concept indicate the count of research papers associated with that concept. To enhance clarity, we pruned the tree by removing branches that did not contain any concepts related to more than 100 research papers. By examining the hierarchical concept tree, we can observe that genetic studies of stroke encompass a wide range of research topics from the perspectives of basic medical sciences, clinical medicine, and public health. These topics encompass various indicators, conditions, research methods, and subjects that contribute to understanding the onset, progression, and prognosis of stroke. Furthermore, the branch related to biology reveals the emergence of computational biology and bioinformatics, signifying the increasing significance of data-driven genetic knowledge discovery in recent years. This development underscores the value and impact of integrating computational approaches in advancing genetic research on stroke.

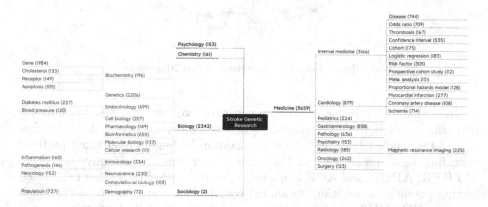

Fig. 3. Hierarchical concept tree of stroke genetic research

3.3   Gene Maps and Biomedical Entity Rankings

Gene Co-occurrence Map. In order to provide a comprehensive overview of gene interactions from a literature-based standpoint, we present a gene co-occurrence map in Fig. 4. This map displays the top 20 genes along with their co-occurrence links. The width of the ribbons connecting two genes represents the strength of their co-occurrence.

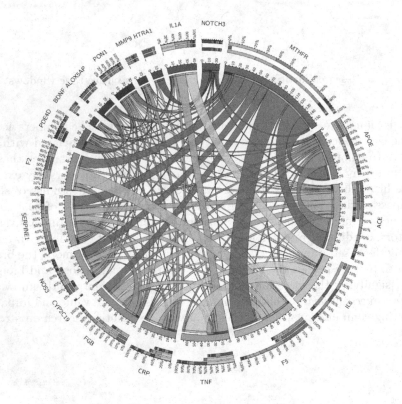

Fig. 4. Co-occurrence map of top 20 genes

By examining this gene co-occurrence map, we can gain insights into the potential interactions and relationships between different genes within the context of the studied literature. The visualization highlights interesting patterns regarding gene interactions in the studied literature. Specifically, the genes **MTHFR**, **APOE**, and **ACE** frequently appear together with other genes, suggesting potential associations or shared research interests. On the other hand, the gene **NOTCH3** stands out as being relatively studied alone, possibly due to its distinctive associations with CADASIL, a condition linked to stroke.

Further analysis of relevant papers provides insights into specific gene pairs: (1) Prothrombotic factors: The genes **MTHFR** and **F5** are commonly studied together in genetic association studies due to their shared genetic variants, such as Factor V Leiden and C677T, which are known prothrombotic factors associated with increased stroke risks [2]. Additionally, mutations in the gene **F2** (prothrombin G20210) are frequently observed in such studies. (2) Inflammatory cytokine: The genes **IL6** and **TNF** play significant roles in inflammatory responses that occur in the brain, which can be triggered by tissue damage or injuries following a stroke [1]. Upregulation of these genes and the subsequent release of corresponding proteins contribute to the immune response and inflammatory cascade observed in the brain after a stroke. (3) Other possible risk factors: Mutations in the genes **ACE** and **APOE** are more commonly associated with heart diseases and Alzheimer's disease. However, their associations with stroke have been investigated, yielding inconsistent evidence [4]. These findings highlight the relationships and potential roles of these gene pairs in stroke and related conditions, providing valuable insights into ongoing research in the field.

Gene Importance-Specificity Map. To overcome the potential bias towards frequently studied genes and to identify genes that play significant but less explored roles in the onset and progression of stroke, we employed two indicators, importance and intersection ratio as introduced in Sect. 2.4, to profile all the identified genes. Figure 5 presents the gene profiling results, where the x-axis represents the centrality dominating score of genes, and the y-axis indicates the intersection ratio of genes specific to stroke.

By examining the gene profiling plot, we can identify genes that have lower frequencies but are more specifically associated with stroke. In addition to well-studied genes such as IL6, TNF, and NOS3, the map highlights a few genes that are relatively low-ranked but possess high dominating scores and specificity, denoted by red markers in Fig. 5. To gain further insights into their associations with stroke, we delved into relevant research papers and summarized the findings in Table 3. The results reveal that mutations in these genes potentially have associations with different subtypes of stroke in diverse populations. However, it is important to note that the exploration of such associations is limited, necessitating additional case studies and experiments to establish and comprehend the underlying mechanisms. These genes warrant further investigation and may provide novel insights into the mechanisms and treatment of stroke.

Overall Rankings of All Biomedical Entities. Additionally, the dominating scores of the three centrality measures and the intersection ratio were computed for all entities, resulting in overall rankings across four categories. These rankings, presented in Table 3, provide a comprehensive integration of the four measurement dimensions. Notably, they highlight several emerging low-frequency entities across the four categories (Table 2).

The overall rankings provide valuable insights into entities that warrant further investigation in future stroke studies. In the list of diseases, the majority are conditions, complications, or risk factors associated with stroke. The gene ranking reveals that the top two entities are both MicroRNAs, and the analysis of relevant papers suggests their potential as biomarkers for ischemic stroke [8].

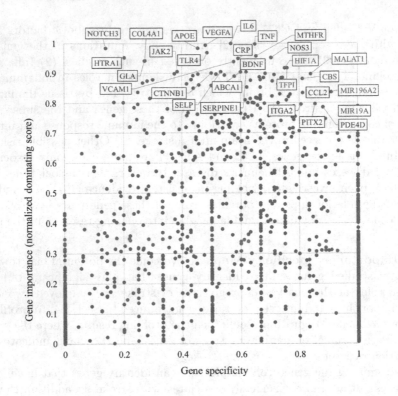

Fig. 5. Gene importance-specificity map

Table 2. Low-frequency genes highlighted by the gene importance-specificity map

Gene	Findings and evidence
HIF1A	A gender-based gene regulation comparison on stroke patients indicates that HIF1A is associated with female-specific stroke genes [12]
CBS	CBS is found to influence poststroke homocysteine metabolism which is associated with recurrent stroke [6]
TFPI	It was found that plasma TFPI level shows a significant effect as an environmental factor in addition to heritable factors [11]
MALAT1	Serum MALAT1 level and the mutant rs3200401 in MALAT1 are identified to be independent predictors of cerebral ischemic stroke [3]
MIR196A2	The combination of miR-146aG/-149T/-196a2C/-499G allele is found to be associated with the pathogenesis of ischemic stroke [7]
MIR19A	The expression of MIR19A is found to be significantly decreased in acute ischemic stroke patients [8]

Among the chemicals, ginkgolides emerge as a potential therapy for preventing stroke progression, although the evidence remains limited and conflicting [13]. Additionally, there is evidence suggesting that the level of methionine can pos-

Table 3. Overall rankings of four categories of biomedical entities

Disease	Gene	Chemical	Mutation
intracerebral hemorrhage	MIR19A	aspirin	rs2292832
coronary artery disease	MIR125A	homocysteine	rs6265
neurological disease	MAF	clopidogrel	rs710446
atherosclerosis	SHMT1	triglyceride	rs579459
venous thromboembolism	MIRLET7I	lipid	rs6843082
hypertension	ANXA3	polyacrylamide	rs243865
myocardial infarction	SLC22A4	technetium	rs1126579
atrial fibrillation	CST12P	ginkgolides	rs3200401
inflammation	IFNG	arachidonic acid	rs320
bleeding	FOS	methionine	rs28933697

sibly be associated with increased stroke risk. The mutation list highlights less frequently studied mutations, such as rs2292832 and rs579459, which may hold potential associations with stroke and thus require further investigation.

4   Conclusions and Further Study

This paper presents BiblioEngine, a biomedical literature analysis platform designed to aid researchers in efficiently and effectively extracting disease genetic knowledge from research papers. The platform integrates two AI-empowered data sources and employs a heterogeneous network analysis framework to facilitate biomedical entity ranking and gene prioritization. Its effectiveness is demonstrated by a case study on stroke genetic research analysis.

This platform is subject to certain limitations. Efforts are underway to enhance its functionalities in three key directions: First, the current network does not distinguish between positive and negative associations in gene and disease pairs. Future iterations of network construction will incorporate sentiment scores as edge attributes, enabling the indication of positive and negative associations. Second, The prediction of gene-disease associations holds significant value and will be prioritized as the next step in network analysis, treating it as a link prediction problem. Last, The interpretation of the obtained results can be further enhanced through real-world experimental validation, which may require ethical considerations [15]. To pursue this objective, collaboration with researchers specializing in this field is being actively sought.

Acknowledgements. This work is supported by the Australian Research Council Linkage Project LP210100414.

References

1. Banerjee, I., Gupta, V., Ahmed, T., Faizaan, M., Agarwal, P., Ganesh, S.: Inflammatory system gene polymorphism and the risk of stroke: a case-control study in an Indian population. Brain Res. Bull. **75**(1), 158–165 (2008)
2. Curry, C.J., Bhullar, S., Holmes, J., Delozier, C.D., Roeder, E.R., Hutchison, H.T.: Risk factors for perinatal arterial stroke: a study of 60 mother-child pairs. Pediatr. Neurol. **37**(2), 99–107 (2007)
3. Fathy, N., Kortam, M.A., Shaker, O.G., Sayed, N.H.: Long noncoding RNAs MALAT1 and ANRIL gene variants and the risk of cerebral ischemic stroke: an association study. ACS Chem. Neurosci. **12**(8), 1351–1362 (2021)
4. Gao, X., Yang, H., ZhiPing, T.: Association studies of genetic polymorphism, environmental factors and their interaction in ischemic stroke. Neurosci. Lett. **398**(3), 172–177 (2006)
5. Guo, K., et al.: Artificial intelligence-driven biomedical genomics. Knowl.-Based Syst. (2023, accepted)
6. Hsu, F.C., et al.: Transcobalamin 2 variant associated with poststroke homocysteine modifies recurrent stroke risk. Neurology **77**(16), 1543–1550 (2011)
7. Jeon, Y.J., et al.: Association of the miR-146a, miR-149, miR-196a2, and miR-499 polymorphisms with ischemic stroke and silent brain infarction risk. Arterioscler. Thromb. Vasc. Biol. **33**(2), 420–430 (2013)
8. Jickling, G.C., Ander, B.P., Zhan, X., Noblett, D., Stamova, B., Liu, D.: microRNA expression in peripheral blood cells following acute ischemic stroke and their predicted gene targets. PLoS ONE **9**(6), e99283 (2014)
9. Lu, J., Behbood, V., Hao, P., Zuo, H., Xue, S., Zhang, G.: Transfer learning using computational intelligence: a survey. Knowl.-Based Syst. **80**, 14–23 (2015)
10. Lu, J., Wu, D., Mao, M., Wang, W., Zhang, G.: Recommender system application developments: a survey. Decis. Support Syst. **74**, 12–32 (2015)
11. Nowak-Göttl, U., Langer, C., Bergs, S., Thedieck, S., Sträter, R., Stoll, M.: Genetics of hemostasis: differential effects of heritability and household components influencing lipid concentrations and clotting factor levels in 282 pediatric stroke families. Environ. Health Perspect. **116**(6), 839–843 (2008)
12. Tian, Y., et al.: Effects of gender on gene expression in the blood of ischemic stroke patients. J. Cerebral Blood Flow Metab. **32**(5), 780–791 (2012)
13. Wang, T.J., et al.: Multiple mechanistic models reveal the neuroprotective effects of diterpene ginkgolides against astrocyte-mediated demyelination via the PAF-PAFR pathway. Am. J. Chin. Med. **50**(06), 1565–1597 (2022)
14. Wu, M., Zhang, Y., Zhang, G., Lu, J.: Exploring the genetic basis of diseases through a heterogeneous bibliometric network: a methodology and case study. Technol. Forecast. Soc. Chang. **164**, 120513 (2021)
15. Zhang, Y., Wu, M., Tian, G.Y., Zhang, G., Lu, J.: Ethics and privacy of artificial intelligence: understandings from bibliometrics. Knowl.-Based Syst. **222**, 106994 (2021)

Enhancing Clustering Performance in Sepsis Time Series Data Using Gravity Field

Rui Hao[1](✉), Ming Sheng[2], Yong Zhang[3], Huiying Zhao[4], Chenxiao Hao[4], Wenyao Li[5], Luoxi Wang[6], and Chao Li[3]

[1] Beijing University of Posts and Telecommunications, Beijing 100876, China
haorui@bupt.edu.cn
[2] School of Computer Science and Technology, Beijing Institute of Technology, Beijing 100081, China
[3] BNRist, DCST, RIIT, Tsinghua University, Beijing 100084, China
{zhangyong05,li-chao}@tsinghua.edu.cn
[4] Department of Critical Care Medicine, Peking University People's Hospital, No. 11 Xizhimen South Street, Xicheng District, Beijing 100044, China
zhaohuiying109@sina.com, 1410122922@pku.edu.cn
[5] Software school of Henan university, Kaifeng, Henan, China
[6] The Experimental High School Attached to Beijing Normal University, Beijing 100032, China

Abstract. Sepsis, a severe systemic response to infection, represents a pressing global public health challenge. Time series research, including the analysis of medical data, encounters significant obstacles due to the high dimensionality, complexity, and heterogeneity inherent in the data associated with sepsis. To address these obstacles, this paper proposes a novel approach for enhancing time series datasets. The primary objective of this approach is to enhance clustering performance and robustness without requiring modifications to existing clustering techniques. Specifically, this approach can improve the clustering performance in sepsis patients. The effectiveness of the proposed approach is validated through comprehensive experiments conducted on both non-medical and medical sepsis datasets, showcasing its potential to advance time series analysis and significantly contribute to the effective management of sepsis medical conditions. In addition, we use this approach to establish three subtypes in the clustering of sepsis patients, which provide meaningful interpretations in terms of medical significance and we further explore the therapeutic heterogeneity among the three subtypes.

Keywords: Clustering · Spesis · Gravity Field

1 Introduction

Sepsis, a critical global public health problem, arises from an imbalanced immune response to infection, leading to life-threatening organ dysfunction. Its incidence

© The Author(s), under exclusive license to Springer Nature Singapore Pte Ltd. 2023
Y. Li et al. (Eds.): HIS 2023, LNCS 14305, pp. 199–212, 2023.
https://doi.org/10.1007/978-981-99-7108-4_17

and mortality rates are persistently on the rise, making it the foremost cause of death among critically ill patients. In 2017, there were an alarming 48.9 million new cases of sepsis worldwide, resulting in approximately 11 million associated deaths [2,7]. Mortality rates for sepsis vary depending on disease severity and the specific population studied. It is estimated that among hospitalized patients, the mortality rates for sepsis and septic shock are approximately 17% and 26%, respectively [8]. Furthermore, a comprehensive multicenter study conducted in China revealed that around one-fifth of ICU patients suffered from sepsis, with mortality rates as high as 35.5% for sepsis and 51.9% for septic shock [20].

Sepsis, as a heterogeneous disease, can greatly benefit from the identification of its subtypes to enhance and optimize clinical management. More importantly, precise treatment strategies can be developed for different subtypes, leading to improved outcomes for sepsis patients [10,15]. Currently, research on sepsis subtypes is still in its early stages, and clustering analysis has emerged as a valuable tool that has gained significant attention. Unsupervised clustering methods have been utilized to identify sepsis subtypes and have been shown to be associated with outcomes [16,17]. Clustering analysis will play an irreplaceable role in the research process [9], although the quality of clustering results can be influenced by the choice of clustering methods and datasets.

Time series clustering analysis holds significant value in the field of medical research, particularly in the context of sepsis. By clustering similar time series patterns, researchers can uncover meaningful subgroups of septic patients with distinct clinical characteristics, treatment responses, or prognoses. However, the inherent challenges of high dimensionality, complexity, and heterogeneity in time series data have hindered the extraction of meaningful insights. Nowadays, although there are some good systems and methods for collecting and analyzing data [6,12,14,19,21], there are few methods that can cluster more effectively by changing the data distribution.

To address these challenges, this paper presents a novel approach to enrich time series datasets with the explicit objective of enhancing the performance and robustness of clustering techniques. Notably, this method does not necessitate any modification to the existing clustering techniques, thereby offering the flexibility to be employed in conjunction with a wide range of established algorithms.

The contributions of this article are as follows:

1. We propose a new method to enhance time series datasets in this paper. It addresses the challenges posed by data associated with sepsis, aiming to improve clustering performance and robustness without requiring modifications to existing clustering techniques.
2. We conduct comprehensive experiments on both non-medical and medical sepsis datasets to validate the effectiveness of the proposed method. The experimental results demonstrate the method's potential in time series analysis and its ability to significantly facilitate effective management of septic conditions.

3. We discover three subtypes in sepsis patients and explore their treatment heterogeneity using the proposed method in the clustering analysis. This provides meaningful explanations in terms of medical significance.

2   Related Work

2.1   Similarity in Time Series

In the field of time series analysis [4, 13], various methods have been proposed to measure the similarity between time series data. The Euclidean distance calculates the straight-line distance between two points in the data, making it suitable for data with linear trends and similar amplitudes. On the other hand, the Manhattan distance, also known as the L1 distance, measures the sum of absolute differences along each dimension, making it more sensitive to differences in data with varying amplitudes and trends. Another method, DTW (Dynamic Time Warping) [5], aligns the time axes of two time series data elastically and computes the minimum distance between them, allowing for handling time shifts, compressions, and expansions. These popular similarity measures are extensively used in tasks such as clustering, classification, and anomaly detection. The choice of similarity measure depends on the specific characteristics of the data and the analytical requirements. DTW can perform operations like linear scaling on one sequence to better align it with another, enabling a one-to-many relationship suitable for complex time series measurements. In patient time series data, DTW can align similar changes occurring at different times due to patient-specific variations, enhancing patient similarity measurements.

2.2   Using Field to Improve Datasets

Improving the dataset can be a better approach to enhance clustering results. In fact, the impact of the dataset on clustering outcomes has been studied by other researchers for quite some time. Blekas and Lagaris [1] introduced a method called Newton clustering, which forces all objects to tend towards the cluster centers to facilitate the determination of the number of clusters. Shi et al. [11] proposed a shrinkage-based clustering approach (referred to as SBCA) where the dataset is first partitioned into several cells. The cells are then moved along the density gradient direction, effectively detecting clusters of various densities or shapes in noisy datasets of arbitrary dimensions. Wong et al. [18] introduced flock clustering, which continuously drives objects towards the median of their neighbors, providing a friendly feature space for the clustering process. Newton clustering, flock clustering, and SBCA explicitly separate the process of dataset variation from the overall method and treat it as data preprocessing. Researchers have proposed the HIBOG algorithm based on physical analysis [3]. HIBOG focuses on improving the dataset so that various clustering algorithms can achieve faster and more accurate results. The HIBOG algorithm introduces a novel gravity function that incorporates additional attractive forces between objects. This innovative approach enhances the clustering process by considering the interaction and attraction among data points. However, these methods primarily operate on vectors and do not provide explicit steps for handling time series data tensors. In contrast to these methods, we have optimized our approach specifically for time series datasets.

3   Method

According to the definition of sepsis, which refers to the dysregulated host response to infection leading to life-threatening organ dysfunction, we have selected three sets of indicators, namely infection markers, organ function indicators, and basic vital signs, as clustering variables. These variables will be included along with multiple clinical variables for analysis. Therefore, our dataset can be represented as a tensor in the form of (X, Y, Z), where X represents the number of samples, Y represents the time steps, and Z represents the number of different indicators or features being considered. Furthermore, we will divide the patient data with a total count of X into several classes, ensuring that patients within each class possess similar time series characteristics. Below, we will provide a detailed explanation of our method.

3.1   Distance Computation with Dynamic Time Warping

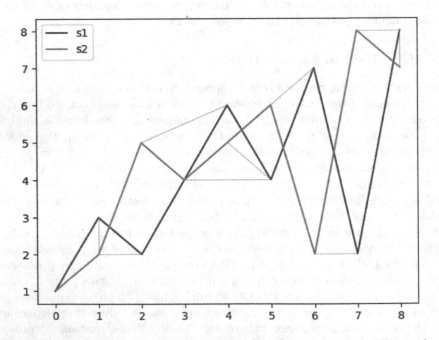

Fig. 1. An example of the DTW algorithm, where S1 and S2 are two time series.

In patient time series data, DTW (Dynamic Time Warping) can align similar changes occurring at different times due to patient-specific variations, thereby enhancing patient similarity measurements. This is particularly valuable because patients may exhibit similar patterns of physiological changes but at different time points. By considering the temporal alignment and allowing for time shifts, DTW enables a more accurate comparison of patient trajectories, capturing the similarity of patterns and changes across different time scales. This ability to align and compare time series data in a flexible manner makes DTW a powerful technique for analyzing patient data and understanding disease progression, enabling more accurate clustering and classification of patients based on their temporal patterns. Figure 1 is an example of the DTW algorithm, where S1 and S2 are two time series, and the corresponding points in the two sequences are connected by lines.

3.2   Preprocess the Dataset with HIBOG Algorithm

HIBOG, an acronym for Highly Improving clustering accuracy by transforming Bad datasets intO Good datasets, is a method proposed with a unique perspective. It recognizes that a good dataset possesses two key properties: small distances between similar objects and large distances between dissimilar objects. By leveraging this understanding, HIBOG aims to transform datasets into improved versions suitable for clustering tasks.

Unlike traditional approaches that treat dataset objects as mere numbers, HIBOG considers them as vectors in a vector space. Its primary focus lies in reducing the distances between similar objects and increasing the distances between dissimilar objects. By effectively restructuring the dataset, HIBOG significantly enhances clustering accuracy, offering a powerful tool for data analysis and exploration.

After computing the pairwise distances between objects using DTW, we use HIBOG which can highly improve clustering accuracy by transforming Bad datasets into good datasets to preprocess the dataset. The HIBOG algorithm treats each object as a vector in space, computing a "gravitational" force between each object and its k-nearest neighbors. Unlike the original HIBOG method, our method is designed specifically for temporal tensor data. We consider the factor of temporal data requiring more processing time and therefore perform only one iteration. The entire process is illustrated in the Fig. 2. In this paper, we use the gravitation function created by HIBOG. The function considers the interaction between each object and its k nearest neighbors. It is widely acknowledged that an object is likely to be similar to its nearest neighbors, as seen in methods like KNN (K-Nearest Neighbors). However, we introduce an innovative approach in representing distances. While HIBOG utilizes the 2-Norm of vectors, we employ the DTW matrix. The gravitation between object i and its j-nearest neighbor (where $j \leq k$) is defined as follows:

$$F_{ij} = G \frac{DTW(o_i, o_{i1})}{DTW(o_i, o_{ij})^2}(o_i - o_{ij}) \tag{1}$$

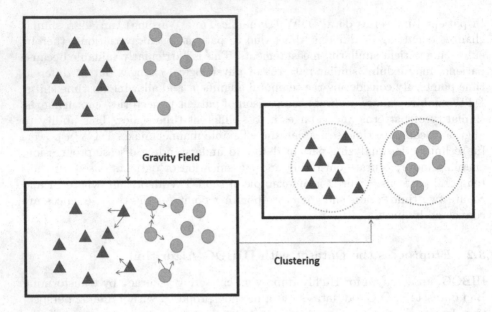

Fig. 2. This is an example of the process of clustering with HIBOG, where Different shapes in the diagram represent data points that potentially belong to different categories.

Each object is gravitationally influenced only by its k nearest objects. The total force exerted on object i is determined by the following equation:

$$F_i = \sum_{j=1}^{k} G \frac{DTW(o_i, o_{i1})}{DTW(o_i, o_{ij})^2}(o_i - o_{ij}) \tag{2}$$

In this paper, we make use of the formula for uniform speed movement to compute the displacement. Based on the physical theory, when a force is applied to an object, it results in displacement. To simplify the operation, we assume that the force F_i remains constant during the movement of object i. According to Newton's law, an object subjected to an external force will undergo uniformly accelerated linear motion. In the above scenario, object i will experience acceleration due to the force. $F_i = ma$ and $x = \frac{1}{2}at^2$, where F_i is the force acting on the object. For the object i we assume its mass to be 1, and t is artificially determined. Therefore, we can consider $x = F_iT$, where T is the motion coefficient, representing the duration of time that can be sustained after calculating F_i.

$$o_i' = o_i + x = o_i + F_iT \tag{3}$$

The specific algorithm is shown as Algorithm 1.

Algorithm 1. HIBOG Algorithm with DTW distance

Input: The medical dataset O; k:the number of nearest neighbors to be selected; T:a parameter that controls the degree of data transformation.

2: **Output:** The improved dataset O'

Optional: data normalization

4: **Step 1:** Computing D_{DTW} of data objects

$distance\_matrix \leftarrow$ compute $D_{DTW}(O)$ //Calculate the DTW distance of any two objects in O and store them in $distance\_matrix$

6: $dis\_sort \leftarrow$ sort($distance\_matrix$, axis = 1)

$dis\_argsort \leftarrow$ argsort($distance\_matrix$, axis = 1)

8: **Step 2:** Data changing

$G \leftarrow$ mean($dis\_sort[:,1]$)

10: **for** i in $range(N)$ **do**

$neighbors \leftarrow dis\_argsort[i, : k]$

12: Initialize $gravitation\_total$

for j in $neighbors$ **do**

14: $gravitation \leftarrow G \times (\|O[j] - O[i]\| \times \frac{dis\_sort[i,1]}{\|dis\_sort[i,j]\|^2})$

$gravitation\_total \leftarrow gravitation\_total + gravitation$

16: **end for**

$O'[i] \leftarrow O[i] + gravitation\_total \times T$

18: **end for**

Return: O'

3.3 Clustering Method

K-means is one of the most popular clustering methods and commonly employed algorithm for clustering or grouping data points. K-means is known for its simplicity and efficiency, making it a popular choice in various fields such as data analysis, machine learning, and pattern recognition. It aims to partition the data points into K clusters by iteratively assigning each point to the nearest cluster centroid and updating the centroids based on the mean of the assigned points. The algorithm continues to refine the clusters until convergence is reached, resulting in a final clustering solution.

This study utilizes the TimeSeriesKMeans Clustering algorithm available in the tslearn package within the PyCharm software for conducting cluster analysis on time series data. TimeSeriesKMeans Clustering is an extension of the K-means clustering algorithm specifically designed for handling time series data. It is primarily employed to partition data points with similar temporal patterns into distinct clusters.

In the TimeSeriesKMeans Clustering algorithm, each time series data point is represented as a vector, and all vectors have a fixed dimensionality. These vectors are arranged in chronological order, thereby capturing the sequential nature of time series data. The objective of this algorithm is to divide the time series data points into k different clusters, where data points within the same cluster exhibit similar temporal patterns.

During the clustering process, the TimeSeriesKMeans algorithm considers the temporal aspect of the data by employing a distance matrix based on DTW.

By utilizing the DTW distance matrix, the algorithm can capture the nuanced similarities and dissimilarities among time series data points, leading to more accurate clustering results.

4   Experiment

We are conducting experiments on two non-medical time-series datasets, and the results have confirmed the effectiveness of our method. The results indicate that our method enhances the performance of the data analysis compared to previous approaches. Moreover, we have specifically applied our method to a time-series dataset related to sepsis. In addition to evaluating the results using information-theoretic metrics, we have also provided additional medical interpretation and insights. We have categorized sepsis into three subtypes and we have described the medical characteristics of each subtype based on medical knowledge.

4.1   Experiments on Non-medical Datasets

In the experiments, we test the effectiveness of the method on two non-medical datasets that have labels. To evaluate the performance of the method, we use NMI as the evaluation metric.

NMI, an acronym for Normalized Mutual Information, measures the similarity between two clusterings or partitions of a dataset. It is widely used to assess the performance of clustering algorithms. A higher NMI value indicates a stronger agreement or similarity between the clusterings and the true class labels.

By calculating the NMI, we compare the results before and after applying the method. This allows us to assess the improvement achieved by the method in terms of clustering accuracy or alignment with the ground truth labels. A higher NMI score suggests that the method successfully aligns the clusters with the true class labels, indicating improved performance.

EEG Eye State Dataset: This dataset describes individual EEG data and whether their eyes are open or closed. The goal is to predict, based solely on EEG data, whether the eyes are open or closed. This dataset contains instances of EEG measurements indicating whether the eyes are open or closed.

We utilize the dataset to form time series data and perform clustering, calculating the NMI metric. Afterward, we make equidistant transformations to the K and T parameters and use our method to process the dataset. We conduct clustering again and obtain the NMI metric. The final comparison results are shown in the Table 1.

The table shows the changes in the clustering effect of the dataset before and after using our method. From the data in the table, it can be seen that the clustering effect has been improved for almost all parameters K and T. Moreover, in most cases, the NMI index has been improved by more than 50%.

The Ozone Level Detection Dataset: The Ozone Level Detection dataset consists of ground-level ozone concentration observations spanning a period of six years. The primary objective of this dataset is to predict whether a given day is classified as an "ozone day".

We utilize the dataset to compose time series data and conduct clustering, calculating the NMI metric. Subsequently, we apply equidistant transformations to the K and T parameters and employ our method to process the dataset. We then perform clustering again and obtain the NMI metric. The ultimate comparison results are presented in the Table 2.

The table shows the changes in the clustering effect of the dataset before and after using our method. From the data in the table, it can be seen that the clustering effect has been improved for almost all parameters K and T. Moreover, in most cases, the NMI index has been improved by more than 30%.

4.2 Experiments on Medical Dataset

The method was tested using the K-means algorithm on a medical dataset without labels. The Sum of Squares Error (SSE) metric was used to compare the results before and after applying the method.

People's Hospital Dataset: Medical analysis was conducted to observe whether the final clustering results have medical significance, with subsequent elucidation. According to the definition of sepsis, which refers to a life-threatening organ dysfunction caused by a dysregulated host response to infection, three groups of variables were selected as clustering variables for analysis. These groups include infection indicators, organ function indicators, and basic vital signs. In total, 17 clinical variables were included.

The selected variables encompass a range of clinical measurements, including heart rate (HR), respiratory rate (RR), mean arterial pressure (MAP), temperature (T), white blood cell count (WBC), and others. These variables provide insights into the patient's physiological responses, infection status, and organ function.

By incorporating these variables into the analysis, researchers aim to gain a deeper understanding of the clustering patterns and potential subtypes within sepsis. This comprehensive approach allows for a more comprehensive assessment of the clinical presentation and progression of sepsis, ultimately contributing to improved diagnosis and management strategies. Based on medical knowledge of sepsis, we selected various medical indicators at 15 time points (1, 2, 3, 4, 5, 6, 8, 10, 12, 14, 16, 18, 20, 22, and 24 h) for each patient as temporal data in this study.

To begin with, we need to determine the optimal number of clusters for clustering. We consider the following factors:

1. Avoiding excessive number of clusters: We aim to have a reasonable number of clusters to ensure meaningful groupings without creating an unnecessarily large number of categories.

Table 1. Comparison of clustering effect before and after using our method on EEG Eye State dataset

	K	T	NMI	(After-Before)/Before
Before			0.0063	
After	K = 1	0.3	0.008964	42.29%
		0.6	0.008964	42.29%
		0.9	0.008964	42.29%
		1.2	0.009993	58.62%
		1.5	0.008009	27.13%
		1.8	0.011343	80.05%
	K = 2	0.3	0.008964	42.29%
		0.6	0.009993	58.62%
		0.9	0.009993	58.62%
		1.2	0.009993	58.62%
		1.5	0.009993	58.62%
		1.8	0.009993	58.62%
	K = 3	0.3	0.009993	58.62%
		0.6	0.009993	58.62%
		0.9	0.009993	58.62%
		1.2	0.011097	76.14%
		1.5	0.011097	76.14%
		1.8	0.012518	98.70%
	K = 4	0.3	0.011343	80.05%
		0.6	0.009993	58.62%
		0.9	0.009993	58.62%
		1.2	0.011343	80.05%
		1.5	0.012518	98.70%
		1.8	0.0105	66.67%
	K = 5	0.3	0.011343	80.05%
		0.6	0.011343	80.05%
		0.9	0.012518	98.70%
		1.2	0.009739	54.59%
		1.5	0.014228	125.84%
		1.8	0.009993	58.62%

2. Identifying the elbow point in the SSE metric: We analyze the SSE values for different cluster numbers and look for a point where the SSE decreases significantly, indicating that additional clusters may not contribute significantly to the overall clustering quality.

Table 2. Comparison of clustering effect before and after using our method on the Ozone Level Detection dataset

	K	T	NMI	(After-Before)/Before
Before			0.068567	
After	K = 1	0.3	0.087175	27.14%
		0.0	0.092893	35.48%
		0.9	0.098715	43.97%
		1.2	0.090965	32.67%
		1.5	0.090965	32.67%
		1.8	0.092893	35.48%
	K = 2	0.3	0.082015	19.61%
		0.6	0.096756	41.11%
		0.9	0.09881	44.11%
		1.2	0.082015	19.61%
		1.5	0.107228	56.38%
		1.8	0.100696	46.86%
	K = 3	0.3	0.08906	29.89%
		0.6	0.107228	56.38%
		0.9	0.108838	58.73%
		1.2	0.121913	77.80%
		1.5	0.102698	49.78%
		1.8	0.096756	41.11%
	K = 4	0.3	0.094818	38.29%
		0.6	0.109261	59.35%
		0.9	0.115652	68.67%
		1.2	0.099519	45.14%
		1.5	0.091502	33.45%
		1.8	0.073079	6.58%
	K = 5	0.3	0.098715	43.97%
		0.6	0.100829	47.05%
		0.9	0.109146	59.18%
		1.2	0.087638	27.81%
		1.5	0.08906	29.89%
		1.8	0.061176	−10.78%

Table 3. Comparison of clustering effect before and after using our method on the People's Hospital dataset

	SSE	(After-Before)/Before
Before	22.707	
After	15.249	−32.84%

3. Ensuring an adequate number of instances in each cluster: We aim to avoid having clusters with too few instances, as this can lead to unreliable or inconclusive results. Having a balanced distribution of instances across clusters helps ensure meaningful and robust clustering outcomes.

By considering these factors, we can determine the optimal number of clusters for our clustering analysis. Figure 3 describes the trend of SSE changes. We can see from it that there is an inflection point in the change of SSE when it is divided into three categories. In the case of clustering with three clusters, we conducted comparative experiments. The Table 3 illustrates the significant reduction in SSE before and after applying our clustering method, demonstrating its effectiveness. Based on the features of the three patient subtypes resulting from our clustering, we further analyze the medical interpretations of the patients as follows:

– Type A: This subtype exhibits relatively stable vital signs and organ function.
– Type B: This subtype shows prominent inflammatory response, characterized by high body temperature, rapid heart rate, and fast respiratory rate.
– Type C: This subtype experiences severe organ dysfunction, manifested by deteriorated liver and kidney function, impaired coagulation function, and worsened respiratory function.

The mortality rate is highest in Type C, followed by Type B, while Type A has the lowest mortality rate.

These three subtypes exhibit certain treatment heterogeneity. For all subtypes (A, B, and C), it is necessary to maintain an average arterial pressure of ≥ 65 mmHg in the early stages. Type A patients require adequate fluid resuscitation, whereas Type C patients need restricted fluid resuscitation. Both Type B and Type C patients require early central venous catheter placement.

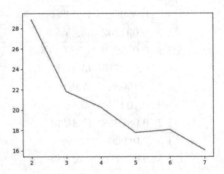

Fig. 3. The trend of the SSE index of clustering as the number of clusters increases.

5   Conclusion

In conclusion, the challenges posed by the complexity of sepsis time series data require innovative approaches to enhance the dataset and improve clustering performance. The proposed physics-based method for manipulating time series datasets offers a promising solution to enhance the robustness and effectiveness of clustering algorithms. By leveraging the principles of physics, this approach provides a unique perspective that improves the quality and reliability of clustering results. Through comprehensive experiments on diverse datasets encompassing both non-medical and medical domains, we have demonstrated the potential of this approach to enhance information extraction, especially in the medical field. Furthermore, we have successfully applied this method to classify sepsis patients and provide valuable medical interpretations, highlighting its practical applicability in the medical domain. Overall, this research contributes to the advancement of time series analysis and offers valuable insights for the effective management of sepsis medical conditions.

References

1. Blekas, K., Lagaris, I.: Newtonian clustering: an approach based on molecular dynamics and global optimization. Pattern Recognit. **40**(6), 1734–1744 (2007). https://doi.org/10.1016/j.patcog.2006.07.012, https://www.sciencedirect.com/science/article/pii/S0031320306003463
2. Fleischmann, C., et al.: Assessment of global incidence and mortality of hospital-treated sepsis. Current estimates and limitations. Am. J. Respir. Crit. Care Med. **193**(3), 259–272 (2016). https://doi.org/10.1164/rccm.201504-0781OC
3. Li, Q., Wang, S., Zhao, C., Zhao, B., Yue, X., Geng, J.: HIBOG: improving the clustering accuracy by ameliorating dataset with gravitation. Inf. Sci. **550**, 41–56 (2021). https://doi.org/10.1016/j.ins.2020.10.046, https://www.sciencedirect.com/science/article/pii/S0020025520310392
4. Mudelsee, M.: Trend analysis of climate time series: a review of methods. Earth-Sci. Rev. **190**, 310–322 (2019)
5. Rakthanmanon, T., et al.: Searching and mining trillions of time series subsequences under dynamic time warping. In: Proceedings of the ACM SIGKDD International Conference on Knowledge Discovery and Data Mining (KDD), pp. 262–270 (2012). https://doi.org/10.1145/2339530.2339576
6. Rehman, O., Al-Busaidi, A.M., Ahmed, S., Ahsan, K.: Ubiquitous healthcare system: architecture, prototype design and experimental evaluations. EAI Endors. Trans. Scalable Inf. Syst. **9**(4) (2022). https://doi.org/10.4108/eai.5-1-2022.172779
7. Rhee, C., et al.: Incidence and trends of sepsis in us hospitals using clinical vs claims data, 2009–2014. JAMA **318**(13), 1241–1249 (2017). https://doi.org/10.1001/jama.2017.13836
8. Rudd, K.E., et al.: Global, regional, and national sepsis incidence and mortality, 1990–2017: analysis for the global burden of disease study. Lancet **395**(10219), 200–211 (2020). https://doi.org/10.1016/S0140-6736(19)32989-7
9. Sarki, R., Ahmed, K., Wang, H., Zhang, Y., Wang, K.: Convolutional neural network for multi-class classification of diabetic eye disease. EAI Endors. Trans. Scalable Inf. Syst. **9**(4) (2021). https://doi.org/10.4108/eai.16-12-2021.172436
10. Seymour, C.W., et al.: Precision medicine for all? Challenges and opportunities for a precision medicine approach to critical illness. Crit. Care **21**(1), 257 (2017). https://doi.org/10.1186/s13054-017-1836-5

11. Shi, Y., Song, Y., Zhang, A.: A shrinking-based clustering approach for multidimensional data. IEEE Trans. Knowl. and Data Eng. **17**(10), 1389–1403 (2005). https://doi.org/10.1109/TKDE.2005.157
12. Siddiqui, S.A., Fatima, N., Ahmad, A.: Chest X-ray and CT scan classification using ensemble learning through transfer learning. EAI Endors. Trans. Scalable Inf. Syst. **9**(6) (2022). https://doi.org/10.4108/eetsis.vi.382
13. Stoffer, D., Ombao, H.: Editorial: special issue on time series analysis in the biological sciences. J. Time Ser. Anal. **33**(5), 701–703 (2012). https://doi.org/10.1111/j.1467-9892.2012.00805.x
14. Schmierer, T., Li, T., Li, Y.: A novel empirical wavelet SODP and spectral entropy based index for assessing the depth of anaesthesia. Health Inf. Sci. Syst. **10**(1), 10 (2022). https://doi.org/10.1007/s13755-022-00178-8
15. Vincent, J.L.: The coming era of precision medicine for intensive care. Crit. Care **21**(Suppl 3), 314 (2017). https://doi.org/10.1186/s13054-017-1910-z
16. Wong, H.R., et al.: Identification of pediatric septic shock subclasses based on genome-wide expression profiling. BMC Med. **7**, 34 (2009). https://doi.org/10.1186/1741-7015-7-34
17. Wong, H.R., et al.: Validation of a gene expression-based subclassification strategy for pediatric septic shock. Crit. Care Med. **39**(11), 2511–2517 (2011). https://doi.org/10.1097/CCM.0b013e3182257675
18. Wong, K.C., Peng, C., Li, Y., Chan, T.M.: Herd clustering: a synergistic data clustering approach using collective intelligence. Appl. Soft Comput. **23**, 61–75 (2014). https://doi.org/10.1016/j.asoc.2014.05.034, https://www.sciencedirect.com/science/article/pii/S1568494614002610
19. Pang, X., Ge, Y.F., Wang, K., Traina, A.J., Wang, H.: Patient assignment optimization in cloud healthcare systems: a distributed genetic algorithm. Health Inf. Sci. Syst. **11**(1), 30 (2023). https://doi.org/10.1007/s13755-023-00230-1
20. Xie, J., et al.: The epidemiology of sepsis in Chinese ICUs: a national cross-sectional survey. Crit. Care Med. **48**(3), e209–e218 (2020). https://doi.org/10.1097/CCM.0000000000004155
21. Zhang, Y., et al.: A heterogeneous multi-modal medical data fusion framework supporting hybrid data exploration. Health Inf. Sci. Syst. **10**(1), 22 (2022). https://doi.org/10.1007/s13755-022-00183-x

Multi-modal Medical Data Exploration Based on Data Lake

Tao Zhao[1], Nan Hai[2(✉)], Wenyao Li[2], Wenkui Zheng[2], Yong Zhang[3], Xin Li[4], and Gao Fei[5]

[1] Shangqiu Institute of Technology, Shangqiu 476000, China
zhaotao123666@163.com
[2] School of Software, Henan University, Kaifeng 475004, China
dgfzz0602@163.com, lwymuelsyse@gmail.com, zhengwenkui@126.com
[3] BNRist, DCST, RIIT, Tsinghua University, Beijing 100084, China
zhangyong05@tsinghua.edu.cn
[4] Beijing Tsinghua Changgung Hospital, School of Clinical Medicine,
Tsinghua University, Beijing 100084, China
Horsebackdancing@sina.com
[5] Henan Justice Police Vocational College, Zhengzhou 450018, China
heracles113@126.com

Abstract. In the field of medicine, the rapid increase of medical devices has generated a substantial volume of multi-modal data, encompassing structured, semi-structured, and unstructured formats. Data fusion and exploration are crucial to enable medical professionals to integrate and locate specific datasets efficiently. However, traditional relational databases exhibit poor query performance when dealing with large-scale data, and data warehouse platforms struggle to effectively integrate diverse and comprehensive multi-source heterogeneous medical data while maintaining efficiency. This paper proposes a distributed computing and storage strategy based on Data Lake technology to address these challenges. The data lake platform offers a solution for storing and integrating multi-modal data from various sources and powerful data exploration capabilities that facilitate the rapid identification of desired datasets. Experimental results indicate that data lake technology outperforms traditional relational databases, significantly reducing storage space requirements and query processing time. As a result, it enables the rapid processing of large-scale medical data, demonstrating excellent performance in medical data management and analysis tasks.

Keywords: Multi-modal data · Federated query · Data exploration · Data lake

1 Introduction

With the rapid advancement of information technology, most hospitals and medical institutions have undergone large-scale digitization. However, medical data exists in various types and structures due to the need for a unified standard for information systems across these institutions, which includes structured data stored in databases such as MySQL, Oracle, and SQL Server, semi-structured data in formats such as CSV, JSON, and XML, as well as unstructured data such as EMRs, ECGs and CTs [1]. The diverse data sources, originating from hospital information systems, imaging systems, and biosensors, contribute to the complexity and challenges associated with processing and analyzing the data. However, the use of data exploration techniques on this data can go a long way in assisting physicians to make accurate medical decisions [2,3]. According to healthcare research, imaging data generated in modern hospital environments can reach hundreds of terabytes [4]. Query operations are often required to extract relevant information from these datasets efficiently. Consequently, this paper aims to explore efficient methods for processing and analyzing large-scale medical data [5].

The Join operation is a fundamental operation that combines data from multiple tables into a single result dataset. It allows for more complex data analysis by providing consolidated information from various tables. However, the Join operation may impact query performance, especially when dealing with large datasets. Joining such datasets may require more computation time and system resources to complete the operation effectively.

Traditional databases and data warehouses have limitations and shortcomings when handling large-scale data queries. These limitations include performance constraints due to hardware resources, data scale, and restricted query functionality. In managing a vast amount of multi-source heterogeneous medical data, the key challenge lies in establishing an efficient method for obtaining, storing, and providing unified management [6]. Databases play a crucial role in early medical data management, offering capabilities for fast insertion, deletion, and querying of smaller datasets. However, when it comes to tasks involving the retrieval of significant amounts of data, database technology falls short in handling complex and multi-table join queries. While traditional data warehouses can address scalability and data fragmentation issues, the associated costs can be prohibitively high. Moreover, the existing data storage approaches are inadequate for efficient joint queries [7].

Contributions. In order to optimize the joint query problem of multi-modal data, this paper proposes a solution based on data lake technology applied to medical data management. Based on this solution, our contributions are summarized as follows:

1. This paper presents a solution that leverages data lake for medical data management through distributed computing and storage strategies.
2. Utilizing various open-source softwares, we successfully integrate multi-modal data, transform it into a unified data model, and store data within data Lake. This approach enables efficient exploration of medical data.

The rest of this paper is organized as follows. Section 2 describes the related work. Section 3 gives the functional structure of the data lake platform. Section 4 shows the storage of data. Section 5 shows the experiments and results analysis. Section 6 summarizes the paper and indicates future research directions.

2   Related Work

Given the diverse sources of data, mixed queries are common in the medical field. Ren et al. [8] proposed an efficient framework for fusing heterogeneous medical data, converting structured and unstructured data into a unified format. They also introduced a dynamic index management strategy for unstructured data, offering enhanced convenience for users conducting mixed queries. Meriem Amina Zingla et al. [9] proposed a hybrid query extension model that explores incorporating external resources into association rule mining. This approach improves the generation and selection of extension items. Joint queries involving medical data enable doctors and researchers to simultaneously query and analyze data from multiple sources, thus facilitating more informed clinical, research, and management decisions.

Ding et al. [10] presented a distributed migration storage and computation method for medical data. They utilized Sqoop to migrate data to a Hadoop cluster and optimized queries by partitioning data tables using converted file storage structures. Additionally, some researchers have introduced a hybrid query framework that leverages original vocabulary resources and embedded information related to question-and-answer processes [11]. However, in the field of mixed query research, these studies alone are still insufficient. Through joint queries, they verified that column data has better efficiency when the amount of data is large.

To harness the vast amount of medical data effectively, medical institutions require a centralized, unified data platform for querying and analyzing. This need has given rise to the development of data warehouses. Begoli et al. [12] discussed the implementation of data warehouses in biomedical research and health data analysis, highlighting some unique and innovative features. Farooqui et al. [13] proposed a method for constructing a medical information system data warehouse using data mining technology and presented a clinical data warehouse model based on data mining techniques. This system serves as a repository for storing medical information. Neamah et al. [14] utilized data warehouse technology to enhance performance in electronic health technology.

Zhang et al. [15] introduced a framework based on data lake technology to facilitate the fusion of multi-modal medical data and hybrid data exploration. Dynamic methods are employed to establish and manage indexes for these diverse data sources, effectively managing multi-modal data. Ren et al. [16] proposed an efficient multi-source heterogeneous data lake platform to handle such data efficiently. This platform ensures persistent storage of different types and sources of data, maintains data source traceability, and implements methods for fusing multi-source heterogeneous data and efficient data querying strategies.

3   Architecture Design

Our system is built on a heterogeneous medical data fusion framework (HMDFF) that supports multi-modal queries. It utilizes Apache Hudi as the data lake platform and Apache Spark as the computational engine. Based on this framework, we propose a multi-modal data fusion query optimization strategy based on Apache Hudi to improve the performance of the multi-modal query layer. In this section, we present the key system design.

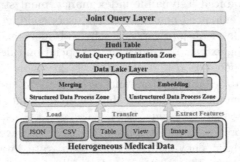

Fig. 1. System architecture overview

3.1   Architecture Overview

The architecture of the system is shown in Fig. 1. It comprises four modules: the joint query optimization zone, the structured data process zone, the unstructured data process zone, the joint query layer. The data is transformed into DataFrame for structured and semi-structured data, and the merged dataset is stored as a Hudi table by the Hudi engine. The Hudi table is partitioned into multiple data partitions, each containing various files. This approach enhances data read and write performance while facilitating data management and maintenance. When querying data, the Spark SQL API can be utilized along with Spark's Hudi data source to retrieve data from the Hudi table. In the unstructured data processing zone, feature vectors are extracted from unstructured data with pre-trained deep learning model, and these vectors are converted into columns within the DataFrame.

4   Data Migration and Optimization Method

As a persistent data storage system, HDFS provides underlying storage support for large-scale data processing and analysis. As a cluster computing system, Spark provides a comprehensive interface for accessing and managing structured and semi-structured data. Our big data platform has integrated Hudi as a data management framework to generate high-quality data with a unified data model. By utilizing the cluster computing capabilities of Spark, our platform enables the fusion of multi-modal data while also delivering efficient data federation query capabilities.

4.1 Data Migration

For structured and semi-structured data such as CSV files and JSON files, Spark can read them from the database. However, for unstructured data, different feature vectors are generated using different embedding models according to the requirements, and the information, such as the address and size of the original data, is stored in a structured manner.

Spark provides a data structure Dataframe with rows and columns, different data types can be accommodated. Hudi framework provides a distributed table based on columnar storage Hudi Table, which has advanced features such as data partitioning and indexing; these features can improve data query and access speed, reduce the overhead of data scanning, and support more efficient data processing and analysis. DataFrame and Hudi Table can be converted to each other by Spark DataSource API. This provides a more flexible means of data processing and management for Hudi. The process is shown in Fig. 2.

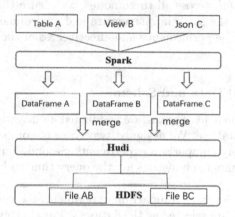

Fig. 2. Data migration process.

4.2 Data Exploration and Optimization Scheme

Hudi adopts the Parquet format, which offers several advantages: First, columnar storage, which is a data storage method that stores the data of each column separately. This method can improve query efficiency because only the required columns need to be read during queries, rather than reading the entire row of data. Second, parquet file supports multiple compression encoding methods. Using special compression encoding methods can reduce file storage space and disk I/O, thus improving data read and write speed.

We can find that tables with a large amount of data have two characteristics: First, the number of columns is fixed, but the number of rows far exceeds the number of columns; secondly, a table containing a large amount of data has billions of rows, but the value of a column is hundreds of fixed values. We choose COW tables to store data. To ensure the uniqueness of the data, we have designed a method to generate a unique UUID. Data partitioning is a commonly used data grouping method. If there are no suitable columns in the table, we have designed a UDF function to achieve controllable setting of the number of data partitions.

5   Experiment and Analysis

5.1   Experimental Environment

To ensure fairness and consistency in our experimental environment, we have set up a cluster comprising three nodes with identical hardware and software configurations. Each node is equipped with an Intel Gen X 16-core processor and 16GB of RAM. In addition, we can leverage the scalability and parallel processing capabilities of the distributed PostgreSQL database. By adopting this consistent configuration across all three nodes, we ensure that our experiments are conducted under the same infrastructure and environment. This allows for a fair comparison of the performance and effectiveness of the methods proposed in this paper.

5.2   Experimental Data and Scheme

During research in the field of sepsis, we conducted an investigation and analysis of the MIMIC-IV database. We designed two types of comparison experiments: first, single-table query comparison experiments. Second, multi-table join query. The experimental comparison metrics are the query time and the amount of data read.

For the single-table query comparison experiment, the chartevents table and the inputevents table are selected as the datasets. The chartevents table contains 329,499,789 rows of data, with a storage size of 27.8 GB in text format. The labevents table, on the other hand, has 123,715,424 rows of data, with a storage size of 12.8 GB in text format. To highlight the approach of porting the data to the data lake with improved query efficiency, the comparison is conducted using three dimensions: distributed PostgreSQL, Hudi with no partitioning, and Hudi with set partitioning. Table 1 presents the list of query statements for both PostgreSQL and Hudi.

For the purpose of data exploration through federated queries based on Data Lake, we designed two groups of experiments. First, we select the chartevents table and the inputevents table as the two datasets for the joint query. Considering the huge amount of data after joining and the performance of our cluster, we select 1,000,000 rows of data from each of these two tables. They are respectively denoted as chartevents_1M and inputevents_1M. Secondly, we select the chartevents table with complete data and the erqi_fanganyi table for the join

Table 1. List of executed queries.

Query No.	Query
Q1	Select * from chartevents;
Q2	Select hadm_id from chartevents;
Q3	Select * from labevents;
Q4	Select hadm_id from labevents;

query. The three dimensions are compared in distributed PostgreSQL, the join function in Spark, and our method. The query schema and data volume are shown in Table 2.

Table 2. Query scheme and data volume.

Experimental No.	Datasets	Amount of data after join
S1	chartevents_1M, inputevents_1M	534,152,359
S2	chartevents, erqi_fanganyi	45,471,544

5.3 Experimental Results and Analysis

Whether a single table query or a federated query, each query is executed three times, and the average execution time is calculated as the experimental result. The final results are shown in Table 3, Table 4, Fig. 3, Fig. 4.

Table 3. Execution time (min) using different methods of Single Table

Query No.	Distributed PG	Hudi no partition	Hudi partition
Q1	26.2	8.6	3.6
Q2	20.3	7.5	3.0
Q3	8.6	3.2	2.5
Q4	6.5	2.2	1.4

As shown in Table 3, with distributed PostgreSQL, the average execution time of Q1 is 26.2 min, if Hudi Table is not partitioned, its query time is 8.6 min. However, the query time for Hudi Table is 3.6 min with reasonable partitioning.

As shown in Table 4, the average execution time is 25 min for PostgreSQL, while the average execution time for the join function of Spark and merge operations are 7.55 min and 3.25 min. When the data volume becomes larger, the execution time of the method proposed in this paper will still be shorter than PostgreSQL, and the optimization effect of our proposed in this paper will be better.

Table 4. Execution time (min) using different methods of joint query

Experimental No.	PostgreSQL	Join	Merge
S1	44	12.6	5.3
S2	6	2.5	1.2
Average	25	7.55	3.25

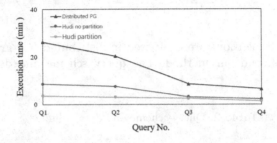

Fig. 3. Time consuming comparison of different methods of single table.

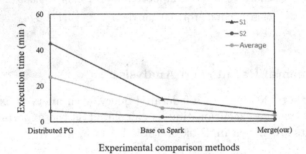

Fig. 4. Time consuming comparison of different methods of joint query.

As depicted in Fig. 4, regardless of the data volume, the joint query performed after the fusion of multiple tables consistently exhibited superior query efficiency. Spark, with its parallel computing capabilities, plays a crucial role in the data lake platform. During the querying process, the query engine assigns the query task to various nodes, enabling parallel processing of data within each block. Additionally, when data is written to the Hudi Table, it is partitioned to optimize query performance. Consequently, the query efficiency achieved by the data lake platform is significantly higher than PostgreSQL when executing identical queries.

The reason why data lake can quickly meet the query requirements of large-scale data is that it can store massive data and support parallel processing. Based on this advantage, querying large-scale data in the data lake will save more time than PostgreSQL. On the one hand, the reason is that our data format is a columnar storage database that stores and retrieves data in a column-by-column manner, unlike row storage. It means that columnar storage has higher scanning efficiency for large amounts of data. In contrast, row storage requires scanning the entire row to obtain the required data, making it slower to process large amounts of data. On the other hand, we partition sepsis-related tables to reduce datasets, and improve query speed and performance.

6   Conclusion and Future Work

In this paper, we leverage multiple open-source big data frameworks to transform multi-modal medical data into a unified data model, enabling migration to data Lake for distributed storage and querying. By merging and storing the data in the data lake, we have achieved the optimization of multi-table federated queries. Moving forward, our future work will focus on enhancing the data layout approach during data writing to the Hudi Table and improving its indexing mechanism, aiming to optimize query efficiency further.

Acknowledgements. This work was supported by National Key R&D Program of China (No.2020AAA0109603), National Natural Science Foundation of China (No.62202332), Diversified Investment Foundation of Tianjin (No.21JCQNJC00980) and key funding from National Natural Science Foundation of China (No.92067206)

References

1. Li, T.: Enabling precision medicine by integrating multi-modal biomedical data. Georgia Institute of Technology, Atlanta, GA, USA (2021)
2. Pandey, D., Wang, H., Yin, X., Wang, K., Zhang, Y., Shen, J.: Automatic breast lesion segmentation in phase preserved DCE-MRIS. Health Inf. Sci. Syst. **10**(1), 9 (2022)
3. Pan, L., et al.: MFDNN: multi-channel feature deep neural network algorithm to identify covid19 chest x-ray images. Health Inf. Sci. Syst. **10**(1), 4 (2022)
4. Xiao, Q., et al.: MHDML: construction of a medical lakehouse for multi-source heterogeneous data. In: Traina, A., Wang, H., Zhang, Y., Siuly, S., Zhou, R., Chen, L. (eds.) HIS 2022. LNCS, vol. 13705, pp. 127–135. Springer, Cham (2022). https://doi.org/10.1007/978-3-031-20627-6_12
5. Mesterhazy, J., Olson, G., Datta, S.: High performance on-demand de-identification of a petabyte-scale medical imaging data lake. arXiv preprint arXiv:2008.01827 (2020)
6. Faludi, B., Zoller, E.I., Gerig, N., Zam, A., Rauter, G., Cattin, P.C.: Direct visual and haptic volume rendering of medical data sets for an immersive exploration in virtual reality. In: Shen, D., et al. (eds.) MICCAI 2019. LNCS, vol. 11768, pp. 29–37. Springer, Cham (2019). https://doi.org/10.1007/978-3-030-32254-0_4
7. Kalkman, S., Mostert, M., Udo-Beauvisage, N., Van Delden, J., Van Thiel, G.: Responsible data sharing in a big data-driven translational research platform: lessons learned. BMC Med. Inform. Decis. Mak. **19**(1), 1–7 (2019)
8. Ren, P., et al.: HMDFF: a heterogeneous medical data fusion framework supporting multimodal query. In: Siuly, S., Wang, H., Chen, L., Guo, Y., Xing, C. (eds.) HIS 2021. LNCS, vol. 13079, pp. 254–266. Springer, Cham (2021). https://doi.org/10.1007/978-3-030-90885-0_23

9. Zingla, M.A., Latiri, C., Mulhem, P., Berrut, C., Slimani, Y.: Hybrid query expansion model for text and microblog information retrieval. Inf. Retrieval J. **21**, 337–367 (2018)
10. Ding, S., Mao, C., Zheng, W., Xiao, Q., Wu, Y.: Data exploration optimization for medical big data. In: Traina, A., Wang, H., Zhang, Y., Siuly, S., Zhou, R., Chen, L. (eds.) HIS 2022. LNCS, vol. 13705, pp. 145–156. Springer, Cham (2022). https://doi.org/10.1007/978-3-031-20627-6_14
11. Esposito, M., Damiano, E., Minutolo, A., De Pietro, G., Fujita, H.: Hybrid query expansion using lexical resources and word embeddings for sentence retrieval in question answering. Inf. Sci. **514**, 88–105 (2020)
12. Begoli, E., Goethert, I., Knight, K.: A lakehouse architecture for the management and analysis of heterogeneous data for biomedical research and mega-biobanks. In: 2021 IEEE International Conference on Big Data (Big Data), pp. 4643–4651. IEEE (2021)
13. Farooqui, N.A., Mehra, R.: Design of a data warehouse for medical information system using data mining techniques. In: 2018 Fifth International Conference on Parallel, Distributed and Grid Computing (PDGC), pp. 199–203. IEEE (2018)
14. Neamah, A.F.: Flexible data warehouse: towards building an integrated electronic health record architecture. In: 2020 International Conference on Smart Electronics and Communication (ICOSEC), pp. 1038–1042. IEEE (2020)
15. Zhang, Y., et al.: A heterogeneous multi-modal medical data fusion framework supporting hybrid data exploration. Health Inf. Sci. Syst. **10**(1), 22 (2022)
16. Ren, P., et al.: MHDP: an efficient data lake platform for medical multi-source heterogeneous data. In: Xing, C., Fu, X., Zhang, Y., Zhang, G., Borjigin, C. (eds.) WISA 2021. LNCS, vol. 12999, pp. 727–738. Springer, Cham (2021). https://doi.org/10.1007/978-3-030-87571-8_63

Multi-model Transfer Learning and Genotypic Analysis for Seizure Type Classification

Yue Yang[1], Kairui Guo[1], Zhen Fang[1], Hua Lin[2], Mark Grosser[2], and Jie Lu[1(✉)]

[1] Faculty of Engineering and IT University of Technology Sydney, Sydney, NSW, Australia
yue.yang-4@student.uts.edu.au, {Kairui.guo,zhen.fang,Jie.Lu}@uts.edu.au
[2] 23Strands, Suite 107, 26-32 Pirrama Rd, Pyrmont NSW 2009, Sydney, Australia
{hua.lin,mark.grosser}@23strands.com

Abstract. The recent progress in phenotypic information and machine learning has led to a remarkable development in the accuracy of binary seizure detection. Yet the performance of classifying specific seizure types remains suboptimal due to the limited availability of annotated data with accurate seizure type labels. Transfer learning is promising to mitigate data scarcity to improve classification accuracy on smaller datasets. However, finding the best transferable model based on the specific training and testing dataset can be a complex and repetitive process, and a single-modelled approach may not fully capture the best feature representation of the input data. Moreover, genotypic data is often neglected in previous AI-based seizure detection studies, where analyses like Polygenic Risk Scores (PRS) could offer insights into genetic predispositions to seizures. To mitigate these challenges, we propose a seizure-type classification framework incorporating a multi-model weighting system designed to assign weights to different models, thus reducing computational complexity and processing time. In addition, we carry out a PRS analysis, aiming to bridge the gap between genotypic and phenotypic data, further enhancing the comprehensiveness and precision of seizure detection. Our model outperformed similar classifiers by more than 13–16% on the Temple University Hospital EEG Seizure Corpus dataset. This study represents a pioneering examination of the multi-source transfer learning framework in the field of type-specific seizure classification.

Keywords: Genomics · Transfer learning · Machine learning · Seizure genetic

1 Introduction

Seizure, a manifestation of abnormal brain activity, is one condition that demands immediate detection for effective management. Electroencephalogram (EEG), a form of phenotypic data, is commonly employed for this purpose.

Y. Li et al. (Eds.): HIS 2023, LNCS 14305, pp. 223–234, 2023.
https://doi.org/10.1007/978-981-99-7108-4_19

Since the 1970s, artificial intelligence (AI) has substantially explored the connection between biomedical traits and phenotypes, notably exemplified by the development of automated seizure detection (ASD). Despite the recent progress in the detection accuracy of standard ASD, difficulties such as detecting the specific seizure type due to the limitation of data availability and the labelling issue remain to be solved [9]. To mitigate this, a variety of strategies such as Deep Learning and Riemann geometry have been introduced for the phenotypic study of seizure traits [15]. However, conventional methodologies presume that the training and testing datasets are derived from a uniform distribution, which might not hold true in real-world conditions. Furthermore, due to limitations in data collection and labelling processes like time, ethical considerations, and cost constraints, acquiring source data or target labels sufficient for deep learning algorithms often poses a challenge in seizure trait studies, leading to potential issues of overfitting and sampling bias.

To mitigate this problem, transfer learning can be a suitable solution. It involves leveraging knowledge and models obtained from a source domain to improve performance in a related but distinct target domain [7]. Several transfer learning methods, such as semi-supervised [5] and model-based transfer learning [8], have been investigated in phenotypic seizure classification to mitigate the data scarcity problem. However, in single-model-based seizure classification, due to the necessity of processing such massive labelled data, the computing complexity and time of finding the best transferable model may be tremendously high, and the process can be highly repetitive. Thus, using a multi-model network allows the system to capture multiple aspects of the input data and make more informed predictions. Therefore, researchers have focused on a practical problem known as multi-source domain adaptation [3]. This study explores the possibility of transferring knowledge from multiple source domains to a target domain. Based on this idea, we propose a framework wherein multiple pre-trained source models can be transferred and accessed simultaneously.

Moreover, the historical focus of AI research in seizures has predominantly utilized phenotypic data, with genotypic information often overlooked. This constraint can be attributed to the inherent complexity and interpretive challenges posed by genomic data. Yet, the recent advancements in genomic analysis tools have enabled a more profound exploration into the genetic aspects of seizures. One such genomic tool is the Polygenic Risk Score (PRS), which aggregates the effects of genetic variants to estimate an individual's genetic susceptibility to a particular trait or condition [1]. While phenotypic data like EEG recordings capture the manifestations of seizures, the integration of genotypic data and tools, such as PRS offers a genetically informed probability that may predispose an individual to these conditions. Consequently, integrating genotypic data and PRS into AI research on seizures could significantly augment predictive accuracy and enable the development of more personalized treatment strategies. As such, our study aims to fill this gap by proposing a novel framework that integrates AI models with PRS for enriched and more precise seizure detection,

In light of this, the present paper introduces a novel multi-model framework that employs ten pre-trained transferable models. Our approach aims to capture and integrate transferable knowledge from multiple sources, thereby enhancing the prediction accuracy in the target domain. To complement phenotypic data with genotypic information, we incorporate a PRS analysis, designed to bridge the genotype-phenotype divide in seizure detection. To validate the performance of the proposed algorithm, we conduct extensive experiments on the largest publicly available dataset on seizure EEG, the Temple University Hospital EEG Corpus [11]. By combining AI and polygenic analysis, our study strives to push the boundaries of current seizure detection methods, offering a more integrated and precise approach to diagnosing this complex neurological condition.

The contributions of this paper are summarized as follows:

- A multi-model-based transfer learning approach was applied to capture transferable information to enhance the performance of the seizure classification performance. To our best knowledge, this study represents a pioneering examination of the multi-source domain adaptation in the field of type-specific seizure classification.
  A novel self-attention (SA) mechanism was designed to assign weight to each model, picking up the key information extracted from different models. The classifier developed using the combination of pre-trained networks outperformed other machine-learning-based classifiers.
- As an innovative approach to enriching phenotypic data with genotypic information, we incorporated PRS analysis into seizure detection, bridging the genotype-phenotype divide.

This manuscript is organized as follows. Section 2 reviewed the related work in automated seizure classification, transfer learning, and SA mechanism. Section 3 explained the feature extraction, multi-model system, and PRS methods. Next, Sect. 4 described the dataset, baseline model, and the results of our classifiers. The clinical applications and significance were also discussed in Sect. 5. Lastly, a conclusion of this work was drawn in Sect. 6.

2   Related Work

The following areas need to be studied to establish the multi-model seizure classification system: automated seizure classification, transfer learning of convolutional neural networks, and SA mechanism.

2.1   Automated Seizure Classification

Generalized seizures include absence, myoclonic, tonic, clonic, tonic-clonic, and atonic. In clinical practice, trained individuals evaluate phenotypic and clinical information to identify seizure types. With the development of AI, the application of ASD in medical fields has had significant success. The majority of ASD applications focus on tonic-clonic seizures, and the classifiers' outputs are either binary (normal, ictal), or three-class (normal, interictal, ictal stages). Despite reaching 95%–100% accuracy in these scenarios, several issues still need to be solved before clinical deployment. First, a specific type is needed after detecting seizures' start and end times. Knowing the seizure type is the first step of personalized healthcare [9]. Second, the complexity, redundancy and significance of the phenotypic features need to be considered, especially in real-world applications. More importantly, the limited publicly available datasets with a relatively small number of participants pose the issue of poor performance for deep learning algorithms. Each step of the automated seizure type classification must be carefully designed to overcome these issues.

2.2 Transfer Learning of Convolutional Neural Network

Recently, Convolutional Neural Networks (CNN) have demonstrated remarkable outcomes in seizure classification. Several studies have applied transfer learning on CNN to mitigate the distribution difference between the source and target domains of the seizure phenotypic data [4]. Yang et al. [16] applied large-margin projection combined with Maximum Mean Discrepancy to identify essential knowledge between the source and target domains, resulting in better performance in seizure detection using EEG signals as the phenotypic data. Furthermore, Jiang et al. [5]adapted domain adaptation with the Takagi-Sugeno-Kang fuzzy system as the base classifier. The result showed higher classification accuracy. From the model-based transfer learning perspective, Raghu et al. [8] transferred 10 pre-trained CNN models separately with fine-tuning, among which GoogleNet yielded the highest classification accuracy of 82.85%. However, for such single-model-based studies, finding the best model can be highly complex and time-consuming. Using a multi-model network allows the system to capture multiple aspects of the input data and make more informed predictions. As this paper presents the first study using deep learning for the classification of multi-class seizure type, our framework was compared with this approach in the result section.

2.3 Self-attention Mechanism

The concept of SA was initially introduced in the research by [14] and applied in machine translation. It aimed to capture global input dependencies. In recent years, it has been applied to the field of seizure classification. Tao et al. [13] used SA to model long-range dependencies in the phenotypic information and to weigh the importance of each feature for classification, achieving improved performance compared to traditional CNNs. Choi et al. [2] combined SA with a bidirectional gated recurrent unit network for seizure classification. The authors found that the SA mechanism improved the ability of the model to identify important features in the input signals, leading to improved classification performance. These studies proved that the SA mechanism has the potential to capture the complex and dynamic patterns of EEG as the phenotypic data in deep learning models. Inspired by this, we applied the SA mechanism to look for critical information in multi-model transfer learning.

3   Proposed Methodology

In this section, we introduce the methodology employed in this study, which involves pre-processing and feature extraction of the phenotypic data, the implementation of a multi-model weighting system and the calculation of the PRS.

3.1   Phenotypic Analysis: Pre-processing and Connectivity Analysis

Due to its exceptional ability to capture real-time brain activity, EEG signal is selected as the phenotypic data utilized for seizure-type classification in our proposed framework. The raw data from the Temple University Hospital EEG Seizure Corpus underwent a sequence of pre-processing stages, including bandpass filtering and segmentation of seizure and non-seizure events. We also reduced the number of channels to optimize the performance of our deep learning systems, employing both four (T3, F7), (C3, Cz), (O2, P4), (Fp2, F8) and eight-channel strategies (T3, T5), (F8, T4), (T4, T6), (P3, O1), following the findings by Shah [10]. As a key part of the data transformation, we implemented effective connectivity to generate image-based features for the classifiers. For this, we used Multivariate Auto-Regressive models and linear Kalman filtering method. The pre-processed recordings were treated as univariate time series, with consecutive measurements modeled as a weighted linear sum of their previous values. This approach was extended to multivariate time series in the Multivariate Auto-Regressive models. The model order, p, was determined using the Bayesian-Schwartz's criterion:

$$SC(p) = ln[det(V)] + \frac{ln(N) * p * n^2}{N} \tag{1}$$

where V is the noise covariance matrix, and N is the total number of the data. n indicates the number of channels. The normalized Directed Transfer Function (DTF) represents the ratio between the inflow from the source channel to the destination channel to the sum of all inflows to this channel. The value of the normalized DTF is from 0 to 1, where 0 means no influence and 1 means the maximum influence. The calculation is shown as follows:

$$\gamma_{ij}^2(\lambda) = \frac{(|H_{ij}^2(\lambda)|^2)}{\sum_{m=1}^{n}(|H_{im}^2(\lambda)|^2)} \tag{2}$$

where i is the destination channel and j is the source channel that is used to calculate the influences compared with the total influence from all channels for both direct and indirect flows. To distinguish between the direct and indirect transmissions, Partial Directed Coherence (PDC) is utilized to show the direct relations only in the frequency domain. It is defined as:

$$\pi_{ij}^2(\lambda) = \frac{(|A_{ij}^2(\lambda)|^2)}{\sum_{m=1}^{n}(|A_{im}^2(\lambda)|^2)} \tag{3}$$

This function describes the ratio between outflows from channel j to channel i to all the outflows from channel j. In this project, PDC and DTF were computed with the idea of a short-term 1-second window and 25% overlap to address the immediate direct dynamic frequency domain link between the various time series and expose the links from one time series to another regardless of the influence pathway.

3.2 Multi-model Weighting System

A multi-model weighting system is designed to investigate the contribution of the extracted feature from each model. We introduce it at the end of the output layer of the pre-trained models. It takes the model's feature embeddings em as input and outputs the weights W of all models based on the contribution of the extracted information. We utilize several paralleled SA mechanisms to capture the relationships between these embeddings from multiple aspects. A multi-attention mechanism is used to concatenate the multi- attention's weight. As the calculated weight ω now has the same dimension as em, a fully connected fc layer is introduced at the end to obtain the vector output W, which has 1 single value representing the weight of each model. The structure of the system is shown in Fig. 1.

The SA mechanism is used in deep learning models that compute a set of attention scores to weigh the importance of different elements when making predictions [14]. Note that unlike the original SA algorithm proposed in [14], the Value Weight is not used in this paper as the main purpose of this system is not to update the original embedding vector, but instead computes and outputs the models' weights. The Query (Q) represents the current model that is being weighted and the Key (K) is the other model (including Q) that is being weighted against. Because multiple paralleled SA mechanisms are used, we introduce a multi-head attention algorithm, shown in Fig. 1 to concatenate the paralleled outputs into 1 linear vector W, which is the final output of the multi-model weighting system. Based on the previous experience from [14], the experiment set $h = 2$.

The dot product of Q and K is then calculated by Eq.(4).

$$S_{qk} = Q * K^T \tag{4}$$

where S_{qk} represents the similarity vector of the current model Q against model K.

The obtained score S is then normalized using SoftMax function:

$$\sigma(S_i) = \frac{e^{S_i}}{\sum_{j=1}^n e^{S_j}} \tag{5}$$

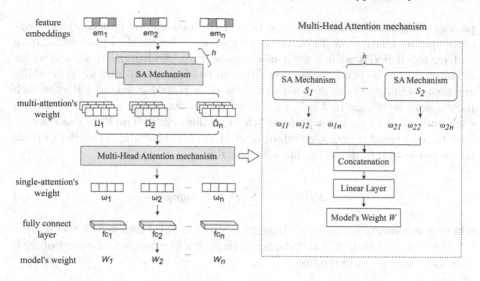

Fig. 1. The multi-model weighting system consists of multiple paralleled SA mechanisms, which compute the multi-attention weight and a multi-head mechanism that outputs the single-attention weight. The structure of the multi-head attention mechanism concatenates the paralleled outputs into one linear vector W is shown on the right. In this study, h was set as 2

where $\sigma(S_i)$ represents the normalized score of the i_{th} model, n is the length of the feature embedding of Q_i. The final output of the SA mechanism ω is then computed by scaling $\sigma(S_i)$ as shown below:

$$\omega(S_i) = \frac{\sigma(S_i)}{\sqrt{d_k}} \tag{6}$$

where d_k is the dimension of the vector K. The final output ω is scaled by the square root of d_k to prevent the attention scores from becoming too large and overwhelming the other components of the model.

3.3   Genotypic Analysis: PRS Calculation

Our seizure-type classification framework integrates genotypic data through a PRS analysis. In this study, we focused on 29 Single Nucleotide Polymorphisms (SNPs) derived from the NHGRI-EBI GWAS Catalog [12]. Linkage disequilibrium metrics (0.4, 0.6, 0.8) and significance thresholds ($Pvalue = 0.5, 0.05, 5 \times 10^{-4}$) were employed to further refine this selection. The chosen SNPs were independently significant, presenting low collinearity (< 0.05) and maintaining a distance of more than 2000 kilobases apart. We estimated the squared correlation coefficient (r^2) among these SNPs, utilizing genotype data from the summary statistics to understand their genetic relationship and potential impact on seizure predispositions. These analyses were executed using the PLINK software package, version 1.9. Before proceeding to PRS analysis, we first conducted rigorous quality control checks on the genotype data. We checked for missing data and excluded SNPs with a high missingness rate. Additionally, we tested for deviations from Hardy-Weinberg equilibrium to identify and exclude potentially erroneous genotype calls. Subsequently, we constructed weighted PRS for each participant according to Eq. 7, calculated as the weighted sum of risk alleles, each multiplied by its corresponding trait-specific weight. The PRS was normalized to a mean of 0 and a standard deviation of 1, enabling reporting of odds ratios per standard deviation increase in PRS.

$$PRS(k) = \sum_{j}^{N} \beta_j * dosage_{jk} \qquad (7)$$

where k represents an individual sample, N is the total number of SNPs, β_j is the effect size of variant j and $dosage_{jk}$ indicates the number of copies of SNP j in the genotype of individual k.

4   Experiments

In this section, we introduce the phenotypic and genotypic data used in this study and list the parameter, baseline models and seizure classification results.

4.1   Phenotypic and Genotypic Dataset

The Temple University Hospital EEG Seizure Corpus version 2.0.0 [11] was used as the phenotypic data in this study. It contains EEG data with sampling frequency of 250 Hz, and the standard 10–20 system was used as the sensor placement guideline. Two annotation files were created for each data file to demonstrate the seizure types, channel indices, and the start/end time of seizure events. The seizure types are determined by certified professionals with both phenotypic and clinical information for absence, complex partial, simple partial, tonic-clonic, and tonic seizures, phenotype only for focal non-specific and generalized non-specific seizures. Due to the limited number of phenotypic information for atonic and myoclonic seizures, these two types are excluded from this work. It is worth noting that the clinical information is not provided in the public dataset. The issue of unmatched resources between the neurophysiologists who labelled the seizure events and the proposed framework is further addressed in the classifier design and the clinical significance of this framework.

The genotypic data used in this study was obtained from the Medical Genome Reference Bank [6]. It is a high-quality genomic database comprising sequence data from 4,011 healthy older individuals. This data, stored in the Variant Call Format, provides an industry-standard notation for storing gene sequence variations. Variant Call Format files are an efficient and compact way of storing and sharing genomic data, accommodating from SNPs to large structural variants, along with rich annotations. Additionally, the seizure summary statistics, which provides the association strengths and significances of different genetic variants to seizure incidents, was downloaded from the NHGRI-EBI GWAS Catalog [12].

4.2   Parameter Setup and Baseline Methods

Two classifiers were developed to verify the seizure type classification framework: the three-class (FN, GN and normal) and the six-class (AB, CP, SP, TC, TN and normal). The experiment was conducted using a LR decay with a staring LR of $1e-2$, the batch size was set to 32 and the epoch was set as 50. Based on the result from [8], we selected GoogleNet as the baseline model when running the single-model task. To compare the performance of the phenotypic features, short-time Fourier transform (STFT) [17] was used as the baseline as it is a common imaged-based feature in CNN-related EEG applications.

4.3   Seizure Classification Results

Table 1. three-class seizure type classification results using the single-model and multi-model system, key values are highlighted in bold for emphasis.

Seizure Type	Features	Precision		Recall		F1-score	
		Single model	Multi-model	Single model	Multi-model	Single model	Multi-model
FN	STFT	**0.6906**	0.7810	0.8298	0.8120	0.7562	0.7979
	8-Ch connectivity	0.7969	0.7803	0.8266	0.9510	0.8730	0.8435
	4-Ch connectivity	0.9293	**0.9862**	0.9730	0.9235	0.9177	**0.9561**
GN	STFT	**0.7827**	0.7931	0.6293	0.789	0.6922	0.7888
	8-Ch connectivity	0.8215	0.8893	0.7817	0.7563	0.7961	0.8149
	4-Ch connectivity	0.9385	**0.9282**	0.9293	0.9768	0.9288	**0.9567**
Normal	STFT	1	1	1	1	1	1
	8-Ch connectivity	1	1	1	1	1	1
	4-Ch connectivity	0.9797	0.9802	1	1	0.9843	0.9977

The results indicate that eight out of nine F1-Score pairs showed improved or maintained performance in three-class seizure classification using our multi-model system. It improved FN and GN seizure F1-scores by 3.84% and 2.79% respectively, using 4-channel features. Similarly, 15 out of 18 F1-scores were sustained or boosted in six seizure-type tasks. The optimal feature shown in this experiment is the four-channel connectivity images, presenting 98.62% and 92.82% precision with 0.956 F1-score in Table 1 for both focal and generalized seizures, demonstrating a balanced precision and sensitivity of the classifier. The STFT's performance for tonic seizures in the six-type classifier shows imbalances due to fewer participant numbers, resulting in low sensitivity. Meanwhile, the multi-model approach with four-channel connectivity achieves 100% precision, recall, and F1-score, demonstrating stability even with smaller sample classes. Our method surpasses a similar classifier [8] where tonic seizures had the lowest accuracy. The multi-model approach enhances the F1 score substantially for both STFT and connectivity features. Using ten weighted pre-trained networks, we see an approximately 50% recall increase for STFT, 15% precision rise with eight channels, and around 45% F1-score improvement with four channels. This illustrates that our system effectively uses model-extracted key information, boosting detection performance and robustness (Table 2).

Table 2. six-class seizure type classification results using the single-model and multi-model system, the key improvements and values are highlighted in bold for emphasis.

Seizure Type	Features	Precision		Recall		F1-score	
		Single model	Multi-model	Single model	Multi-model	Single model	Multi-model
AB	STFT	1	1	0.9910	0.9060	0.9582	0.9544
	8-Ch connectivity	0.8700	0.9139	1	1	0.9305	0.9584
	4-Ch connectivity	0.9514	1	1	1	0.9841	1
CP	STFT	0.8117	0.9720	0.9724	0.9474	0.8889	0.9681
	8-Ch connectivity	1	0.9340	0.9564	0.9581	0.9794	0.9307
	4-Ch connectivity	1	1	1	1	1	1
SP	STFT	1	0.7727	0.965	1	0.9596	0.8721
	8-Ch connectivity	0.9591	0.9518	0.9584	0.9583	0.9574	0.9595
	4-Ch connectivity	0.9538	1	0.9564	0.9594	0.9566	0.9790
TC	STFT	0.7543	0.8341	0.5810	0.8396	0.6160	0.8377
	8-Ch connectivity	1	1	0.9283	0.8394	0.9620	0.9104
	4-Ch connectivity	1	0.9234	0.9235	1	0.96270	0.9644
TN	STFT	1	1	**0.2568**	**0.7541**	**0.4110**	**0.8603**
	8-Ch connectivity	0.7158	0.8644	0.6283	0.7551	0.6720	0.8620
	4-Ch connectivity	0.8800	1	0.8804	1	0.8819	1

The three-class classifier using four-channel connectivity and ten pre-trained networks achieved the best performance with an average accuracy of 96.33%. With only four channels (eight electrodes), this classifier could be used in emergencies for efficient patient triage. Using the same configuration, the six-class classifier delivered 99.00% average accuracy, surpassing the highest accuracy from a similar work by over 13–16% [8].

5   Discussion

This result confirms that multi-model transfer learning is an excellent solution to the small dataset challenge often faced in clinical applications. Both classifiers exhibited exceptional precision and recall using the transfer learning approach, showing that transferring knowledge from large datasets to epileptic seizures can achieve excellence in detection tasks in clinical settings. Moreover, In the phenotypic dataset, seizure types were labelled using both EEG and clinical data, yet our framework solely relied on phenotypic data. Despite a relatively small participant count, this finding suggests that with appropriate processing techniques and deep learning, an accurate differentiation of epileptic seizure types is possible with phenotypic data only. This could be particularly useful in situations where clinical data isn't readily available, such as telehealth in remote areas or rescue missions in challenging conditions. To capitalize on our classifier system in diagnosing various seizure types, we further expanded our research to target stroke epilepsy, a subtype posing complex diagnostic challenges. Stroke-induced seizures have complex mechanisms, making stroke epilepsy difficult to distinguish from other seizure types clinically, thereby complicating patient management. This underpins the necessity for better diagnostic tools to assist clinicians in accurately diagnosing stroke epilepsy. While age is a known risk factor for stroke and subsequent seizures, genetic factors introduce considerable risk variation among individuals of the same age group. Hence, a more comprehensive approach considering genetic predisposition is vital. To address this challenge, we conducted a PRS analysis, identifying 371 individuals presenting a heightened genetic risk for seizures. This approach of using genetic risk profiling serves as a proactive screening method for individuals at elevated risk for stroke epilepsy. When integrated with our high-performing machine learning model as a diagnostic tool, we provide a comprehensive solution promising enhanced diagnostic accuracy and improved patient outcomes, particularly for older individuals at risk of stroke-induced seizures. Given the precision of this approach, it has significant potential to aid in clinical decision-making and early intervention strategies.

6   Conclusion and Future Work

This study explores the potential of enhancing seizure classification by integrating multi-model transfer learning and genotypic data analysis. Our unique approach amalgamates multiple sources of transferable knowledge, effectively bridging the genotype-phenotype divide in seizure detection. Using four-channel EEG features with a ten-network model, we achieved 96.33% and 99.00% accuracy for the three-type and six-type classifiers with over 0.95 F1-score. This work improved the accuracy and robustness of the seizure-type classifiers compared with others' work. In the future, expanding the knowledge base by adding genetic data in this multi-source domain adaptation framework can potentially further enhance the performance.

Acknowledgement. This research is supported by the Australian Research Council Linkage scheme: LP210100414.

References

1. Choi, S.W., Mak, T.S.H., O'Reilly, P.F.: Tutorial: a guide to performing polygenic risk score analyses. Nat. Protoc. **15**(9), 2759–2772 (2020)
2. Choi, W., Kim, M.J., Yum, M.S., Jeong, D.H.: Deep convolutional gated recurrent unit combined with attention mechanism to classify pre-ictal from interictal EEG with minimized number of channels. J. Personalized Med. **12**(5), 763 (2022)
3. Dong, J., Fang, Z., Liu, A., Sun, G., Liu, T.: Confident anchor-induced multi-source free domain adaptation. In: Advances in Neural Information Processing Systems, vol. 34, pp. 2848–2860 (2021)
4. Guo, K., et al.: Artificial intelligence-driven biomedical genomics. Knowl. Based Syst. 110937 (2023)
5. Jiang, Y., et al.: Seizure classification from EEG signals using transfer learning, semi-supervised learning and tsk fuzzy system. IEEE Trans. Neural Syst. Rehabil. Eng. **25**(12), 2270–2284 (2017)
6. Lacaze, P., et al.: The medical genome reference bank: a whole-genome data resource of 4000 healthy elderly individuals. Rationale and cohort design. Eur. J. Hum. Genet. 27(2), 308–316 (2019)

7. Lu, J., Zuo, H., Zhang, G.: Fuzzy multiple-source transfer learning. IEEE Trans. Fuzzy Syst. **28**(12), 3418–3431 (2019)
8. Raghu, S., Sriraam, N., Temel, Y., Rao, S.V., Kubben, P.L.: EEG based multi-class seizure type classification using convolutional neural network and transfer learning. Neural Netw. **124**, 202–212 (2020)
9. Roy, S., Asif, U., Tang, J., Harrer, S.: Seizure type classification using EEG signals and machine learning: setting a benchmark. In: 2020 IEEE Signal Processing in Medicine and Biology Symposium (SPMB), pp. 1–6. IEEE (2020)
10. Shah, V., Golmohammadi, M., Ziyabari, S., Von Weltin, E., Obeid, I., Picone, J.: Optimizing channel selection for seizure detection. In: 2017 IEEE signal Processing in Medicine and Biology Symposium (SPMB), pp. 1–5. IEEE (2017)
11. Shah, V.: The temple university hospital seizure detection corpus. Front. Neuroinform. **12**, 83 (2018)
12. Sollis, E., et al.: The NHGRI-EBI GWAS catalog: knowledgebase and deposition resource. Nucleic Acids Res. **51**(D1), D977–D985 (2023)
13. Tao, W., et al.: EEG-based emotion recognition via channel-wise attention and self attention. IEEE Trans. Affect. Comput. (2020)
14. Vaswani, A., et al.: Attention is all you need. In: Advances in Neural Information Processing Systems, vol. 30 (2017)
15. Wan, Z., Yang, R., Huang, M., Zeng, N., Liu, X.: A review on transfer learning in EEG signal analysis. Neurocomputing **421**, 1–14 (2021)
16. Yang, C., Deng, Z., Choi, K.S., Jiang, Y., Wang, S.: Transductive domain adaptive learning for epileptic electroencephalogram recognition. Artif. Intell. Med. **62**(3), 165–177 (2014)
17. Yuan, Y., Xun, G., Jia, K., Zhang, A.: A multi-view deep learning method for epileptic seizure detection using short-time Fourier transform. In: Proceedings of the 8th ACM International Conference on Bioinformatics, Computational Biology, and Health Informatics, pp. 213–222 (2017)

Requirement Survey in Thai Clinician for Designing Digital Solution of Pain Assessment

Noppon Choosri[1]([✉]) [iD], Pattama Gomutbutra[2] [iD], Adisak Kittisares[2] [iD],
Atigorn Sanguansri[1], and Peerasak Lettrakarnon[2] [iD]

[1] College of Arts, Media, and Technology, Chiang Mai University, Chiang Mai, Thailand
noppon.c@cmu.ac.th
[2] Faculty of Medicine, Chiang Mai University, Tiergartenstr. 17, 69121 Heidelberg, Germany

Abstract. To successfully implement a digital solution for pain assessment using the User Centred Design (UCD) approach, one must have an in-depth understanding of the requirements of clinicians and synchronize these needs with real practices. This paper presents the findings from the survey research conducted to understand the overall operations of Maharaj Nakorn Chiang Mai Hospital in Thailand. Clinicians from multiple departments who have their roles involved with pain management participated in the research. The key findings are that the majority of the participants are more familiar with the numeric scale of 10 for rating patients' pains; Clinicians usually take approximately 1 min to determine the pain level; the major issue is the informed pain scores are not related to pain symptoms. When clinicians treat patient's pains, their clinical decision is based on patient's symptoms and their reactions rather than the measured score; and participants preferred to have a tool to assist their decision rather than an automated tool to make smart decisions for them.

Keywords: Pain assessment · Pain management · Requirement · User research

1 Introduction

The official definition of pain in a clinical context is recently proposed as "a distressing experience associated with actual or potential tissue damage with sensory, emotional, cognitive, and social components [1]. Pain is a significant cause impacting the quality of life because when it is persistent and severe, it has a great impact on patients on both the emotional and physical health of an individual [2]. Also, Pain is the most common symptom in several diseases such as Atopic Dermatitis [3], chronic venous insufficiency [4].

The significance of pain management was substantialized by the American Pain Society (APS) which has advocated pain as "the fifth" vital sign [1]. That campaign set to amplify the importance of pain assessment which must be accurate and timely [2].

Due to pain being individually subjective [3], accurately determining pain severity is a challenge in a clinical setting. Among several existing pain assessment approaches, the

Y. Li et al. (Eds.): HIS 2023, LNCS 14305, pp. 235–244, 2023.
https://doi.org/10.1007/978-981-99-7108-4_20

self-reported approach has been shown to have strong validity [4], yet the common issue is patients overstate or understate their pain [5]. Meanwhile, assessing pain using an observational approach by nurses is found is under-triaged in paediatric patients when the self-report approach was used [6, 7]. Therefore, researchers and clinicians have always quested for objective solutions.

Several digital-based solutions have been proposed to assist clinicians in the diagnosis of pain as their pain assessment approaches are rigorous. Hammel and Cohn [8] investigated an automatic pain detection solution using Support Vector Machine (SVM) technique to determine pain intensity from facial expressions. It was shown that this approach delivers some promising results in participants with orthopaedic injuries. Jacob et al. [9] proposed a solution that utilizes a smartphone application that functions as a pain diary to support pain monitoring in Children with sickle cell disease (SCD). The usability study found that children were able to use smartphones to access a web-based e-Diary for reporting pain and symptoms successfully. Game-based pain assessment system was proposed by Stinson et al. [10] to improve the compliance of adolescents with cancer patients. Patients feel minimum bothersome, resulting high compliance score produced up to 81% from the evaluation.

Although several studies reported positive results from adopting digital tools to assist pain assessment, the researcher barely gave details or the process of acquiring or formulating a list of requirements before turning them into the features of the system. Co-design, Participatory- design, User centre design, and Design thinking are the design approaches that targets user and ultimately gain better user experiences. Those methods share the common key success to the requirement acquisition phase. In fact, the review of pain management applications reported that 86% of 111 pain management applications even do not have healthcare professional involvement [11].

The aim of this research is to investigate the positioning of pain assessment and management from the clinical practice of the target users. The study also has the objective to explore the basic needs of the users to define the overview character of the proposed solution.

2 Method

The research selectively recruited participants who have experience in pain assessment and management from the Maharaj Nakorn Chiang Mai Hospital, a teaching hospital operated by Chiang Mai University. The research team hosted the technical pain management symposium. The invitation was sent to target wards and clinical units that should involve patient pain assessment and management. The keynote speaker of the seminar is a member of this research team who is considered defined in this research as a pain management expert (PG). She is a neurologist who specialized in palliative care in which pain management is a major part of routine care. Questionnaires about the experience in pain assessment were prepared. The questionnaire was designed by the pain expert; on the occasion that the questionnaire or the provided choice refers to the specific episode in pain assessment or management, information was from her experience co-working with several clinicians. The questionnaire was distributed to all participants who attended the symposium, and statistical analysis was made after the event. Each question in a questionnaire has the objective to understand the pain assessment experience of the participant from different perspectives. The outcomes of the research are to be used to design a digital tool for pain assessment and management that inclusively considers the user's viewpoint from the beginning of the design process. The details of six major research questions in the questionnaire are elaborated as follows:

2.1 RQ1 What are the Pain Assessment Methods that Clinicians Acknowledge?

According to a vast variety of pain assessment methods, the objective of this research question is to investigate the approaches that the participants of this research are familiar with. The development of pain management solutions in digital platforms is expected to include the standard pain assessment feature, the findings of this research question will inform the solution designer to adopt the approach that the participant found practical to use. In the questionnaires, the participants are asked to select the pain assessment approach that they know from the given choices multiple selections can be made from the list of common pain assessment methods identified by the pain physiologists who are the co-authors of this paper. The choices of pain assessment methods that include in this question are:

- visual analogue
- PAINAD
- Numeric scale
- face pain scale
- CHEOP
- NIPS
- CPOT
- BPS
- BPI

2.2 RQ2: What are the Pain Scale Systems that Clinicians Usually Use?

In this research question, the focus is to understand how fine the pain scale is measured and referred to in pain management. There are 3 levels of fine scale asking the participants to identify commonly in use which are:

- 2 scales of pain which is pain and not pain.
- 3 scales of pain which is mild, moderate, and severe.
- 10 scale of pain which is the magnitude of pain from 1 to 10.

2.3 RQ3: How Long Do Clinicians Take to Assess a Patient's Pain?

This question is to survey how long approximately the participants spent assessing the patient's pain. This information can imply how sophisticated pain assessment clinicians perceived and set up referencing expected time spent to complete the assessment process; the developing solution should require the approximate amount of time to complete but provide more accuracy or more useful functionality added. The participants are asked to fill in the approximate time spent on one assessment.

2.4   RQ4: What Factors Impact the Clinician's Decision to Adjudge Pain Relievers?

In this survey question, the research focuses on understanding the current practice that what information clinicians consider adjudging prescribing pain relievers. The common reasons are listed based on the experience of the pain management experts who identified these common reasons from the experience of working with a number of colleagues. The common reason listed for selections are:

- frequency of requesting pain relievers
- Patient's suffering
- Pain score
- Pain pattern and position of pain

2.5   RQ5: What are the Common Challenges When Asking Patients to Level Pain to Scores?

This question targets to explore the faced challenges when clinicians assess patient's pain. So, potential solutions can be envisaged to address the problem. The assumption was that the challenges were the majority from two commonly known issues; the study verified that the assumptions were correct and in which frequency clinicians found the issues happened. The questionnaire also asks if there were other challenging issues that they used to encounter. Participants can add that issue to the survey. Those two known issues are:

- Informed pain scores are not related to pain symptoms.
- Patients are unable to assess their pain to scores.

2.6   RQ 6: What are the Preferred Characteristics of the Application for Pain Management?

The focus of this research question is to investigate the expected outlook of the solution from the clinician's viewpoint. The research defined three characters of the application and asked participants to rank them to show that indicate the level of significance of each character.

- Character 1: The solution is a kind of decision support tool. For example, the system collects pain information from patients manually. No artificial intelligence module to synthesize decisions or advice. The focus is to help clinicians systematically record and retrieve/visualize pain information to support clinicians' decisions.
- Character 2: The solution is Artificial Intelligent oriented. The solution is focused on assisting clinicians determine pain levels automatically from the given contextual information.
- Character 3: The solution focuses on treatment recommendations such as giving advice on pain reliever prescriptions and assisting calculate medication doses for individual cases.

3 Results

3.1 Participants

There were 25 participants participating in the research. It is optional for the participant to disclose or undisclosed their identity in the questionnaire. Classifying participants by role found that of the participant who disclosed their role identity, there were 3 doctors, and 17 nurses, while 5 of the participants undisclosed their role. The classification of the participants by role is summarized in Table 1.

Classifying participants by departments found that there were participants from 7 different departments participating in the research. The largest number of participants was from the Department of Obstetrics and Gynecology (Ob/GYN). The summary of the participants by department is shown in Table 2.

Table 1. Participants by roles

Role	Number of participants
Doctors	3
Nurses	17
Undisclosed	5

Table 2. Participants by roles

Department	Number of participants
General Nurse	8
Internal medicine	1
ICU	1
OB/GYN	11
Family medicine	1
Orthopaedics	1

3.2 What are the Pain Assessment Methods that Clinicians Acknowledge?

The best-known pain assessment is the numeric scale (f = 17), while the visual analogue and face pain scale are the second and the third best-known methods, (f = The rest of the pain assessment methods and f = 10, respectively. The other pain assessment methods are only little known by the participants. The frequency of the pain assessment methods that the participants know is illustrated in Fig. 1.

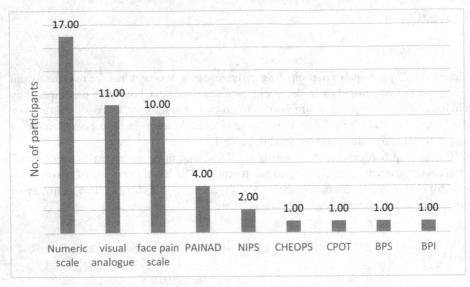

Fig. 1. The pain assessment method that participants acknowledge.

3.3 What are the Pain Scale Systems that Clinicians Usually Use?

The result found the participants have a consensus on the scale of measuring pain. The 10 scale is the only scale that the clinician in this research uses for communicating patients' pain as shown in Fig. 2.

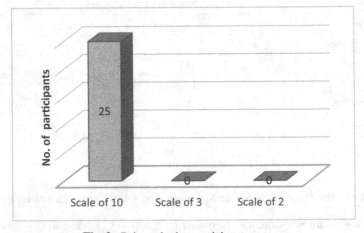

Fig. 2. Pain scale that participant measure

3.4   How Long Do Clinicians Take to Assess a Patient's Pain?

The pain assessment is usually done in 5 min. In most cases, participants take approximately 1 min to assess the patient's pain as shown in Fig. 3.

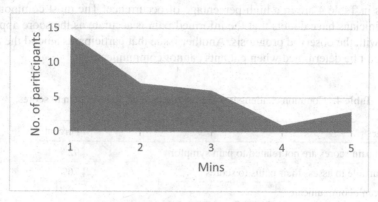

Fig. 3. Time spent in pain assessment.

3.5   RQ4: What Factors Impact the Clinician's Decision to Adjudge Pain Relievers?

When clinicians treat patients' pains, their clinical decisions are based on the patient's prognosis and reactions rather than the measured score. The result has shown that two major reasons impact clinicians' decision to adjust the prescription of the pain relievers which are the frequency that patients make their request for pain relievers and the patient's sufferings from the observation. The findings from this research question are shown in Table 3.

Table 3. The factors impact clinician's decision to adjudge pain relievers.

Factors	Percent
frequency of requesting pain relievers	37.03%
Patient 's suffering	33.33%
Pain score	11.11%
Pain pattern and position of pain	7.40%

3.6 What are the Common Challenges When Asking Patients to Level Pain to Scores?

The survey result confirms the assumptions that the two major issues when asking patients to level pain to scores accurately are common. Both of them depicted in the first two rows in Table 4 are in a high percentage of occurrence. The most common cause is that clinicians have doubts that the informed pain is accurate as the score appears to contrast with the observed prognosis. Another issue that participants amend the answer is pain can't be determined when patients cannot communicate.

Table 4. Common challenges when asking patients to level pain to scores.

Challenges	Percent
Informed pain scores are not related to pain symptom	92%
Patients unable to assess their pains to scores	76%
Patients can't communicate	8%

3.7 What are the Preferred Characteristics of the Application for Pain Management?

The survey results show that most participants highly agree that the pain management solution should predominate character 1 - It should act as a decision support tool. Also, it shows that character 1 is mandatory because all participants rated this character either highly or moderately significant. Meanwhile, some participants have not rated character 2 and character 3 which can be interpreted as these characters are not even important for pain management.

The majority of the participants rated character 2 as moderately significant and rated character 3 as low significant. The survey result showing the expected characteristics of the digital pain management system is illustrated in Fig. 4.

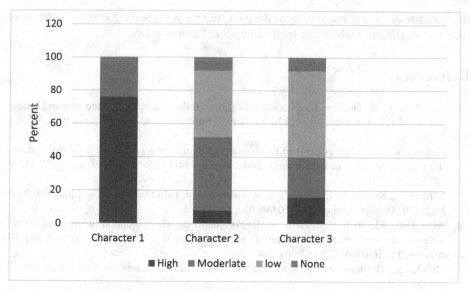

Fig. 4. The preferred character of the pain management tool

4 Discussion and Conclusion

Pain assessment is commonly required in treatment. It is common and significant to several healthcare specialists. One piece of evidence shown by the result of this study is a variety of backgrounds of healthcare professionals showing their interest and registering to participate in the research. From this research, it is found that the pain management topic attracted the largest number of participants from the OB/GYN department.

The findings from the survey inform some useful implications for designing digital solutions for pain management through the UCD approach. First, participants are familiarized with the numeric scale using a scale of ten to grade the pain level the most when assessing a patient's pain. The experience and the view related to the pain assessment shared by the participants of this research could be subject to this pain assessment method. For example, we can imply that when using the numeric pain assessment scale, clinicians usually take approximately 1 min and it can extend up to 5 min (RQ2), and the problem with this pain assessment method is the curiosity that the informed pain score is trustable and whether patients is able to assess their pain in number precisely (RQ5).

Next, it was found from the survey that pain management usually starts with a pain assessment. Although the pain assessment that delivers objective outcomes, i.e., levelling pain into a score, is measured, in clinical practice clinicians rely a lot on the subjective expression of patients and use this information to prescribe pain medication (RQ4).

Finally, the research explored the preferred character of digital solutions that clinicians prefer to have. The result found that the participants prefer a tool to support their justification rather than a tool for making decisions for them in pain management. An automated feature that employs intelligent module can be useful, but it should be a supplement feature as most of the participants rated this character the second priority. While the majority of the participants rated the pain treatment supporting features defined as only low significance which can imply an optional functionality.

References

1. Max, M.B., et al.: Quality improvement guidelines for the treatment of acute pain and cancer pain. JAMA: J. Am. Med. Assoc. **274**(23) (1995). https://doi.org/10.1001/jama.1995.035302 30060032
2. Lichtner, V., et al.: Pain assessment for people with dementia: a systematic review of systematic reviews of pain assessment tools. BMC Geriatr. **14**(1) (2014). https://doi.org/10.1186/1471-2318-14-138
3. Tripathi, L., Kumar, P.: Challenges in pain assessment: pain intensity scales. Indian J. Pain **28**(2) (2014). https://doi.org/10.4103/0970-5333.132841
4. Price, D.D., McGrath, P.A., Rafii, A., Buckingham, B.: The validation of visual analogue scales as ratio scale measures for chronic and experimental pain. Pain **17**(1) (1983). https://doi.org/10.1016/0304-3959(83)90126-4
5. Mogil, J.S.: The history of pain measurement in humans and animals. Front. Pain Res. **3** (2022)
6. Shavit, I., Kofman, M., Leder, M., Hod, T., Kozer, E.: Observational pain assessment versus self-report in paediatric triage. Emerg. Med. J. **25**(9) (2008). https://doi.org/10.1136/emj.2008.058297
7. Rajasagaram, U., Taylor, D.M.D., Braitberg, G., Pearsell, J.P., Capp, B.A.: Paediatric pain assessment: differences between triage nurse, child and parent. J. Paediatr. Child Health **45**(4) (2009). https://doi.org/10.1111/j.1440-1754.2008.01454.x
8. Hammal, Z., Cohn, J.F.: Automatic detection of pain intensity. In: ICMI 2012 - Proceedings of the ACM International Conference on Multimodal Interaction (2012). https://doi.org/10.1145/2388676.2388688
9. Jacob, E., et al.: Usability testing of a smartphone for accessing a web-based e-diary for self-monitoring of pain and symptoms in sickle cell disease. J. Pediatr. Hematol. Oncol. **34**(5) (2012). https://doi.org/10.1097/MPH.0b013e318257a13c
10. Stinson, J.N., et al.: Development and testing of a multidimensional iPhone pain assessment application for adolescents with cancer. J. Med. Internet Res. **15**(3) (2013). https://doi.org/10.2196/jmir.2350
11. Rosser, B.A., Eccleston, C.: Smartphone applications for pain management. J. Telemed. Telecare **17**(6) (2011). https://doi.org/10.1258/jtt.2011.101102

Predictive Analysis and Disease Recognition

A Comprehensive Approach for Enhancing Motor Imagery EEG Classification in BCI's

Muhammad Tariq Sadiq[1]([⊠])(iD), Siuly Siuly[2], Yan Li[3], and Paul Wen[4]

[1] Advanced Engineering Center, School of Architecture, Technology and Engineering,
University of Brighton, Brighton BN2 4AT, UK
m.t.sadiq@brighton.ac.uk
[2] Institute for Sustainable Industries and Liveable Cities, Victoria University,
Melbourne, VIC 3011, Australia
siuly.siuly@vu.edu.au
[3] School of Mathematics Physics and Computing, University of Southern
Queensland, Toowoomba Campus, Toowoomba 4350, Australia
Yan.Li@usq.edu.au
[4] School of Engineering, University of Southern Queensland, Toowoomba Campus,
Toowoomba 4350, Australia
Paul.Wen@usq.edu.au

Abstract. Electroencephalography (EEG) based on motor imagery has become a potential modality for brain-computer interface (BCI) systems, allowing users to control external devices by imagining doing particular motor activities. The existence of noise and the complexity of the brain signals, however, make it difficult to classify motor imagery EEG signals. This work suggests a systematic method for classifying motor imagery in the EEG. A technique known as Multiscale Principal Component Analysis (MSPCA) is used for efficient noise removal to improve the signal quality. A unique signal decomposition technique is proposed for modes extraction, allowing the separation of various oscillatory components related to motor imagery tasks. This breakdown makes it easier to isolate important temporal and spectral properties that distinguish various classes of motor imagery. These characteristics capture the dynamism and discriminative patterns present in motor imagery tasks. The motor imagery EEG signals are then classified using various machine learning and deep learning-based models based on the retrieved features. The findings of the classification show how well the suggested strategy works in generating precise and trustworthy classification success for various motor imaging tasks. The proposed method has enormous potential for BCI applications, allowing people with motor limitations to operate extrasensory equipment via brain signals.

Keywords: Motor Imagery EEG · Brain-Computer Interface · MSPCA · Signal Decomposition · Classification

Supported by organization x.

1   Introduction

Brain-computer interface (BCI) systems have numerous applications [1] and can enable disabled individuals to interact with the real world using their thoughts alone [2,3]. These systems collect electrical signals generated by brain activity and translate them into control outputs through nonmuscular channels [6]. Motor imagery (MI) imagery is a commonly used mental rehearsal technique in BCI applications [4,5,7], where participants imagine themselves performing specific motor actions without physical muscle activation [8]. BCIs based on MI have attracted extensive interest in recent years [9,28], and various clinical methods such as electroencephalography (EEG) [29], magnetoencephalography (MEG) [30], functional magnetic resonance imaging (fMRI) [31], positron emission tomography (PET) [32], and single-photon emission computed tomography (SPECT) [33] have been employed to monitor brain activities during motor rehearsal. Among these methods, EEG signal analysis is the most widely used due to its affordability, ease of use, excellent temporal information, and non-invasive nature [9–15].

Currently, most motor imagery BCIs operate as pattern recognition systems. They initially identify EEG signals using feature extraction and detection schemes and subsequently translate these signals into corresponding task commands. Capturing and classifying EEG signals with high accuracy is crucial for BCI development, and various signal processing techniques have been proposed in the literature [34–40]. These techniques can be categorized into Fourier transform (FT)-based methods, autoregressive (AR) model-based methods, common spatial pattern (CSP)-based methods, sparse representation (SR) methods, and signal decomposition (SD)-based methods. FT-based methods are typically used for EEG signal power spectral analysis but lack time domain information [34,35]. AR model-based methods are computationally efficient and suitable for online systems, but they suffer from artifacts that reduce BCI system reliability [36–40]. Spatial pattern-based methods, which employ appropriate spatial filtering techniques for analyzing oscillatory EEG components, have also been proposed [42–50]. These methods have improved the overall classification accuracy of EEG signals but are often limited by small sample sizes and may suffer from overfitting issues.

To further improve classification accuracy, clustering-based least square support vector machine (LS-SVM) classifiers [51], iterative spatio-spectral pattern learning (ISSPL) methods [52], and feature extraction techniques such as covariance-based second-order dynamic features [53] and constraint-based independent component analysis [54] have been proposed. These methods have achieved higher accuracy but often neglect the selection of optimal regularization parameters. Higher order statistics (HOS) features, including signal skewness (Sk) and kurtosis (Kt), have also gained popularity for analyzing biomedical signals [41,55].

Recently, deep learning approaches based on convolutional neural networks (CNNs), recurrent neural networks (RNNs), and sparse Bayesian extreme learning schemes have been applied to EEG signal feature extraction and classification

[56–59]. While these methods show promise, their classification accuracies are often limited by the lack of extensive training data, and their practical application is hindered by high computational requirements and system complexity [24–27].

Signal decomposition (SD)-based methods are relatively new for MI task classification. These methods decompose EEG signals into different sub-bands and extract desired coefficients separately. Empirical mode decomposition (EMD), discrete wavelet transform (DWT), and wavelet packet decomposition (WPD) are three SD-based methods that have been proposed [41]. While they have achieved classification accuracies of 62.8%, 81.1%, and 92.8%, respectively, they suffer from relatively low success rates and challenges in selecting the appropriate number of decomposition levels, especially for WPD [41]. Empirical wavelet transform (EWT) is a relatively new SD-based method for signal analysis [61] and has applied to MI-based EEG signal classification. However, it required large number of modes, restricting its practical applicability [16–23].

This paper focuses on the feasibility of Sliding Singular Spectrum Analysis (SSA) for classifying motor imagery (MI) electroencephalography (EEG) signals. We introduce a new data adaptive decomposition method to analyze the nonstationary and nonlinear characteristics of MI EEG signals. By applying SSA, we decomposed the signals into adaptive frequency modes. From these modes, we extract statistical features that capture meaningful information of the SSA decomposition. Additionally, we employed a wide range of classifiers to assess the effectiveness of our approach. To evaluate the proposed SSA-based framework, we conducted experiments using the benchmark dataset IVa from BCI competition III. The results of our experiments validate the efficacy of the proposed SSA-based framework for MI EEG signal classification.

2   Materials

The study utilized the publicly available benchmark dataset IVa, which is obtained from BCI competition III [62]. This dataset was generously provided by the Institute of Medical Psychology and Behavioral Neurobiology at the University of Tübingen, headed by N. Birbaumer, the Max-Planck-Institute for Biological Cybernetics in Tübingen, headed by B. Schökopf, and the Department of Epileptology at Universität Bonn. The IVa dataset comprises two motor imagery (MI) tasks: right hand (RH, class 1) and right foot (RF, class 2). The recordings were conducted with five healthy participants who were seated in a relaxed state in a chair throughout the experiment. EEG signals were acquired using BrainAmp amplifiers and a 128-channel Ag/AgCl electrode cap manufactured by ECI. The EEG channels were positioned according to the extended international 10/20 system [63].

3   Methods

In this study, a Sliding Singular Spectrum Analysis (SSA)-aided automated framework is proposed for the identification of right hand and right foot motor imagery (MI) EEG signals. The framework consists of dataset preparation, noise removal, SSA for generating dominant components, extraction of statistical features, and classification models. The proposed framework is illustrated in Fig. 1 as,

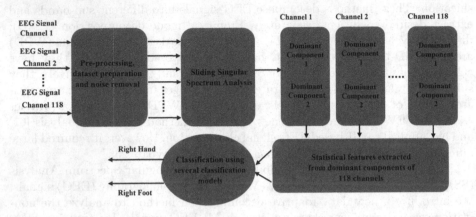

Fig. 1. Block diagram of the proposed automated SSA framework for Motor Imagery EEG Classification

3.1   Module 1: Pre-processing

The IVa dataset that we used comes with position indicators determining the data points from 280 sessions with 118 EEG electrodes for every single subject. The participants "aa", "al", "av", "aw", and "ay" in both groups had initial data lengths that were the following: 298458×118, 283574×118, 283042×118, 282838×118, and 283562×118. The EEG segments that matched particular MI (motor imagery) activities were the focus of our attention. To identify these segments, we relied on the position markers that indicated the start of each trial. The original dataset was recorded with a sampling frequency of 1000 Hz Hz. However, for consistency with previous studies, we used a down-sampled version of the dataset that was available at a rate of Fs=100 Hz. For our analysis, we selected a duration of 4 s from each EEG segment in both classes, resulting in 400 samples (4xFs). Consequently, we obtained a data matrix of size 400×118 for each EEG segment of a specific class, which was used for each participant in our study. We used a multiscale principal component analysis method to remove noise due to the fragile and vulnerable traits of EEG data acquired from the subject's scalp.

3.2   Module 2: Sliding Singular Spectrum Analysis for Meaningful Components Extraction

Sliding Singular Spectrum Analysis (SSA) is a technique used for extracting meaningful components from time series data, such as EEG (Electroencephalogram) signals, particularly those related to motor imagery tasks. It applies Singular Value Decomposition (SVD) to decompose the time series into a set of basis functions called singular vectors, which capture the dominant patterns present in the data.

The motivation behind using SSA for EEG analysis, specifically for motor imagery tasks, is to identify and extract relevant brain activity patterns associated with the imagination of movement. Motor imagery EEG signals capture the brain's electrical activity when an individual mentally simulates or imagines performing a specific motor action, without actually executing the movement. Analyzing these signals can provide insights into the brain's motor processes and assist in developing brain-computer interfaces and rehabilitation techniques.

Let's delve into the mathematical equations involved in the Sliding SSA algorithm in the context of motor imagery EEG signals:

1. Given a time series of EEG data for 5 subjects, represented by matrices X_1, X_2, X_3, X_4, X_5 of size $(n \times m)$, where n is the number of time steps and m is the number of electrodes or channels. In this case, $m = 118$ according to the 10–20 framework.

2. Sliding SSA applies a sliding window of length L to the time series. The window moves step-by-step, extracting segments of length L from the EEG data for further analysis.

3. For each window, the Singular Value Decomposition (SVD) is performed on the windowed matrix. SVD decomposes the windowed data matrix W into three matrices: U, Σ, and V.
   $W = U\Sigma V^T$ Here, U represents the left singular vectors, which capture the spatial patterns or topographies of the EEG components related to motor imagery. Σ is a diagonal matrix containing the singular values, which represent the magnitudes or strengths of the corresponding singular vectors. V consists of the right singular vectors, which describe the temporal dynamics or time courses of the EEG components associated with motor imagery.

4. To extract the dominant components, we retain only the first k singular values and their corresponding singular vectors. The value of k is determined based on the desired level of decomposition or the explained variance.
   U_k, Σ_k, and V_k represent the truncated matrices that retain the first k singular vectors and singular values from U, Σ, and V, respectively.

5. The reconstructed window is obtained by multiplying the retained left and right singular vectors with their corresponding singular values: Reconstructed Window $RW = U_k\Sigma_k V_k^T$ Here, U_k represents the truncated matrix of left singular vectors, Σ_k represents the truncated diagonal matrix of singular values, and V_k^T represents the transpose of the truncated matrix of right singular vectors.

6. The reconstructed windows from each sliding window are collected and concatenated to obtain the final SSA reconstructed time series.

The Sliding SSA algorithm enables the identification and isolation of meaningful EEG components related to motor imagery tasks by exploiting the temporal and spatial characteristics of the data. By decomposing the time series into singular vectors through SVD and retaining the most important components, Sliding SSA facilitates the identification of prominent brain activity patterns associated with motor imagery from the noisy EEG signals.

This approach can be valuable for various applications, such as decoding motor intentions from EEG signals, developing neurorehabilitation strategies, and controlling prosthetic devices through brain-computer interfaces, all of which rely on understanding and analyzing the specific brain activity patterns elicited.

3.3   Module 3: Feature Extraction

In this study, a set of statistical features was extracted from the motor imagery EEG signals for the classification of right hand (RH) and right foot (RF) tasks. The following statistical features were computed for each EEG signal segment:

- **Mean:** The average value of the EEG signal.
- **Median:** The middle value of the sorted EEG signal.
- **Std:** The standard deviation of the EEG signal, which measures the dispersion of data points around the mean.
- **Min:** The minimum value of the EEG signal.
- **Max:** The maximum value of the EEG signal.
- **MAD:** The Median Absolute Deviation of the EEG signal, which quantifies the dispersion of data points around the median.
- **Q1:** The first quartile of the EEG signal, representing the value below which 25% of the data points fall.
- **Q3:** The third quartile of the EEG signal, representing the value below which 75% of the data points fall.
- **IQR:** The Interquartile Range, calculated as the difference between the third and first quartiles, indicating the spread of the middle 50% of the data.
- **Skewness:** The measure of the asymmetry of the EEG signal distribution.
- **Kurtosis:** The measure of the "tailedness" of the EEG signal distribution, indicating the presence of outliers or extreme values.

These statistical features provide valuable information about the amplitude, variability, and shape characteristics of the EEG signals. They are commonly used in motor imagery EEG classification tasks to capture relevant patterns and discriminate between different tasks or classes. The extracted statistical features were then used as inputs for the classification models to differentiate between the right hand and right foot motor imagery tasks.

3.4   Module 4: Classification

In this study, several classification models were employed to classify the statistical features extracted from the right hand (RH) and right foot (RF) motor imagery EEG signals. The following classifiers were utilized [13, 64–74]:

- **BayesNet:** BayesNet is a probabilistic classifier based on Bayesian networks. It models the dependencies between features using a directed acyclic graph and calculates the posterior probabilities of class labels using Bayes' theorem.
- **Naïve Bayes:** Naïve Bayes is a simple probabilistic classifier based on the assumption of independence between features. It calculates the posterior probabilities of class labels using Bayes' theorem and the assumption of feature independence.
- **Logistic Regression:** Logistic Regression is a linear classifier that models the relationship between the input features and the class labels using logistic functions. It estimates the probability of each class label and makes predictions based on a decision boundary.
- **Multilayer Perceptron (MLP):** MLP is a feedforward neural network model with multiple layers of nodes. It learns the complex non-linear relationships between the input features and the class labels using backpropagation algorithm.
- **Simple Logistic:** Simple Logistic is a logistic regression classifier that handles multi-class problems by combining multiple binary logistic regression models. It makes predictions based on the maximum posterior probability.
- **SMO:** SMO (Sequential Minimal Optimization) is an efficient algorithm for training support vector machines (SVMs). SVMs construct a hyperplane that maximally separates the data points of different classes in a high-dimensional feature space.
- **K-Nearest Neighbors (KNN):** KNN is a non-parametric classifier that assigns a class label to an input sample based on the majority class labels of its k nearest neighbors in the feature space.
- **Adaboost:** Adaboost is an ensemble learning algorithm that combines multiple weak classifiers to create a strong classifier. It iteratively trains classifiers on different weighted versions of the training data to focus on misclassified samples.
- **Bagging:** Bagging is an ensemble learning technique that trains multiple classifiers on different bootstrap samples of the training data and combines their predictions through voting or averaging.
- **LogitBoost:** LogitBoost is an ensemble learning algorithm that combines multiple weak classifiers using a forward stagewise additive modeling approach. It iteratively fits classifiers to the residuals of the previous iterations.
- **JRIP:** JRIP (Jumping Rule Inference Prism) is a rule-based classifier that generates a set of IF-THEN rules to classify the data. It uses a jumping rule search algorithm to find a compact set of rules that accurately represent the data.

- **J48:** J48 is an implementation of the C4.5 decision tree algorithm, which constructs a decision tree by recursively splitting the data based on the attribute that maximizes the information gain or the gain ratio.
- **LMT:** LMT (Logistic Model Trees) is a decision tree algorithm that combines the advantages of decision trees and logistic regression. It constructs a decision tree and fits logistic regression models at the leaf nodes.
- **Random Forest (RF):** Random Forest is an ensemble learning method that combines multiple decision trees to make predictions. It trains each tree on a random subset of the training data and a random subset of the input features.

These classifiers were chosen for their diverse modeling techniques and ability to handle different types of data. They were trained and evaluated on the extracted statistical features to classify the motor imagery EEG signals into the right hand and right foot tasks.

4   Results and Discussions

In this study we employed several performance evaluation parameters for EEG classification. The details of these parameters is detailed as,

- **Percent Correct:** This metric indicates the overall accuracy of the classifier in correctly classifying the instances. It represents the percentage of correctly classified instances.
- **True Positive Rate:** Also known as sensitivity or recall, this metric measures the proportion of true positive instances (correctly classified as positive) out of all actual positive instances.
- **True Negative Rate:** Also known as specificity, this metric measures the proportion of true negative instances (correctly classified as negative) out of all actual negative instances.
- **IR Precision:** This metric represents the precision or positive predictive value for the class of interest (IR class). It measures the proportion of true positive instances out of all instances classified as positive.
- **IR Recall:** This metric represents the recall or true positive rate for the class of interest (IR class). It measures the proportion of true positive instances out of all actual positive instances.
- **F-Measure:** This metric combines precision and recall into a single score. It provides a balanced measure of the classifier's performance by considering both false positives and false negatives.
- **Matthews Correlation:** This metric evaluates the quality of binary classifications. It takes into account true positives, true negatives, false positives, and false negatives, providing a correlation coefficient that ranges from -1 to 1. Higher values indicate better performance.
- **Area Under ROC:** This metric is a common measure used in evaluating binary classifiers. It represents the area under the receiver operating characteristic (ROC) curve, which illustrates the trade-off between true positive rate and false positive rate at various classification thresholds. A higher value indicates better performance.

By examining these metrics, we can assess the classification performance of each classifier for five subjects and compare their effectiveness in accurately classifying the right hand and right foot signals based on the given statistical features. The results are shown in Fig. 2(a–e).

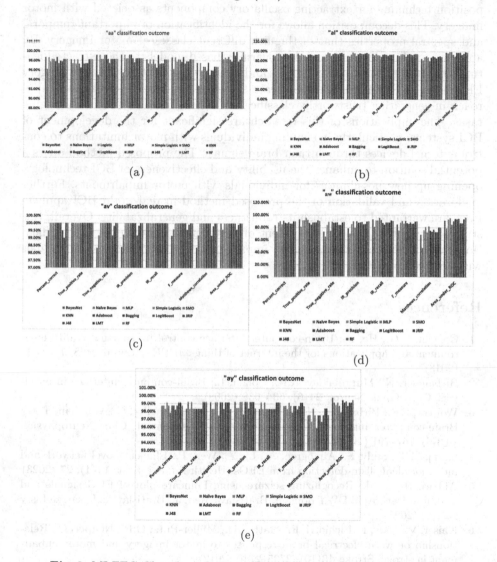

Fig. 2. MI EEG Classification using Sliding Singular Spectrum Analysis

5 Conclusion

In conclusion, this article presents a systematic approach for classifying motor imagery electroencephalography (EEG) signals in the context of brain-computer interface (BCI) systems. The study addresses the challenges posed by the complexity and noise in EEG signals, which make accurate classification of motor imagery tasks difficult. The proposed method utilizes Multiscale Principal Component Analysis (MSPCA) for efficient noise removal and a unique signal decomposition technique for extracting oscillatory components associated with motor imagery. This decomposition allows for the identification of important temporal and spectral properties that distinguish different classes of motor imagery. By applying machine learning and deep learning-based models to the extracted features, the researchers achieved precise and reliable classification of motor imagery EEG signals. The findings demonstrate the effectiveness of the suggested approach in generating trustworthy classification results for various motor imaging tasks. The implications of this research are significant for the development of BCI systems, particularly in enabling individuals with motor limitations to control external devices through their brain signals. The proposed method offers a potential solution to enhance the usability and effectiveness of BCI technology, opening up new possibilities for individuals with motor impairments. Further exploration and validation of the proposed method in real-world BCI applications are warranted to establish its robustness and generalizability. Overall, this study contributes to the advancement of EEG-based motor imagery classification and underscores its potential for improving the quality of life for individuals with motor disabilities.

References

1. Coogan, C.G., He, B.: Brain-computer interface control in a virtual reality environment and applications for the internet of things. IEEE Access **6**, 10 840–10 849 (2018)
2. Birbaumer, N., Murguialday, A.R., Cohen, L.: Brain-computer interface in paralysis. Curr. Opin. Neurol. **21**(6), 634–638 (2008)
3. Wolpaw, J.R., Birbaumer, N., McFarland, D.J., Pfurtscheller, G., Vaughan, T.M.: Brain-computer interfaces for communication and control. Clin. Neurophysiol. **113**(6), 767–791 (2002)
4. Sadiq, M.T., Siuly, S., Almogren, A., Li, Y., Wen, P.: Efficient novel network and index for alcoholism detection from EEGs. Health Inf. Sci. Syst. **11**(1), 27 (2023)
5. Akbari, H., et al.: Recognizing seizure using Poincaré plot of EEG signals and graphical features in DWT domain. Bratislava Med. J./Bratislavske Lekarske Listy **124**(1) (2023)
6. Kaiser, V., Daly, I., Pichiorri, F., Mattia, D., Müller-Putz, G.R., Neuper, C.: Relationship between electrical brain responses to motor imagery and motor impairment in stroke. Stroke **43**(10), 2735–2740 (2012)
7. Pfurtscheller, G., Neuper, C.: Motor imagery and direct brain-computer communication. Proc. IEEE **89**(7), 1123–1134 (2001)
8. Alkadhi, H., et al.: What disconnection tells about motor imagery: evidence from paraplegic patients. Cereb. Cortex **15**(2), 131–140 (2004)
9. Pfurtscheller, G., et al.: Graz-BCI: state of the art and clinical applications. IEEE Trans. Neural Syst. Rehabil. Eng. **11**(2), 1–4 (2003)

10. Akbari, H., Sadiq, M.T., Siuly, S., Li, Y., Wen, P.: Identification of normal and depression EEG signals in variational mode decomposition domain. Health Inf. Sci. Syst. **10**(1), 24 (2022)
11. Tufail, A.B., et al.: On disharmony in batch normalization and dropout methods for early categorization of Alzheimer's disease. Sustainability **14**(22), 14695 (2022)
12. Akbari, H., Sadiq, M.T., Payan, M., Esmaili, S.S., Baghri, H., Bagheri, H.: Depression detection based on geometrical features extracted from SODP shape of EEG signals and binary PSO. Traitement du Signal **38**(1) (2021)
13. Akbari, H., Sadiq, M.T., Rehman, A.U.: Classification of normal and depressed EEG signals based on centered correntropy of rhythms in empirical wavelet transform domain. Health Inf. Sci. Syst. **9**(1), 1–15 (2021)
14. Sadiq, M.T., et al.: Exploiting feature selection and neural network techniques for identification of focal and nonfocal EEG signals in TQWT domain. J. Healthcare Eng. **2021**, 24 (2021)
15. Hussain, W., Sadiq, M.T., Siuly, S., Rehman, A.U.: Epileptic seizure detection using 1 d-convolutional long short-term memory neural networks. Appl. Acoust. **177**, 107941 (2021)
16. Sadiq, M.T., Yu, X., Yuan, Z., Aziz, M.Z., Siuly, S., Ding, W.: Toward the development of versatile brain-computer interfaces. IEEE Trans. Artif. Intell. **2**(4), 314–328 (2021)
17. Sadiq, M.T., et al.: Motor imagery BCI classification based on multivariate variational mode decomposition. IEEE Trans. Emerg. Top. Comput. Intell. **6**(5), 1177–1189 (2022)
18. Yu, X., Aziz, M.Z., Sadiq, M.T., Jia, K., Fan, Z., Xiao, G.: Computerized multidomain EEG classification system: a new paradigm. IEEE J. Biomed. Health Inform. **26**(8), 3626–3637 (2002)
19. Sadiq, M.T., Siuly, S., Rehman, A.U.: Evaluation of power spectral and machine learning techniques for the development of subject-specific BCI. In: Artificial Intelligence-Based Brain-Computer Interface, pp. 99–120. Elsevier (2022)
20. Sadiq, M.T., et al.: Motor imagery EEG signals decoding by multivariate empirical wavelet transform-based framework for robust brain-computer interfaces. IEEE Access **7**, 171431–171451 (2019)
21. Sadiq, M.T., et al.: Motor imagery EEG signals classification based on mode amplitude and frequency components using empirical wavelet transform. IEEE Access **7**, 127678–127692 (2019)
22. Sadiq, M.T., Yu, X., Yuan, Z., Aziz, M.Z.: Motor imagery BCI classification based on novel two-dimensional modeling in empirical wavelet transform. Electron. Lett. **56**(25), 1367–1369 (2020)
23. Sadiq, M.T., Yu, X., Yuan, Z., Aziz, M.Z.: Identification of motor and mental imagery EEG in two and multiclass subject-dependent tasks using successive decomposition index. Sensors **20**(18), 5283 (2020)
24. Sadiq, M.T., Aziz, M.Z., Almogren, A., Yousaf, A., Siuly, S., Rehman, A.U.: Exploiting pretrained CNN models for the development of an EEG-based robust BCI framework. Comput. Biol. Med. **143**, 105242 (2022)
25. Sadiq, M.T., Akbari, H., Siuly, S., Yousaf, A., Rehman, A.U.: A novel computer-aided diagnosis framework for EEG-based identification of neural diseases. Comput. Biol. Med. **138**, 104922 (2021)
26. Sadiq, M.T., Yu, X., Yuan, Z., Aziz, M.Z., Siuly, S., Ding, W.: A matrix determinant feature extraction approach for decoding motor and mental imagery EEG in subject-specific tasks. IEEE Trans. Cogn. Dev. Syst. **14**(2), 375–387 (2020)

27. Yu, X., Aziz, M.Z., Sadiq, M.T., Fan, Z., Xiao, G.: A new framework for automatic detection of motor and mental imagery EEG signals for robust BCI systems. IEEE Trans. Instrum. Meas. **70**, 1–12 (2021)

28. Kronegg, J., Chanel, G., Voloshynovskiy, S., Pun, T.: EEG-based synchronized brain-computer interfaces: a model for optimizing the number of mental tasks. IEEE Trans. Neural Syst. Rehabil. Eng. **15**(1), 50–58 (2007)

29. Kosmyna, N., Lécuyer, A.: A conceptual space for EEG-based brain-computer interfaces. PLoS ONE **14**(1), e0210145 (2019)

30. Mellinger, J., et al.: An MEG-based brain-computer interface (BCI). Neuroimage **36**(3), 581–593 (2007)

31. Sitaram, R., et al.: FMRI brain-computer interface: a tool for neuroscientific research and treatment. Comput. Intell. Neurosci. **2007**, 1 (2007)

32. Zhu, Y., et al.: PET mapping for brain-computer-interface-based stimulation in a rat model with intracranial electrode implantation in the ventro-posterior medial thalamus. J. Nuclear Med. jnumed-115 (2016)

33. Fukuyama, H., et al.: Brain functional activity during gait in normal subjects: a SPECT study. Neurosci. Lett. **228**(3), 183–186 (1997)

34. Rodríguez-Bermúdez, G., García-Laencina, P.J.: Automatic and adaptive classification of electroencephalographic signals for brain computer interfaces. J. Med. Syst. **36**(1), 51–63 (2012)

35. Polat, K., Güneş, S.: Classification of epileptiform EEG using a hybrid system based on decision tree classifier and fast Fourier transform. Appl. Math. Comput. **187**(2), 1017–1026 (2007)

36. Pfurtscheller, G., Neuper, C., Schlogl, A., Lugger, K.: Separability of EEG signals recorded during right and left motor imagery using adaptive autoregressive parameters. IEEE Trans. Rehabil. Eng. **6**(3), 316–325 (1998)

37. Schlögl, A., Neuper, C., Pfurtscheller, G.: Estimating the mutual information of an EEG-based brain-computer interface. Biomedizinische Technik/Biomed. Eng. **47**(1–2), 3–8 (2002)

38. Burke, D.P., Kelly, S.P., de Chazal, P., Reilly, R.B., Finucane, C.: A parametric feature extraction and classification strategy for brain-computer interfacing. IEEE Trans. Neural Syst. Rehabil. Eng. **13**(1), 12–17 (2005)

39. Jansen, B.H., Bourne, J.R., Ward, J.W.: Autoregressive estimation of short segment spectra for computerized EEG analysis. IEEE Trans. Biomed. Eng. **9**, 630–638 (1981)

40. Krusienski, D.J., McFarland, D.J., Wolpaw, J.R.: An evaluation of autoregressive spectral estimation model order for brain-computer interface applications. In: International Conference of the IEEE Engineering in Medicine and Biology Society, pp. 1323–1326. IEEE (2006)

41. Kevric, J., Subasi, A.: Comparison of signal decomposition methods in classification of EEG signals for motor-imagery BCI system. Biomed. Signal Process. Control **31**, 398–406 (2017)

42. Ramoser, H., Muller-Gerking, J., Pfurtscheller, G.: Optimal spatial filtering of single trial EEG during imagined hand movement. IEEE Trans. Rehabil. Eng. **8**(4), 441–446 (2000)

43. Yong, X., Ward, R.K., Birch, G.E.: Sparse spatial filter optimization for EEG channel reduction in brain-computer interface. In: 2008 IEEE International Conference on Acoustics, Speech and Signal Processing, pp. 417–420. IEEE (2008)

44. Lu, H., Plataniotis, K.N., Venetsanopoulos, A.N.: Regularized common spatial patterns with generic learning for EEG signal classification. In: Annual International

Conference of the IEEE Engineering in Medicine and Biology Society, pp. 6599–6602. IEEE (2009)

45. Lotte, F., Guan, C.: Regularizing common spatial patterns to improve BCI designs: unified theory and new algorithms. IEEE Trans. Biomed. Eng. **58**(2), 355–362 (2010)

46. Zhang, R., Xu, P., Guo, L., Zhang, Y., Li, P., Yao, D.: Z-score linear discriminant analysis for EEG based brain-computer interfaces. PLoS ONE **8**(9), e74433 (2013)

47. Lu, H., Eng, H.-L., Guan, C., Plataniotis, K.N., Venetsanopoulos, A.N.: Regularized common spatial pattern with aggregation for EEG classification in small-sample setting. IEEE Trans. Biomed. Eng. **57**(12), 2936–2946 (2010)

48. Jiao, Y., et al.: Sparse group representation model for motor imagery EEG classification. IEEE J. Biomed. Health Inform. **23**(2), 631–641 (2018)

49. Zhang, Y., Nam, C.S., Zhou, G., Jin, J., Wang, X., Cichocki, A.: Temporally constrained sparse group spatial patterns for motor imagery BCI. IEEE Trans. Cybern. **49**(9), 3322–3332 (2018)

50. Feng, J.K., et al.: An optimized channel selection method based on multifrequency CSP-rank for motor imagery-based BCI system. Comput. Intell. Neurosci. **2019** (2019)

51. Li, Y., Wen, P.P., et al.: Clustering technique-based least square support vector machine for EEG signal classification. Comput. Methods Programs Biomed. **104**(3), 358–372 (2011)

52. Wu, W., Gao, X., Hong, B., Gao, S.: Classifying single-trial EEG during motor imagery by iterative spatio-spectral patterns learning (ISSPL). IEEE Trans. Biomed. Eng. **55**(6), 1733–1743 (2008)

53. Song, L., Epps, J.: Classifying EEG for brain-computer interface: learning optimal filters for dynamical system features. Comput. Intell. Neurosci. **2007**, 3 (2007)

54. Wang, S., James, C.J.: Extracting rhythmic brain activity for brain-computer interfacing through constrained independent component analysis. Comput. Intell. Neurosci. **2007** (2007)

55. Kutlu, Y., Kuntalp, D.: Feature extraction for ECG heartbeats using higher order statistics of WPD coefficients. Comput. Methods Programs Biomed. **105**(3), 257–267 (2012)

56. Sakhavi, S., Guan, C., Yan, S.: Learning temporal information for brain-computer interface using convolutional neural networks. IEEE Trans. Neural Netw. Learn. Syst. **29**(11), 5619–5629 (2018)

57. Thomas, J., Maszczyk, T., Sinha, N., Kluge, T., Dauwels, J.: Deep learning-based classification for brain-computer interfaces. In: 2017 IEEE International Conference on Systems, Man, and Cybernetics (SMC), pp. 234–239. IEEE (2017)

58. Jin, Z., Zhou, G., Gao, D., Zhang, Y.: EEG classification using sparse Bayesian extreme learning machine for brain-computer interface. Neural Comput. Appl. 1–9 (2018)

59. Zhang, Y., Wang, Y., Jin, J., Wang, X.: Sparse Bayesian learning for obtaining sparsity of EEG frequency bands based feature vectors in motor imagery classification. Int. J. Neural Syst. **27**(02), 1650032 (2017)

60. Zhang, X., Yao, L., Wang, X., Monaghan, J., Mcalpine, D.: A survey on deep learning based brain computer interface: recent advances and new frontiers. arXiv preprint arXiv:1905.04149 (2019)

61. Gilles, J.: Empirical wavelet transform. IEEE Trans. Signal Process. **61**(16), 3999–4010 (2013)

62. Blankertz, B., et al.: The BCI competition III: validating alternative approaches to actual BCI problems. IEEE Trans. Neural Syst. Rehabil. Eng. **14**(2), 153–159 (2006)

63. Jurcak, V., Tsuzuki, D., Dan, I.: 10/20, 10/10, and 10/5 systems revisited: their validity as relative head-surface-based positioning systems. Neuroimage **34**(4), 1600–1611 (2007)

64. Akbari, H., Sadiq, M.T.: Detection of focal and non-focal EEG signals using non-linear features derived from empirical wavelet transform rhythms. Phys. Eng. Sci. Med. **44**(1), 157–171 (2021)

65. Akbari, H., Ghofrani, S., Zakalvand, P., Sadiq, M.T.: Schizophrenia recognition based on the phase space dynamic of EEG signals and graphical features. Biomed. Signal Process. Control **69**, 102917 (2021)

66. Akbari, H., Sadiq, M.T., Siuly, S., Li, Y., Wen, P.: An automatic scheme with diagnostic index for identification of normal and depression EEG signals. In: Siuly, S., Wang, H., Chen, L., Guo, Y., Xing, C. (eds.) HIS 2021. LNCS, vol. 13079, pp. 59–70. Springer, Cham (2021). https://doi.org/10.1007/978-3-030-90885-0_6

67. Sadiq, M.T., Siuly, S., Ur Rehman, A., Wang, H.: Auto-correlation based feature extraction approach for EEG alcoholism identification. In: Siuly, S., Wang, H., Chen, L., Guo, Y., Xing, C. (eds.) HIS 2021. LNCS, vol. 13079, pp. 47–58. Springer, Cham (2021). https://doi.org/10.1007/978-3-030-90885-0_5

68. Sadiq, M.T., Akbari, H., Siuly, S., Li, Y., Wen, P.: Alcoholic EEG signals recognition based on phase space dynamic and geometrical features. Chaos Solitons Fractals **158**, 112036 (2022)

69. Asif, R.M., et al.: Design and analysis of robust fuzzy logic maximum power point tracking based isolated photovoltaic energy system. Eng. Rep. **2**(9), e12234 (2020)

70. Akbari, H., et al.: Depression recognition based on the reconstruction of phase space of EEG signals and geometrical features. Appl. Acoust. **179**, 108078 (2021)

71. Akhter, M.P., Jiangbin, Z., Naqvi, I.R., Abdelmajeed, M., Sadiq, M.T.: Automatic detection of offensive language for Urdu and Roman Urdu. IEEE Access **8**, 91213–91226 (2020)

72. Akhter, M.P., Jiangbin, Z., Naqvi, I.R., Abdelmajeed, M., Mehmood, A., Sadiq, M.T.: Document-level text classification using single-layer multisize filters convolutional neural network. IEEE Access **8**, 42689–42707 (2020)

73. Fan, Z., Jamil, M., Sadiq, M.T., Huang, X., Yu, X.: Exploiting multiple optimizers with transfer learning techniques for the identification of Covid-19 patients. J. Healthcare Eng. **2020** (2020)

74. Sadiq, M.T., Akbari, H., Siuly, S., Li, Y., Wen, P.: Fractional Fourier transform aided computerized framework for alcoholism identification in EEG. In: Traina, A., Wang, H., Zhang, Y., Siuly, S., Zhou, R., Chen, L. (eds.) HIS 2022. LNCS, vol. 13705, pp. 100–112. Springer, Cham (2022). https://doi.org/10.1007/978-3-031-20627-6_10

Image Recognition of Chicken Diseases Based on Improved Residual Networks

Nan Zhang[1,2], Xinqiang Ma[2(✉)], Yi Huang[2], and Jinsheng Bai[3]

[1] School of Computer Science and Engineering, Chongqing Three Gorges University, Chongqing 404020, People's Republic of China
[2] School of Artificial Intelligence, Chongqing University of Arts and Sciences, Chongqing 402160, People's Republic of China
xinqma@cqwu.edu.cn
[3] School of Computer Science and Technology, Southwest University of Science and Technology, Mianyang 621000, People's Republic of China

Abstract. Poultry diseases are one of the significant issues that need to be addressed in poultry farming today. In order to contribute to the prevention and control of poultry diseases and promote the healthy development of poultry farming, this paper focuses on a collected dataset of chicken manure images and proposes an improved chicken disease image recognition model based on ResNet18. The model utilizes ResNet18 as the underlying framework and incorporates attention mechanisms into the ResNet18 network model. It also includes a fully connected layer (Fc1) and Dropout for enhanced performance. Transfer learning is employed to train the model by freezing some layers of the pre-trained model to reduce training time. The Adam optimization algorithm is used to update gradients, and a cosine annealing method is implemented to decay the learning rate. Experimental results demonstrate that the improved ResNet18 network achieves an accuracy of 97.81% in chicken disease image recognition, which is 1.27% higher than the accuracy of the original ResNet18 network. This improved model exhibits superior performance and provides valuable insights for the analysis of chicken disease images.

Keywords: Image recognition · Chicken diseases · Deep learning · ResNet18 model

1 Introduction

As scientific and technological advancements continue to evolve, artificial intelligence (AI) has found applications in poultry farming. Poultry farming technolo-

Supported by the National Natural Science Foundation of China under Grant U22A20102; the Key Science and Technology Research Program of Chongqing Municipal Education Commission, China (Grant No. KJZD-K202101305); Natural Science Foundation of Chongqing, China (Grant No. cstc2021jcyj-msxmX0495, cstc2021jcyj-msxmX0654); the Yingcai Program of Chongqing, China(Grant No. cstc2021ycjh-bgzxm0218).

gies also need to be updated to adapt to new environments and requirements. The construction of intelligent poultry farming systems aims to make monitoring the environment of poultry farming areas and the growth conditions of poultry more convenient, effective, and real-time, enhancing farming efficiency and profitability.

At present, poultry farming faces several challenges: traditional feeding methods, inadequate facilities and equipment, poor sanitary conditions, confined spaces with high poultry density, and susceptibility to diseases. If diseases are not promptly detected and treated, it may lead to the widespread propagation of epidemics, resulting in substantial economic loss. Therefore, this experiment combines AI technology with poultry farming, enabling remote monitoring of poultry health conditions, significantly improving the information technology and intelligent level of poultry farming, reducing production costs, and enhancing labor efficiency.

Digestive system diseases are one of the most common diseases in poultry farming, severely affecting production. Fecal examination and observation are accurate techniques for detecting poultry digestive system diseases. The color, shape, and texture of chicken feces depend on diet and health conditions. With birds defecating over 12 times a day, any changes can be detected in real-time, making fecal testing one of the most effective techniques for detecting digestive system diseases. However, manual observation requires a considerable amount of personnel regularly checking the henhouses, and the speed and accuracy of poultry disease diagnosis mainly depend on the keepers' experience and knowledge. This process is time-consuming and labor-intensive, and diseases may not be detected promptly [1]. Recently, AI has made significant breakthroughs in the field of computer vision, and deep learning, a primary direction of AI, has shown good effects in disease detection.

2   Related Works

2.1   Deep Learning in Agricultural Applications

With the continuous deepening of research on deep learning algorithms, deep learning algorithms have shown many advantages in recognition and have been extensively studied in areas such as image classification, recognition, and detection. In the agricultural field, deep learning technology has achieved good results in crop disease recognition.

Arya et al. [2] applied the AlexNet architecture to the detection of potato and mango leaf diseases, achieving an accuracy of 98.33%, 7.84% higher than the CNN architecture's accuracy of 90.85%.

Zhang Jianhua et al. [3] optimized the complete connection layer based on the VGG-16 network model, proposed an improved VGG network model, which accurately identified cotton diseases with an accuracy rate of approximately 89.5%.

Brahimi et al. [4] compared the effectiveness of AlexNet and GoogLeNet in detecting tomato leaf pests and diseases, and the experiments showed that GoogLeNet performed better.

Tan Yunlan et al. [5] adjusted the model based on GoogLeNet for detecting bacterial wilt disease, achieving an accuracy rate of 93%.

Malathi et al. [6] fine-tuned the hyperparameters and layers of the ResNet-50 model and applied the transfer learning method to the Pest dataset, achieving a precision of up to 95%.

Chen Juan et al. [7] proposed to recognize garden pests by improving ResNet.

At present, there are few poultry disease detection methods based on deep learning as a core technology, and there is still a large room for improvement in detection efficiency and recognition accuracy.

2.2 Attention Mechanism in Deep Learning Models

Xu et al. [8] introduced an attention mechanism based on the NIC model, extracting important information from images to improve the model's accuracy. Most attention mechanisms only simulate spatial attention mechanisms. Chen et al. [9] proposed the SCA-CNN model, which models spatial attention mechanisms and channel attention mechanisms, greatly improving the model's performance, but the model is not portable and flexible enough. Pang bo [10] proposed to classify images using the EfficientNet and Convolutional Block Attention Module (CBAM). This attention mechanism (CBAM) combines spatial attention mechanisms and channel attention mechanisms and uses average pooling and max pooling technology to improve the model's efficiency.

Therefore, to further improve the performance of the chicken disease recognition model, this study uses ResNet18 as the base model and adds a convolutional attention module(CBAM) after the last convolutional layer to enhance the extraction capability of detailed features. We also added a fully connected layer and Dropout to solve overfitting problems and poor generalization capabilities, creating a chicken disease recognition model based on the improved ResNet18.

3   Experiments

3.1   Image Acquisition and Preprocessing

Chicken Excrement Image Acquisition. The dataset used in this experiment is sourced from the open dataset "machine-learning-dataset-for-poultry-diseases-diagnostics" available on the Kaggle platform. This dataset consists of poultry feces images. Kaggle is a platform founded by Anthony Goldbloom in Melbourne in 2010, providing functionalities such as machine learning competitions, data sharing, and programming for developers and data scientists [11]. The dataset comprises a total of 8067 images, mostly captured under natural conditions, and it includes four classes of data: Salmonella, Coccidiosis, New Castle Disease, and Healthy. Some examples of chicken feces image samples are shown in Fig. 1.

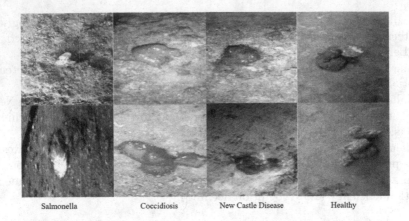

Salmonella   Coccidiosis   New Castle Disease   Healthy

Fig. 1. Samples of chicken manure images.

The distribution of different types of chicken feces image samples in the dataset is shown in Table 1.

Table 1. Distribution of Chicken Feces Image Samples by Category.

Category	Number of Samples
Salmonella	2625
Coccidiosis	2476
New Castle Disease	562
Healthy	2404
Total	8067

Image Data Preprocessing. In order to accelerate the training and convergence speed of the network model and enhance its accuracy, it is necessary to preprocess the image dataset used for model training. In this study, data augmentation was performed on images of chicken feces, utilizing spatial scale transformations, other transformations, and normalization [12]. The spatial scale transformations included random aspect ratio cropping, random rotation, as well as horizontal and vertical flipping of the chicken feces images. The other transformations comprised adjustments to brightness, saturation, and contrast, in addition to the addition of Gaussian blur and salt-and-pepper noise. Normalization was implemented by inputting the mean and standard deviation to standardize the pixel values in the chicken feces images. The normalization process first mapped the single-channel color values of pixels in the chicken feces images from the range [0, 225] to [0, 1], followed by converting the images into tensor format. Subsequently, the pixel value of each channel in the input image was subtracted by the corresponding channel's mean, and then divided by the corresponding channel's standard deviation. The purpose of this procedure was to normalize the pixel values of the images to have zero mean and unit variance, facilitating better adaptation for model training. After preprocessing, the resolution of the chicken feces images was 3 channels × 224 pixels × 224 pixels.

3.2 Model Construction

Improved ResNet18 Model. Convolutional neural networks (CNNs) can automatically extract a large number of spatial visual features from convolutional layers. [13] Furthermore, CNNs also comprise of activation layers that perform solid non-linear mapping, lower sampling layers (i.e., pooling layers), fully connected layers that convert features from two dimensions to one dimension, and loss functions that compute the deviation between output values and true values.

Theoretically, increasing the number of layers in a neural network can extract more complex features and yield better results. However, a substantial amount of experimental evidence suggests that the performance of deep convolutional networks saturates and may even degrade after reaching a certain number of layers. To address the issue of vanishing and exploding gradients in the network, Kaiming He and his colleagues [14] proposed a residual network based on skip connections and identity mapping in 2015.

In this study, we adopt the classical ResNet18 convolutional neural network and make adjustments and optimizations to it, followed by transfer learning and frozen training. The structure of the improved ResNet18 model is illustrated in Fig. 2.

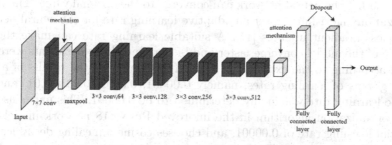

Fig. 2. Improved ResNet18 network structure diagram.

Transfer Learning and Frozen Training. Transfer learning is an extremely effective method for addressing overfitting problems in the learning and training processes of neural networks with small datasets. [15] By storing pre-trained feature parameters from large networks like ImageNet and applying them to new tasks, the transferability of feature model weights between different data enhances the efficiency and accuracy of small data classification problems [16]. This paper uses ResNet18 network as the base architecture, sets the new sample parameters as parameters trained on the ImageNet dataset, and trains the chicken manure image dataset using transfer learning methods.

Frozen training is also an important concept in transfer learning and is widely used in image recognition tasks. If we want the model to achieve a lower loss value, transfer learning alone is not enough; we also need the help of frozen training. We attempt to freeze the training model to further improve its performance. In this paper, due to the small amount of data in the chicken manure dataset, we freeze all the fully connected layers of the model to train the other convolutional layers.

Loss Function. This study chooses cross entropy loss as the loss function for the improved ResNet18 model, which has a larger gradient during network training and optimizes the network faster. Its formula is:

$$L = -\frac{1}{N} \sum_{i}^{N} \sum_{j}^{M} p_{ij} \cdot \log q_{ij} \tag{1}$$

where L is the loss function, N is the number of samples, M is the number of classes, p_{ij} represents the probability distribution value of the jth class of the ith sample in the true value of the label, and q_{ij} represents the probability that sample i belongs to class j in the predicted value.

Optimizer and Learning Rate Decay. Choosing an appropriate learning rate plays a crucial role in classification performance in model training; it determines whether the neural network can converge to the optimal value. The Adam optimization algorithm can set an adaptive learning rate for the neural network during loss gradient updates [17]. A suitable learning rate can make the loss function of the model converge faster and better, and the experiments were conducted according to the exponential scale after comparing the results of a total of five groups of learning rates, namely 0.00001, 0.0001, 0.001, 0.01, and 0.1, and the learning rate was finally determined to be 0.00001. This paper uses the Adam optimization algorithm in the improved ResNet18 network model, with an initial learning rate of 0.00001, and chooses cosine annealing decay learning rate, setting its parameter T_max to the size of the number of iterations. As the number of network iterations increases during the network training process, it gradually decreases, which helps quickly reach the optimal solution and reduces oscillations later.

Fully Connected Layer and Dropout. An additional fully connected layer fc1 is added in the improved ResNet18 model network structure, which can extract more feature information through the neural network. Meanwhile, adding Dropout can avoid the risk of overfitting and reduce the generalization error of classification. The Dropout parameter is set to 0.5, and the network will randomly deactivate half of the neurons during the training process. When the gradient is back-propagated, the neurons that are deactivated and disconnected will not participate in parameter updates.

CBAM Attention Mechanism. To improve the accuracy of the model in extracting image features [18, 19], the CBAM module was added to the base of the ResNet18 network to obtain more key information from the image's spatial attention mechanism and channel attention mechanism.

The CBAM module comprises two parts: the channel attention module and the spatial attention module. The input to CBAM is the intrinsic matrix. The channel attention mechanism performs global average pooling and global max pooling on the incoming feature matrix respectively. The results are then processed through a shared fully connected layer. The two processed results are added together and a sigmoid is taken. At this point, the weights of each channel in the input feature matrix are obtained. After obtaining these weights, the weights are multiplied with the original input feature matrix to get a new feature matrix. Its process formula is:

$$M_c(F) = \sigma(MLP(\text{AvgPool}(F)) + \text{MLP}(\text{MaxPool}(F))) \tag{2}$$

where F is the input feature matrix, MLP is the multilayer perceptron function, AvgPool is the average pooling layer function, MaxPool is the max pooling layer function, and σ is the Sigmoid function.

The new feature matrix obtained is used as the input to the spatial attention mechanism model. The maximum and average values are taken on the channel of each feature point. The two results are then stacked, adjusted by a convolution with a channel count of 1, and a sigmoid is taken to get the weight of each feature point in the input feature matrix. Finally, this weight is multiplied by the original input matrix to get the output, a new feature matrix [20]. Its process formula is:

$$M_s(F) = \sigma\left(f^{7\times7}([\text{AvgPool}(F); \text{MaxPool}(F)])\right) \tag{3}$$

where F is the input feature matrix, $f^{7\times7}$ is the 7×7 convolution kernel, AvgPool is the average pooling layer function, MaxPool is the max pooling layer function, and σ is the Sigmoid function.

4 Results and Analysis

4.1 Model Training and Evaluation

Model Training Environment. The model training environment in this paper is based on the PyTorch deep learning framework, programmed in Python 3.8, running on a Windows 11 operating system, with a GPU featuring 128 GB memory by Nvidia Quadro GP100. The basic configuration includes Anaconda3 and PyCharm.

Performance Comparison of Attention Mechanism Modules at Different Locations. In order to verify the effectiveness of the attention mechanism's placement within the network, we compared the effect of the position and number of attention mechanisms added to the network on model accuracy. Five schemes for adding attention mechanisms were designed in this study.

The five schemes for adding attention mechanisms are: adding an attention mechanism in the Block layer (Scheme 1); adding an attention mechanism after the first convolutional layer (Scheme 2); adding two attention mechanisms after the first and the last convolutional layers (Scheme 3); adding an attention mechanism after the last convolutional layer (Scheme 4); no addition of attention mechanism (Scheme 5). Under the premise of maintaining consistent training parameters, training and verification were carried out in the improved ResNet18 network model. The experimental results are shown in Table 2.

Table 2. Comparison of Different Approaches to Adding Attention.

Attention Mechanism Addition Scheme	Training Set Accuracy	Validation Set Accuracy
Scheme 1	97.49%	97.64%
Scheme 2	97.45%	97.73%
Scheme 3	97.40%	97.81%
Scheme 4	97.59%	97.77%
Scheme 5	96.73%	96.54%

Table 2 shows that adding one attention mechanism slightly improves model performance, and the recognition accuracy reaches the best when two attention mechanisms are added, indicating that the introduction of the attention mechanism effectively improves the accuracy of the validation set.

4.2 Comparative Analysis of the Improved ResNet18 Model and Other Models

In order to verify the recognition effect of the improved model, this study uses the tri-fold validation method to compare the improved ResNet18 model with AlexNet, GoogLeNet, VGG16, ResNet18, ResNet34, and ResNet50 under the condition that the basic settings of preprocessing methods, initialization weights, and optimization algorithms of different models remain the same. The models were evaluated with accuracy. The performance of each model is compared, and the optimal model is selected and saved for each iteration, and the training and verification recognition accuracy results are shown in Table 3.

According to Table 3, the final accuracy of each convolutional network model on the chicken disease recognition dataset is above 95%. Compared to AlexNet, GoogLeNet, VGG16, ResNet18, ResNet34, and ResNet50, the

Table 3. Table captions should be placed above the tables.

Model	Acc(Training)	Acc(Vali)	Size(MB)	TrainingTime(s)
AlexNet	90.51%	95.19%	61.77	8
GoogLeNet	96.59%	96.37%	134.26	16
VGG16	96.35%	96.44%	731.38	63
ResNet18	95.73%	96.54%	107.96	12
Improved ResNet18	**97.40%**	**97.81%**	**114.87**	**15**
ResNet34	97.07%	97.13%	178.06	18
ResNet50	97.54%	97.63%	376.83	31

improved ResNet18 model proposed in this study has a higher test set accuracy, respectively outperforming by 2.62%, 1.44%, 1.37%, 1.27%, 0.68%, and 0.18%. Despite the fact that the ResNet50 utilizes a deeper network structure to ensure strong feature learning capabilities and achieves a test accuracy of 97.63%, it requires a training time of 31 s per iteration, which is not as fast or accurate as the improved ResNet18 model. The improved ResNet18 model is only 6.91 MB larger than the original ResNet18 model, but it greatly improves accuracy. The model size and training time of AlexNet are both smaller than the improved ResNet18, but its accuracy is much lower. Compared to other models, the improved ResNet18 model not only has a smaller model size but also greatly improves recognition accuracy.

5 Conclusion

In order to better contribute to poultry disease control, an improved ResNet18 model is used in this paper to identify and classify four common chicken diseases. With ResNet18 as the base network, the feature extraction capability is enhanced by adding one attention mechanism module after the first convolutional layer and one after the last convolutional layer to focus on chicken droppings; adding a fully connected layer and Dropout to solve the problems of network overfitting and poor generalization ability; introducing a migration learning mechanism and freezing some of the hierarchical parameters of the pre-trained model to reduce the training time. The experimental results show that the improved model has higher recognition accuracy and the model performance has been improved to some extent. The improved method has good classification accuracy and generalization performance, and can provide an effective reference for identifying chickens suffering from a certain disease through chicken feces.

References

1. Yang, J., Sun, R., Jin, C., Yin, B.: Research on the identification method of intestinal diseases in laying hens based on multi-scale convolution. China Agric. Inform. **34**, 14–26 (2022)

2. Arya, S., Singh, R.: A comparative study of CNN and AlexNet for detection of disease in potato and mango leaf. In: 2019 International Conference on Issues and Challenges in Intelligent Computing Techniques (ICICT) (2019)
3. Zhang, J., Kong, F., Wu, J., Zhai, Z., Han, S., Cao, S.: Cotton disease identification model based on improved VGG convolution neural network. J. China Agric. Univ. **23**, 161–171 (2018)
4. Brahimi, M., Boukhalfa, K., Moussaoui, A.: Deep learning for tomato diseases: classification and symptoms visualization. Appl. Artif. Intell. **31**(4–6), 1–17 (2017)
5. Tan, Y., Ouyang, C., Li, L., Liao, T., Tang, P.: Image recognition of rice diseases based on deep convolutional neural network. J. Jinggangshan Univ. (Nat. Sci.) **40**, 31–38 (2019)
6. Malathi, V., Gopinath, M.P.: Classification of diseases in paddy using deep convolutional neural network. In: Journal of Physics: Conference Series, vol. 1964, no. 4, p. 042028 (2021)
7. Chen, J., Chen, L., Wang, S., Zhao, H., Wen, C.: Pest image recognition of garden based on improved residual network. Trans. Chin. Soc. Agric. Mach. **50**, 187–195 (2019)
8. Xu, K., et al.: Show, attend and tell: neural image caption generation with visual attention. Comput. Sci. 2048–2057 (2015)
9. Long, C., Zhang, H., Xiao, J., Nie, L., Chua, T.S.: SCA-CNN: spatial and channel-wise attention in convolutional networks for image captioning. In: 2017 IEEE Conference on Computer Vision and Pattern Recognition (CVPR) (2016)
10. Pang, B.: Classification of images using EfficientNet CNN model with convolutional block attention module (CBAM) and spatial group-wise enhance module (SGE). In: Agyeman, M.O., Sirkemaa, S. (eds.) International Conference on Image, Signal Processing, and Pattern Recognition (ISPP 2022), vol. 12247, p. 1224707. International Society for Optics and Photonics, SPIE (2022)
11. Wei, F., Zhang, Z., Liang, G.: Research on application of insect species image recognition based on convolutional neural network. J. Henan Normal Univ. (Nat. Sci. Ed.) **50**, 96–105 (2022)
12. Wan, P., et al.: Freshwater fish species identification method based on improved ResNet50 model. Trans. Chin. Soc. Agric. Eng. **37**, 159–168 (2021)
13. Sarki, R., Ahmed, K., Wang, H., Zhang, Y., Wang, K.: Convolutional neural network for multi-class classification of diabetic eye disease. EAI Endorsed Trans. Scalable Inf. Syst. e15–e15 (2022)
14. Siddiqui, S.A., Fatima, N., Ahmad, A.: Chest X-ray and CT scan classification using ensemble learning through transfer learning. EAI Endorsed Trans. Scalable Inf. Syst. **9**(6), e8 (2022)
15. He, K., Zhang, X., Ren, S., Sun, J.: Deep residual learning for image recognition. IEEE (2016)
16. Li, L., Tian, W., Chen, L.: Wild plant image recognition method based on residual network and transfer learning. Radio Eng. **51**, 857–863 (2021)
17. Loshchilov, I., Hutter, F.: Decoupled weight decay regularization (2017)
18. Pan, L., et al.: MFDNN: multi-channel feature deep neural network algorithm to identify Covid-19 chest X-ray images. Health Inf. Sci. Syst. **10**(1) (2022)
19. Du, J., Michalska, S., Subramani, S., Wang, H., Zhang, Y.: Neural attention with character embeddings for hay fever detection from Twitter. Health Inf. Sci. Syst. **7**(1), 1–7 (2019)
20. Chen, H., Han, Y.: Tire classification based on attention mechanism and transfer learning. Software **43**, 65–69 (2022)

An Adaptive Feature Fusion Network for Alzheimer's Disease Prediction

Shicheng Wei(✉) , Yan Li, and Wencheng Yang

School of Mathematics, Physics and Computing, University of Southern Queensland,
Toowoomba, Australia
{shicheng.wei,Yan.Li,Wencheng.Yang}@unisq.edu.au

Abstract. Structural Magnetic Resonance Imaging (sMRI) of brain structures has proven effective in predicting early lesions associated with Alzheimer's disease (AD). However, identifying the AD lesion area solely through sMRI is challenging, as only a few abnormal texture areas are directly linked to the lesion. Moreover, the observed lesion area varies when examining two-dimensional MRI slides in different directions within three-dimensional space. Traditional convolutional neural networks struggle to accurately focus on the AD lesion structure. To address this issue, we propose an adaptive feature fusion network for AD prediction. Firstly, an adaptive feature fusion module is constructed to enhance attention towards lesion areas by considering features from three directions and fusing them together. Secondly, a multi-channel group convolution module is designed to improve the network's ability to extract fine-grained features by separating convolutional channels. Finally, a regularized loss function is introduced to combine the Soft-Max loss function and clustering loss function. This helps enhance the network's ability to differentiate between different sample types. Experimental results from binary classification tests on the dataset obtained from Alzheimer's Disease Neuroimaging Initiative (ADNI) demonstrate that our proposed method accurately distinguishes between normal control (NC), progressive mild cognitive impairment (pMCI), stable mild cognitive impairment (sMCI), and AD.

Keywords: Alzheimer's disease · sMRI · convolutional neural network · Deep Learning

1 Introduction

Alzheimer's disease (AD) is a gradually progressing neurodegenerative disorder. Initial symptoms include short-term memory loss, and as the condition advances, individuals may experience language difficulties, confusion, and various behavioral issues. Over time, a patient's physical abilities decline, ultimately resulting in death. Generally, AD can be broadly categorized into four stages, spanning from early to advanced stages: Normal control (NC), stable mild cognitive impairment(sMCI), progressive mild cognitive impairment(pMCI), and AD.

Y. Li et al. (Eds.): HIS 2023, LNCS 14305, pp. 271–282, 2023.
https://doi.org/10.1007/978-981-99-7108-4_23

Currently, there are no efficient therapies and treatments to halt or reverse the progression of the disease. However, if AD is diagnosed at an early stage, doctors can intervene earlier to slow its progression. There are studies [1–4] that show how structural magnetic resonance imaging (sMRI) can be an effective tool for clinical doctors in assessing the state of patients with sMCI, pMCI, and AD. This is because sMRI can provide vital information regarding changes in the brain structure.

Nowadays, deep learning is widely employed for predicting AD using sMRI data [5]. The utilization of sMRI data can be broadly categorized into 2-dimensional (2D) and 3-dimensional (3D) formats. Hoang et al. [6] proposed a method that employed a vision transformer to extract feature maps from three 2D sagittal slices, enabling the classification of Mild Cognitive Impairment (MCI) and AD. Xing et al. [7] introduced a technique that combined fusion attention and residual network, adaptively extracting feature information from 2D sMRI data using the residual network, resulting in effective classification outcomes.

However, contextual information along the depth dimension is lost when a 3D image is sliced into 2D images. To address this issue, the utilization of the entire 3D sMRI data can be explored. Zhang et al. [8] presented an approach incorporating self-attention mechanism and residual learning into a 3D convolutional neural network (CNN). This method intelligently harnesses both global and local information, effectively preventing the loss of crucial context information. Bakkouri et al. [9] introduced a technique that enhanced traditional 3D convolution by incorporating multi-scale convolution. This approach enables the extraction of brain atrophy features across various scales by utilizing convolution modules of different sizes, ultimately enhancing the overall prediction effectiveness. Chen et al. [10] proposed a multi-view slicing attention mechanism that was integrated into a 3D CNN. Initially, 2D slicing was employed to remove redundant information, followed by the use of a 3D network for feature extraction, effectively mitigating the risk of overfitting. Liu et al. [11] proposed a network that leveraged 3D sMRI data to extract feature maps from three distinct perspectives. By employing multi-scale convolution to extract feature information, the obtained results were concatenated in the channel dimension, enabling the acquisition of more comprehensive information regarding lesion regions.

1.1   Motivation and Contribution

Nevertheless, the aforementioned 3D-based methods either overlooked the convolution of 3D data in various directions or struggled to adequately incorporate feature maps acquired from all three dimensions. Consequently, these methods are unable to fully harness the intrinsic feature information embedded within the 3D data. To overcome these limitations, in this paper, we develop a backbone network that excels at extracting focal information from 3D MRI scans across three distinct section directions by leveraging the power of multi-scale and multi-channel group convolution techniques, coupled with an adaptive fusion mechanism. The contributions of this paper are summarised as follows:

1. This paper presents an approach called multi-scale multi-channel group convolution, which isolates information from different groups to ensure a complete fusion of local information. This technique effectively enhances the ability of the network to extract detailed information by allowing a comprehensive integration of local features.
2. An adaptive-attention fusion module is proposed. This module can efficiently extract feature maps from sagittal, coronal, and axial planes. By enabling simultaneous consideration of features from all three directions before classification, this module effectively directs attention towards the crucial lesion atrophy, leading to improved analysis and diagnosis.
3. A regularization loss function is employed. This loss function incorporates a regularization term into a softmax function, encouraging stronger grouping and clustering within the same category.

1.2 Organization of This Paper

The structure of the remaining paper is as follows: Sect. 2 provides a comprehensive overview of the proposed methodology, offering detailed explanations of the key components and techniques employed. Section 3 comprises ablation and competing experiments. Lastly, in Sect. 4, the paper concludes by summarizing the key findings and contributions, emphasizing the significance of the proposed methodology in addressing the research problem at hand.

2 Methdology

This section offers a comprehensive explanation of the proposed network for AD prediction, leveraging multi-channel group convolution and adaptive feature fusion. The initial focus is on introducing the overview of the proposed network. Subsequently, three essential components, namely, multi-scale multi-channel group convolution, adaptive feature fusion module, and regularized loss function, are detailed.

2.1 Overview of the Proposed Network

The overall network is composed of three main parts: multi-scale multi-channel group convolution, adaptive feature fusion module, and a classifier combined with regularized loss function. In this network, sMRI data from three different directions (axial plane, sagittal plane, and coronal plane) are taken as input, and data from different directions will be convolved with convolution kernels of different sizes, respectively, to extract richer feature information. After multi-scale convolution, multi-channel group convolution is performed on the concatenated feature graphs by the proposed network. By employing group convolution, the network is able to isolate and fuse information from different groups, allowing for a clear focus on the details of the focal area.

After obtaining the feature maps from the three different planes, they are first concatenated. The spliced feature map is then input into the adaptive feature fusion module of the proposed network to adaptively learn the clearest feature of the lesion. Then the output was forwarded to the classifier for classification. Figure 1 depicts the architecture of the proposed network.

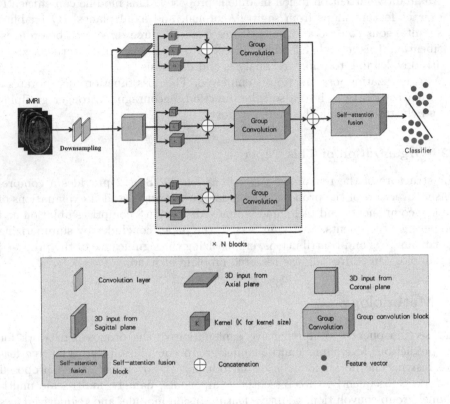

Fig. 1. The Framework of The Proposed Network

2.2   Multi-scale Multi-channel Group Convolution

To extract multi-scale information, this paper simultaneously applies convolution kernels with sizes of $1 \times 1 \times 1$, $3 \times 3 \times 3$, and $5 \times 5 \times 5$ to perform multi-scale convolution on the axial, sagittal, and coronal planes of 3D MRI data, followed by concatenating the obtained feature maps. Although multi-scale convolution can adequately extract features, 3D MRI data contains a wealth of feature information [12], and a simple concatenation operation cannot establish the relationships between features well, therefore hindering the network's ability to consider both local and global feature information during feature assessment. To effectively tackle this challenge, this paper proposes a refinement by introducing a multi-channel grouped convolution operation in conjunction with multi-scale convolution. This approach enhances the synergy among local information within the feature map, enabling a more precise focus on intricate lesion areas while simultaneously extracting comprehensive and information-rich features.

In general, when two convolution kernels are used on the feature map, each kernel should be applied to each channel of the feature mapping. In contrast, when the feature map is grouped with two convolution kernels, each kernel only needs to be applied to the corresponding channel of the feature map. It is evident that using group convolution instead of conventional convolution effectively reduces the number of parameters and computational load by half, thus alleviating the overfitting problem caused by increasing the network's depth.

Following the multi-scale convolution, the feature graph with a certain size is partitioned into three groups. One, two, and four convolution kernels are utilized for group convolution, enabling the extraction of global information from the feature graph. By dividing the feature graphs into two groups using two convolution kernels, separate information exchange between the groups is achieved. This isolation allows for interaction within each group, facilitating the comprehensive extraction of local information and enhancing the network's capacity to capture fine-grained features.

2.3   Adaptive Attention Fusion Module

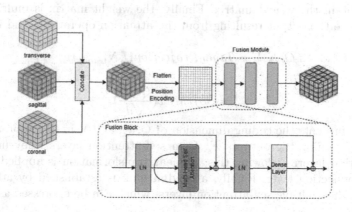

Fig. 2. Structure of Adaptive Fusion Module

After the extraction of the features from the 3D images in each of the three directions using the preceding feature extraction network, it becomes imperative to utilize these features effectively and integrate them across the three directions. To facilitate the complementary nature of features from different directions, an adaptive feature fusion block has been devised in this study. The module's design aims to foster synergistic relationships among features, ensuring that they mutually enhance one another. The details of this adaptive feature fusion module are illustrated in Fig. 2.

Due to the variations in observation angles, and relative positions of features across different directions, directly concatenating feature maps would result in a coarse connection between features, hindering the network's ability to capture precise position and structure information. To address this issue, a series of operations are performed after connecting the feature maps. Specifically, spatial position coding and feature flattening operations transform the 3D feature map into a one-dimensional representation while preserving the original spatial position information. This process not only enhances the network's robustness but also facilitates the input of features into a fusion block, which is responsible for adaptively fusing features from different directions and positions. The calculations involved in this step can be described as follows:

$$F_{out}^0 = Flatten(Concat(F_{Axial}, F_{Sagital}, F_{Coronal}) + Position) \qquad (1)$$

where, $F_{Axial}, F_{Sagital}, F_{Coronal}$ refers to the feature map extracted from different planes of axial, sagittal, and coronal direction.

The fusion block module begins by normalizing the output F_{out} of the previous layer using a Layer Normalization layer. Subsequently, F_{out} undergoes a linear project onto Q (query), K (keys), and V (value), followed by an input into a multi-head self-attention module. The calculation method for the similarity matrix in the self-attention operation is based on the approach proposed in [13]. The similarity matrix, derived from Q and K, is then passed through a SoftMax layer to obtain the weight matrix. Finally, the weight matrix is multiplied by V to produce the output resulting from the attention operation. And it can be described as:

$$Q, K, V = LinerProjection(LN(F_{out}^0)) \qquad (2)$$

$$F_s^1 = SoftMax(\frac{QK^T}{\sqrt{d}}) \qquad (3)$$

where, d represents the coding dimension of Q, K, and V in our approach.

After obtaining the outputs F_s^1 from self-attention layers, they undergo a normalization layer. Following this, a linear transformation is applied through a dense connection layer. Finally, a residual link is established by adding the outputs of the multiple self-attention layers, which can be expressed as:

$$F_{out}^2 = LinearProjection(LN(F_s^1)) + F_s^1 \qquad (4)$$

Adaptive fusion of features in different directions and positions will be achieved by stacking multiple fusion blocks.

2.4   Regularised Loss Function

In this image classification, the primary goal is to minimize the cross-entropy loss, which effectively maximizes the logarithm of the probability with the target labels. This paper introduces the utilization of a clustering loss function, which enables the automatic learning of score centers for each category within the datasets. This is achieved by minimizing the distance between the sample score and the score centers of the corresponding category. The clustering loss function effectively constrains the growth of predicted scores. In the context of tag position scores, it is typically desired that the score accurately reflects the importance of the tag. However, if the score increases infinitely, the network may excessively and overconfidently predict certain tag positions, leading to a decline in generalization ability.

By incorporating score clustering losses, the network is compelled to acquire a smoother label prediction outcome. In other words, if the tag score increases rapidly, the loss function will restrict this situation, encouraging the network to adopt a more gradual score growth approach [14]. This helps to reduce the network's confidence and make it more cautious in its predictions, thereby enhancing the network's generalization ability.

The loss function can be formulated as follows:

$$L_{SC} = \frac{1}{2} \sum_{i=1}^{m} \|\mathbf{S_i} - \mathbf{SC_{yi}}\|_2^2 \tag{5}$$

where m is the number of a batch of training data. S_i is the score vector of i samples, and SC_{y_i} is the score center of class y_i. SC_{y_i} has the same dimension as S_i, equal to the number of categories.

In the training process, SC_{y_i} is initialized as an all-zero vector, which is constantly updated with the training process. The updates of SC_{y_i} are as follows:

$$\Delta SC_j = \frac{\sum_{i=1}^{m} \delta(y_i = j) \cdot (SC_j - S_i)}{1 + \sum_{i=1}^{m}} \tag{6}$$

In the proposed method, the softmax loss function [15] and cluster loss function are combined to train the network, and λ is used to balance the relationship between the two. The formula is expressed as follows:

$$L_{softmax} = -\sum_{i=1}^{m} log \frac{eS_{y_i}}{\sum n_{j=1} eS_{y_i}} \tag{7}$$

$$L_{total} = L_{softmax} + \lambda \cdot L_{SC} = -\sum_{i=1}^{m} log \frac{eS_{y_i}}{\sum n_{j=1} eS_{y_i}} + \frac{\sum_{i=1}^{m} \delta(y_i = j) \cdot (SC_j - S_i)}{1 + \sum_{i=1}^{m}} \tag{8}$$

where S_{y_i} is the score belonging to class y_i in the i_{th} sample.

During each iteration, the network's overall loss, as defined in Eq. (8), is calculated. The weight parameters are then updated using the gradient descent method, and the scoring center is updated according to the formula (6). This iterative training process enforces a constraint on the scores of each category, directing them to stay close to their respective scoring centers. As a result, the problem of overfitting is alleviated by preventing the scores for the correct tag positions from growing infinitely.

3   Experimental Results and Discussion

3.1   Databases Used in This Paper

The experiment utilized a dataset of which the records are selected from the publicly available Alzheimer's Disease Neuroimaging Initiative (ADNI) databases, namely, ADNI-1 and ADNI-2 [16]. The data collection of ADNI-1 was initiated in 2004 and lasted until 2009, while ADNI-2 started in 2011 and continued until 2016. ADNI-2 can be regarded as a continuation or extension of ADNI-1. Because certain records within the ADNI-1 and ADNI-2 databases presented issues such as duplication, missing data, and poor data quality, a selection process was implemented to exclude such records. As a result, the selected dataset comprises 170 AD, 156 pMCI, 202 sMCI, and 206 NC records from the ADNI-1 database, in addition to 102 AD, 101 pMCI, 329 sMCI, and 147 NC records from the ADNI-2 database.

Table 1. Demographic information of the subjects included in this study

Dataset	Category	Gender (Male/Female	Age[a]	Education[b]	CDR[c]	MMSE[d]
ADNI-1	AD	88/82	75.37 ± 7.48	14.61 ± 3.18	0.74 ± 0.24	23.22 ± 2.03
	pMCI	94/62	74.57 ± 7.11	15.74 ± 2.90	0.5 ± 0.0	26.53 ± 1.70
	sMCI	131/71	74.55 ± 7.59	15.54 ± 3.11	0.49 ± 0.03	27.37 ± 1.76
	NC	103/103	75.85 ± 5.10	15.92 ± 2.86	0.0 ± 0.0	29.14 ± 0.98
ADNI-2	AD	58/44	74.44 ± 7.89	15.99 ± 2.51	0.77 ± 0.27	22.99 ± 2.16
	pMCI	55/46	72.54 ± 6.96	15.99 ± 2.58	0.50 ± 0.04	27.55 ± 1.78
	sMCI	174/155	71.11 ± 7.51	16.16 ± 2.67	0.49 ± 0.02	28.18 ± 1.64
	NC	72/75	73.72 ± 6.39	16.68 ± 2.42	0.0 ± 0.0	29.06 ± 1.21

a. Age of subjects, b. Education years of subjects, c. Clinical Dementia Rating (CDR) is a scale used to assess the severity of dementia and cognitive impairment in individuals diagnosed with Alzheimer's disease or other forms of dementia, d. Minimum Mental Status Examination (MMSE) is calculated based on the subjects' performance on a series of questions and tasks that assess the subjects' cognitive abilities.

Table 1 provides an overview of pertinent clinical information about the study subjects, encompassing gender, age, education, CDR, and MMSE scores. Notably, significant disparities in Minimum Mental State Examination scores were observed among the AD, MCI, and NC groups. For example, within the AD group of ADNI-1, there are 88 male and 82 female participants. Their average age is 75.27 years, with a standard deviation of 7.48. On average, they had completed 14.61 years of education, with a standard deviation of 3.18. The mean CDR for this group is 0.74, accompanied by a standard deviation of 0.24. Additionally, the mean score on the MMSE is 23.22, with a standard deviation of 2.03.

The sMR images from selected dataset utilized in this study are initially processed using the Statistical Parametric Mapping (SPM) tool in MATLAB. Subsequently, the images are down-sampled to serve as inputs for the network proposed in this paper. Prior to training, a preconditioning process is employed, which encompasses cranial anatomy, strength correction, and spatial registration. To ensure training results are not skewed, the AD, MCI, and NC data used in the experiments are evenly allocated, guaranteeing an equal representation of each data category during the training phase.

In this paper, experiments are carried out under Windows 10 system, and the proposed network is implemented based on Python3.9 and Pytorch-GPU. Other hardware configurations are listed as follows: CPU(Intel i7-12700K@3.6 GHz), Memory(64 GB), Hard disk(1 TB).

Accuracy (ACC), sensitivity (SEN), specificity (SPE), and area under the ROC curve (AUC) are employed to assess the performance of the network [17]. Furthermore, TP, TN, FP, and FN correspond to true positive, true negative, false positive, and false negative examples, respectively. The calculation formulas for each evaluation metric are as follows [18]:

$$Accuracy = \frac{TP + TN}{TP + TN + FP + FN} \tag{9}$$

$$Sensitivity = \frac{TP}{TP + TN} \tag{10}$$

$$Specificity = \frac{TN}{TN + FP} \tag{11}$$

3.2   Comparison with Related Works

Table 2 presents a comprehensive comparison of the prediction accuracy between our proposed network and other existing studies. This analysis demonstrates the superior performance of our proposed network in identifying key atrophy features, resulting in the highest prediction accuracy among all the evaluated convolutional neural networks.

Table 2. Comparison with the related approaches conducted on the selected dataset

Reference	Method	AD vs. NC				pMCI vs. sMCI			
		ACC	AUC	SEN	SPE	ACC	AUC	SEN	SPE
Nanni et al. [19]	Slice+SVM	0.876	0.903	0.841	–	0.671	0.865	0.345	–
Xing et al. [7]	Slice+CNN	0.953	–	0.889	0.974	–	–	–	–
Zhang et al. [8]	WholeBrain+CNN	0.910	–	0.910	0.920	0.820	–	0.810	0.810
Chen et al. [10]	Slice+WholeBrain+CNN	0.911	0.950	0.914	0.888	0.801	0.789	0.52	0.856
Liu et al. [11]	WholeBrain+CNN	0.977	0.977	0.968	0.985	0.883	0.892	0.840	0.944
Ours	WholeBrain+CNN+ATT	**0.985**	0.946	0.962	0.983	**0.894**	0.887	0.796	0.88

* A part of results listed in this table are cited from [11]. ATT, SVM refers to attention mechanism and supported vector machine, respectively.

3.3   Ablation Experiments

To evaluate the contribution of the multi-scale multi-channel group convolution, adaptive feature fusion module, and regularized loss function used in the network proposed here to its performance, several control groups are designed for ablation experiments. Figure 3 shows the experimental results.

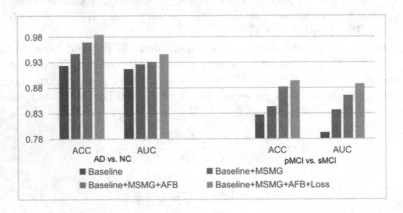

Fig. 3. Results of ablation experiments conducted on different blocks. (Here, MSMG represents multi-scale multi-channel group convolution. AFB represents adaptive feature fusion module. Loss represents regularized loss function.)

The effectiveness of multi-channel group convolution for three-classification tasks is evident in Fig. 3, where it is shown that multi-scale multi-channel group convolution outperforms the backbone network in terms of classification accuracy and AUC. In contrast, single-channel convolution tends to suffer from overfitting issues due to its limited feature extraction capability and insufficient feature expression. Multi-channel group convolution not only reduces the number of parameters but also enhances features and strengthens the integration of global and local information. This improvement in modeling ability allows the network to capture fine-grained features more effectively, leading to improved classification accuracy.

Adaptive feature fusion facilitates a complementary integration of features from all three directions. This enables the network to consider features from all directions simultaneously, leading to a more comprehensive understanding of the data.

The utilization of the regularization loss function significantly improves the classification accuracy and AUC of the backbone, as shown in Fig. 3. This finding confirms that the regularization loss function effectively learns the centroids of each class, reducing the distance between samples within the same class while increasing the distance between different classes. Relying solely on the cross-entropy loss function often causes the network to overly prioritize the prediction label, which can hinder its generalization ability. However, by incorporating a regularization term into the softmax function, the network tends to adopt a smoother scoring growth pattern. As a result, the network avoids making absolute predictions and exhibits enhanced generalization capability. The regularization loss function is therefore crucial in improving the performance of the backbone model and ensuring more accurate and generalized predictions.

4   Conclusion

In this paper, an AD prediction network based on adaptive feature fusion is proposed to overcome challenges in both 2D sections and 3D images. The proposed network addresses limited feature information in 2D sections and the complexities introduced by increased model parameters and inadequate training data in 3D images, enabling a comprehensive analysis of the information from the brain. Experimental results demonstrate the superiority of proposed approach over mainstream methods by achieving a higher classification accuracy. Additionally, the proposed approach effectively distinguishes AD and MCI patients from the NC control group, highlighting its potential for clinical applications.

Acknowledgement. This research is partially supported by the UniSQ Capacity Building Grants with Grant Number 1008313.

References

1. Izzo, J., Andreassen, O.A., Westlye, L.T., van der Meer, D.: The association between hippocampal subfield volumes in mild cognitive impairment and conversion to Alzheimer's disease. Brain Res. **1728**, 146591 (2020). https://doi.org/10.1016/j.brainres.2019
2. Li, Y., Wen, P., Powers, D., Clark, C.R.: LSB neural network based segmentation of MR brain images. In: IEEE SMC 1999 Conference Proceedings. 1999 IEEE International Conference on Systems, Man, and Cybernetics (Cat. No. 99CH37028), vol. 6, pp. 822–825. IEEE (1999)
3. Bashar, M.R., Li, Y., Wen, P.: Study of EEGs from Somatosensory Cortex and Alzheimer's Disease Sources (2011). https://doi.org/10.5281/zenodo.1056719
4. Li, Y., Chi, Z.: MR brain image segmentation based on self-organizing map network. Int. J. Inf. Technol. **11** (2005)
5. Mehmood, A., Maqsood, M., Bashir, M., Shuyuan, Y.: A deep Siamese convolution neural network for multi-class classification of Alzheimer disease. Brain Sci. **10**(2) (2020). https://doi.org/10.3390/brainsci10020084
6. Hoang, G.M., Kim, U.H., Kim, J.G.: Vision transformers for the prediction of mild cognitive impairment to Alzheimer's disease progression using mid-sagittal sMRI. Front. Aging Neurosci. **15** (2023). https://doi.org/10.3389/fnagi.2023.1102869
7. Xing, Y., Guan, Y., Yang, B., Liu, J.: Classification of sMRI images for Alzheimer's disease by using neural networks. In: Yu, S., et al. (eds.) Pattern Recognition and Computer Vision, pp. 54–66. Springer, Cham (2022). https://doi.org/10.1007/978-3-031-18910-4_5

8. Zhang, X., Han, L., Zhu, W., Sun, L., Zhang, D.: An explainable 3D residual self-attention deep neural network for joint atrophy localization and Alzheimer's disease diagnosis using structural MRI. IEEE J. Biomed. Health Inform. **26**(11), 5289–5297 (2022). https://doi.org/10.1109/JBHI.2021.3066832

9. Bakkouri, I., Afdel, K., Benois-Pineau, J., Catheline, G.: Recognition of Alzheimer's disease on sMRI based on 3D multi-scale CNN features and a gated recurrent fusion unit. In: 2019 International Conference on Content-Based Multimedia Indexing (CBMI), pp. 1–6 (2019). https://doi.org/10.1109/CBMI.2019.8877477

10. Chen, L., Qiao, H., Zhu, F.: Alzheimer's disease diagnosis with brain structural MRI using multiview-slice attention and 3D convolution neural network. Front. Aging Neurosci. **14** (2022). https://doi.org/10.3389/fnagi.2022.871706

11. Liu, F., Wang, H., Liang, S.N., Jin, Z., Wei, S., Li, X.: MPS-FFA: a multiplane and multiscale feature fusion attention network for Alzheimer's disease prediction with structural MRI. Comput. Biol. Med. **157**, 106790 (2023). https://doi.org/10.1016/j.compbiomed.2023.106790

12. Hu, K., Wang, Y., Chen, K., Hou, L., Zhang, X.: Multi-scale features extraction from baseline structure MRI for MCI patient classification and AD early diagnosis. Neurocomputing **175**, 132–145 (2016). https://doi.org/10.1016/j.neucom.2015.10.043

13. Vaswani, A., et al.: Attention is all you need. In: Guyon, I., et al. (eds.) Advances in Neural Information Processing Systems, vol. 30. Curran Associates, Inc. (2017)

14. Liang, D., et al.: Combining convolutional and recurrent neural networks for classification of focal liver lesions in multi-phase CT images. In: Frangi, A.F., Schnabel, J.A., Davatzikos, C., Alberola-López, C., Fichtinger, G. (eds.) MICCAI 2018. LNCS, vol. 11071, pp. 666–675. Springer, Cham (2018). https://doi.org/10.1007/978-3-030-00934-2_74

15. Banerjee, K., Gupta, R.R., Vyas, K., Mishra, B.: Exploring alternatives to softmax function (2020)

16. Petersen, R.C., et al.: Alzheimer's disease neuroimaging initiative (ADNI). Neurology **74**(3), 201–209 (2010). https://doi.org/10.1212/WNL.0b013e3181cb3e25

17. Fawcett, T.: An introduction to roc analysis. Pattern Recogn. Lett. **27**(8), 861–874 (2006). https://doi.org/10.1016/j.patrec.2005.10.010

18. Zheng, B., Gao, A., Huang, X., Li, Y., Liang, D., Long, X.: A modified 3D efficientnet for the classification of Alzheimer's disease using structural magnetic resonance images. IET Image Proc. **17**(1), 77–87 (2023). https://doi.org/10.1049/ipr2.12618

19. Nanni, L., Brahnam, S., Salvatore, C., Castiglioni, I.: Texture descriptors and voxels for the early diagnosis of Alzheimer's disease. Artif. Intell. Med. **97**, 19–26 (2019). https://doi.org/10.1016/j.artmed.2019.05.003

A Review on Predicting Drug Target Interactions Based on Machine Learning

Wen Shi[1], Dandan Peng[1], Jinyuan Luo[1], Guozhu Chen[1], Hong Yang[1(✉)], Linhai Xie[2(✉)], Xiao-Xia Yin[1], and Yanchun Zhang[1]

[1] The Cyberspace Institute of Advanced Technology, Guangzhou University, Guangzhou, China
hyang@gzhu.edu.cn, Yanchun.Zhang@vu.edu.au
[2] State Key Laboratory of Proteomics, National Center for Protein Sciences (Beijing), Beijing 102206, China
xielinhai@ncpsb.org.cn

Abstract. The prediction of drug-target interactions (DTIs) is a key preliminary step for drug discovery and development due to the high risk of failure as well as the long validation period of in vitro and in vivo experiments. Nowadays, with the swiftly growing power in solving scientific problems, machine learning has become an important tool in DTI prediction. By simply categorizing them into traditional machine learning-based approaches and deep learning-based ones, this review discusses some representative approaches in each branch. After a brief introduction on traditional methods, we firstly pay large attention to the data representation of deep learning-based methods, which can be summarized with 5 different representations for drugs and 4 for proteins. Then we introduce a new taxonomy of deep neural network models for DTI prediction. Furthermore, the commonly used datasets and evaluation metrics were also summarized for an easier hands-on practice.

Keywords: drug-target interactions · machine learning · data representation · deep neural network models

1 Introduction

Drug development is a complex and time-consuming process, typically taking more than a decade to bring a new drug to the market. In order to develop safe, reliable, and effective drugs, researchers need to conduct extensive experiments to screen potential drug molecules from a vast chemical space. Classical methods such as computational simulations and chemical-biological experiments are often time-consuming and require significant resources and manpower [1].

In recent years, there has been a growing interest among scientists in using computational approaches to efficiently and rapidly predict drug-target interactions, rather than relying solely on expensive and time-consuming in vitro and in vivo experiments. With the rapid advancement of artificial intelligence

(AI) technology and the increasing demand for efficiency and accuracy in drug development, machine learning has become an indispensable tool in the field. Researchers can focus on the target molecules selected through computer-aided screening, validate their rationality, safety, and efficacy, and make necessary adjustments and optimizations based on the results obtained, thereby accelerating the cycle of drug development and inference [26].

Currently, there are three major categories of computational methods for predicting drug-target interactions (DTI): docking simulation, ligand-based, and chemogenomics methods [16]. While ligand-based and docking simulation methods have achieved promising prediction results, they often require high-quality data for drug molecules and proteins, making them less suitable for DTI prediction tasks involving a wide range of drug molecules and proteins. Chemogenomics provides rich feature information, including the chemical properties and structural characteristics of drug molecules, as well as sequence and structural information of protein targets. Machine learning methods can utilize chemical and genomic features to train models for identifying and predicting the interactions between drugs and targets.

It has been reported that there are excellent reviews on chemogenomics methods for DTI prediction [3,14,45]. In comparison to previous work, our focus is specifically on the topic of machine learning methods used in DTI prediction. While the comprehensive overviews [14] provide a broader perspective on chemogenomics methods, our emphasis is on machine learning. In recent years, machine learning has made significant breakthroughs and garnered widespread attention. Discussing state-of-the-art DTI prediction strategies from this important and popular standpoint allows for a more in-depth exploration of methodological details. The review [45] provides a brief overview of similarity-based machine learning methods for DTI prediction. While reviews [3,14] also cover learning-based methods, their focus is primarily on supervised learning.

In contrast, in this review, we categorize machine learning methods into two main types: traditional machine learning and deep learning. Traditional machine learning can be further divided into supervised learning and semi-supervised learning, with supervised learning being further classified into similarity-based and feature-based subclasses. For deep learning, we elaborate on data representation and neural network models: in the "data representation" section, we introduce several data representations used in deep learning-based drug-target interaction prediction, including representations for drug molecules and proteins. In the "neural networks" section, we discuss three types of neural network models: "Y-shaped", "interaction network" and "3D spatial". Lastly, we present evaluation methods for both traditional machine learning models and deep learning models. We discuss the current challenges and future prospects, particularly the challenges and further prospects of deep learning in the field of DTI prediction.

2   Traditional Machine Learning

2.1   Supervised Learning

Similarity-Based Method. The central idea of similarity-based machine learning methods is that similar drugs often share similar targets, and vice versa. In this approach, various similarity measures are used to calculate the similarity between drugs or targets. In [24], drug-target interactions were predicted based on five types of drug similarity measures: chemical-based, ligand-based, expression-based, side effect-based, and annotation-based. In [20], sequence similarity between proteins can be calculated using the Smith-Waterman alignment algorithm. Paper [9] introduced a method based on Gradient Boosting Decision Tree, which takes molecular descriptors of compounds and sequence information of proteins as inputs to the classifier and calculates the similarity score of each training example using similarity measures.

Feature Vector-Based Method. Feature vector-based methods have been used in DTI prediction to capture long-range dependency effectively. This approach represents drugs and targets as feature vectors and utilizes common classification algorithms such as support vector machines, random forests, etc., to train classification models. These traditional machine learning models can predict the interaction class of drug-target pairs, such as positive or negative, based on the combination of feature vectors. In a systematic approach [8], chemical descriptors were computed using the DRAGON software, resulting in a set of 2160-dimensional feature vectors for each drug-target pair. Subsequently, the random forest algorithm was employed, which introduces random training sets (bootstrap) and random input vectors into trees for prediction.

2.2   Semi-supervised Learning

Given that the selection of negative samples greatly affects the accuracy of DTI prediction results, some researchers have proposed semi supervised methods to address this issue. Xia et al. [39] proposed a manifold regularization semi-supervised learning method, which considers that the more common targets two drugs have, the more similar the two drugs are. Van et al. [31] constructed a regression prediction model by introducing Gaussian Interaction Profiles (GIP). Wang et al. [37] used a general two-layer undirected graph model to represent the multidimensional drug-target interaction network and encoded different types of interactions. They trained the Restricted Boltzmann Machine (RBM) method using a contrastive divergence approach to obtain the final prediction results. In Table 1, we have categorized a portion of the mentioned papers into three categories: Similarity-based Method, Feature vector based Method, and Semi-supervised Learning.

Table 1. DTI prediction methods under traditional machine learning.

Reference	Models	Types	Metrics	Year
Kevin et al. [24]	BLM	Similarity-based	AUC, AUPR	2009
Shi et al. [20]	KNN	Similarity-based	AUC, AUPR	2015
T. Pahikkala et al. [9]	KronRLS	Similarity-based	CI, AUC-PR	2014
Faulon et al. [7]	SVM	Future vector-based	ROC	2008
Wang et al. [33]	Adaboost-SVM	Future vector-based	EF, ROC	2016
Wang et al. [37]	RBMs	Semi-supervised	AUC, AUPR	2012
Laarhoven et al. [31]	RLS-Kron	Semi-supervised	AUC, AUPR	2011

3 Deep Learning

The development of representation techniques has directly contributed to the diversity in the input part of deep learning models, attracting extensive attention and in-depth research into various molecular representation methods. At the same time, the algorithms used in deep learning models for DTI prediction have become increasingly diverse and complex. The deep learning models themselves have also become highly diversified to the extent that it is challenging to classify them into appropriate categories [32]. Therefore, we provide a comprehensive overview of recent works that utilize deep neural networks as DTI prediction models, focusing on both data representation and deep learning models.

3.1 Data Representation

Drug: SMILES. The most commonly used representation for drugs is Simplified Molecular Input Line Entry System (SMILES), which is composed of a series of characters representing atoms and bonds. It allows drug molecules to be represented in a text format. SMILES offers the advantages of being concise and easy to handle, ensuring consistency and uniqueness in representation, which makes it directly compatible with deep learning models [28,31,37]. Due to its ability to explicitly represent the topology and connectivity of molecules as a sequence-based feature, SMILES has been widely applied in drug-target interaction prediction.

Drug: Fingerprints. In traditional machine learning approaches based on feature vectors, each element of the molecular fingerprint corresponds to a specific molecular feature or descriptor. These features can be utilized as input feature vectors to train traditional machine learning models. In traditional machine learning methods based on similarity, molecular fingerprints can be employed to compute the similarity measure between drug molecules. The binary or sparse representation of molecular fingerprints enables the calculation of molecular similarity. Many deep learning-based DTI prediction models also employ fingerprints as input features [36,47]. Several widely used molecular fingerprints

(FPs) include: topological structure-based FPs, physicochemical property-based FPs, and pharmacophore-based FPs.

Drug: Graph. Drug molecular diagram is a commonly used method for drug characterization, which captures the chemical characteristics and topological information of drug molecules by representing them as graph structures. In the drug molecular graph, atoms and chemical bond are represented as nodes and edges of the graph, and the interactions and connections in molecules are clearly shown. The construction of drug molecular diagrams can utilize the structural information of drugs, including molecular formula, atomic type, bond type, and spatial arrangement. This characterization method can effectively preserve the structural characteristics of drug molecules and provide rich information for further analysis and prediction.

Drug: Learned Representations. In this approach, the structure and features of drug molecules are encoded as points in a low-dimensional vector or embedding space. These embedding vectors are obtained through training deep learning models, which can capture important structural and property information of molecules. Moreover, this approach possesses strong expressive power, enabling it to extract high-order features and capture nonlinear relationships, thus providing a more accurate description of the properties and behaviors of molecules. This data-driven approach allows the models to adapt to different types of molecules and complex structural features, resulting in a broader applicability.

Drug: 3D Spatial. Researchers are exploring new methods for representing drug molecules to accurately capture their structural information. In these methods, the mesh representation divides the three-dimensional space into regular mesh units, where each unit represents a volume element. The point cloud representation method converts the three-dimensional structure of molecules into a set of discrete points, where each point represents the position of atoms. This representation can comprehensively describe the structure and characteristics of molecules. Voxel representation divides three-dimensional space into a series of small cube units, each representing a voxel. By mapping atoms in molecules to the nearest voxel and recording important information on the voxel.

Protein: Sequence-Based. The sequence based method takes the amino acid sequence of a protein as input and captures sequence patterns and structural information in the protein sequence by learning the relative positions and interactions between amino acids. Zhang et al. [44] discussed three protein sequence representation methods based on physical properties, Fourier transform, and PROFEAT network servers. The paper [4] emphasizes the similarity between sequence based protein prediction tasks and natural language processing (NLP) problems, and outlines the main methods for representing protein sequence data (such as amino acid sequence coding or embedding).

Protein: Structure-Based. Structure-based methods utilize the structural information of proteins, such as 3D coordinates or secondary structures, as input to represent protein molecules. Proteins with 3D structure rely on the spatial organization of amino acids to perform their functions. Inspired by the Word2Vec approach, Zhang et al. [46] introduced the concept of a word vector space, where each vector can be seen as a point in space. The vocabulary or semantic similarity between them can be inferred by the "distance" between points. For known protein structures, these methods are commonly used for target representation to identify ligands that match the structure or to design new ligands for proteins.

Protein: Graph-Based. This method represents proteins in graphical form, where nodes represent amino acids, atoms, or residues, and edges represent their relationships. By defining the characteristics of nodes and edges, their connectivity, and the topological structure of the graph, one can learn the representation of protein graphs. Graph neural networks are commonly used methods for graph based feature learning. In [11], GNN technology is used to model the structure of drug molecules and protein targets. In addition, Wang et al. [34] not only use the protein sequence information, but also use the adjacency matrix (contact graph) of proteins.

Protein: Networks-Based. Many studies have adopted protein-protein interaction (PPI) networks, which are generated as network-based features using node2vec or autoencoders (AE). The key challenge in drug-target interaction is how to extract important features of drug binding sites and how to predict their potential space. Paper [13] not only utilizes sequence information but also incorporates pathway member information. [29] addressed the DTI link prediction problem in heterogeneous networks using graph embedding and ensemble learning techniques.

3.2 Deep Learning Models

This section introduces the DTI prediction model based on deep learning from three perspectives, and classifies several common models as shown in Table 2: (1) The classical Y-shaped architecture model is introduced first. The two branches of the Y-shaped architecture encode the drug molecule and the protein, respectively, to obtain their corresponding embedding representations. These features are then fused and input into a prediction layer for prediction. (2) The models based on interaction networks are then outlined, focusing on the analysis from the perspectives of bipartite graphs and heterogeneous graphs. (3) Next, deep learning methods based on three-dimensional space are introduced for predicting drug-target interactions.

Classic "Y". Figure 1 provides a "Y" shaped deep learning framework for CPI prediction. Two branches are used to represent the data of drug molecules and protein molecules respectively, and the neural network module extracts features and embeds representations of fusion compounds and proteins, and finally outputs the prediction results of drug-target affinity. DeepDTA [19], GraphDTA [18] and MGraphDTA [41] are the three examples of Classic Y.

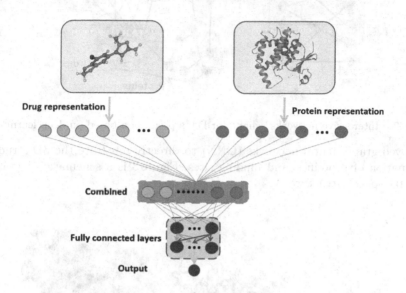

Fig. 1. Classic "Y" shape for DTIs prediction based on deep learning.

"Interactive Network". Bipartite graphs consist of two disjoint and independent node sets, such as drugs and target sets. Edges only connect between the two sets, meaning that a neighbor of a drug can only be a target and vice versa. There are no drug-drug or target-target edges within these two parts. Eslami et al. [5] proposed constructing a semi-bipartite graph by utilizing known DTIs and drug-drug and protein-protein similarity. Heterogeneous graphs integrate various networks such as drug side effects, drug-disease associations and protein function data. In [22], features were extracted from seven networks of drugs and proteins using Jaccard similarity coefficient and RWR algorithm. Figure 2 is a schematic diagram of the "Interaction network" structure.

"3D Space". The advancements in protein structure prediction, such as AlphaFold2 [30] and RoseTTA [2], have the potential to accelerate various stages of the drug discovery process. The use of AlphaFold2 for structure prediction can provide accurate templates for target proteins, enabling the exploration of protein pockets and functionally relevant regions through accessing the target's three-dimensional structure. To learn accurate three-dimensional structural information of proteins, [12] utilizing three-dimensional convolutional neural network or graph neural networks have also been applied for protein structure learning. Thereby improving the accuracy of DTI prediction. Jaechang Lim et al. [15]

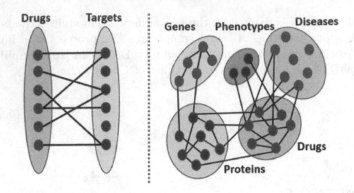

Fig. 2. "Interactive networks" shape for DTIs prediction based on deep learning.

employed graph neural networks (GNN) to directly integrate the 3D structure information of protein-ligand binding sites. Figure 3 is a schematic diagram of the "3D Space" structure.

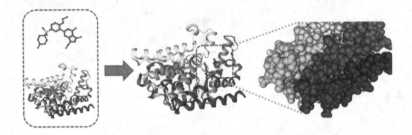

Fig. 3. "3D space" shape for DTIs prediction based on deep learning.

Table 2. DTI prediction methods under traditional machine learning.

Reference	Models	Types	Metrics	Year
Ozturk et al. [19]	CNN, CNN	Classic "Y"	MSE, CI	2018
Jiang et al. [11]	GNN, GNN	Classic "Y"	MSE, CI, Pearson	2020
Nguyen et al. [18]	CNN, GNN	Classic "Y"	MSE, CI	2021
Yang et al. [41]	CNN, CNN	Classic "Y"	MSE, CI, r_m^2 Index	2022
Mukherjee et al. [17]	LSTM,GCN	Classic "Y"	MSE, CI, r_m^2 Index	2022
Peng et al. [23]	GCN	"Interactive Network"	AUROC, AUPR	2021
Wang et al. [35]	CNN	"Interactive Network"	ACC, F1, AUROC	2022
Wu et al. [38]	GraphSAGE	"Interactive Network"	AUROC, AUPR	2022
Lim et al. [12]	GNN	"3D space"	AUROC, AUPR	2019
Jiménez et al. [15]	3D CNN	"3D space"	RMSD, R	2018
Stärk et al. [27]	SE(3)	"3D space"	L/K-RMSD, CD	2022

4   Datesets and Evaluation Metrics

With the advancement of molecular biology, a wealth of information about drugs and targets has been accumulated. So far, there are many different specialized databases covering potential cellular targets of various compound families. In Table 3, we list commonly used databases, their URLs, the number of compounds, targets, and compound-target interactions.

Table 3. Databases used in drug-target interaction prediction

Database and URL	No. of targets	No. of drugs	No. of int.
BinddingDB: https://www.bindingdb.org/	9,021	1,160,301	2,701,247
ChEMBL: https://www.ebi.ac.uk/chembl/	15,139	2,354,965,	20,038,828
DrugBank: https://go.drugbank.com/	5,296	15,550	29,466
PDBbind: http://www.pdbbind.org.cn/	1,469	41,847	–
STITCH: http://stitch.embl.de/	9,600,000	430,000	–
TTD: https://db.idrblab.net/ttd/	3,578	38,760	–
Davis: (DAVIS et al. 2011)	442	68	30,056
Kiba: (He et al. 2017)	229	2,111	118,254

Prediction DTI tasks can be divided into two types: predicting Drug-Target Pairs (DTP) using a classification model and predicting drug-target affinity (DTA) using a regression model. In the former, a classification model is employed to classify DTPs as positive or negative, while in the latter, a regression model is used to predict the binding affinity between drugs and targets.

4.1   Classification Metrics

Several evaluation metrics commonly used in DTP prediction research include accuracy, precision, recall, specificity, F1-Score and area under the precision-recall curve (AUPR). Accuracy is a direct measure of classifier performance, but it may not be suitable for imbalanced datasets where the number of positive and negative samples differs significantly. Sensitivity and specificity are introduced as additional metrics to evaluate the model's ability to identify positive and negative samples. The F1 score, AUPR and the ROC curve offer more comprehensive insights into the usefulness, rationality, and effectiveness of the model.

4.2   Regression Metrics

DTA (Drug-Target Affinity) prediction models can be evaluated using several metrics, including mean squared error (MSE), root mean squared error (RMSE), Pearson correlation coefficient, squared correlation coefficient (r_m^2), confidence interval count (CI), and Spearman correlation coefficient. MSE is defined as the average squared difference between the predicted and actual binding affinity scores. r_m^2 measures the goodness of fit, indicating the degree of match between predicted and actual values. Confidence interval count, applicable for regression tasks with continuous output, evaluates the ranking performance of the model.

5   Conclusion and Outlook

We have categorized the prediction methods of drug-target interactions (DTIs) into two main branches: traditional machine learning methods and deep learning methods. In this review, we discuss some representative approaches from each of these branches. After providing a brief introduction to traditional methods, we then shift our focus to the data representation in deep learning-based methods. And we introduce a novel taxonomy for classifying deep neural network models for DTI prediction, categorizing them into three classes: Classic "Y", "Interactive network", and "3D Space".

This article provides a new perspective for DTI prediction, and the review aims to systematically classify the early and outstanding technologies in DTI prediction. However, despite the utilization of machine learning, particularly deep learning, in these methods, there are still existing challenges and potential strategies that can be explored to address them. (1) Imbalanced datasets: Sampling methods impact predictive accuracy in addressing imbalanced datasets. Semi-supervised methods are proposed instead of random selection of negative samples. Ensemble learning treats data-level and algorithm-level strategies as sub-classes of imbalanced data classification strategies [6]. One can also draw inspiration from the ensemble strategies presented in the paper by [25]. (2) Lack of standard benchmarks: Limited testing of drugs and proteins makes it impossible to guarantee their performance under the same conditions. Pre-training with multi-task learning [40], and Extended Stein Unbiased Risk Estimator (eSURE) [42] can be considered for unsupervised learning of drug-target affinity prediction. Knowledge fusion with transfer learning [21,43], and integrating multi-modal and multi-channel information enhance generalization capability. (3) Black box nature of deep learning makes result explanation challenging. Developing interpretable deep learning and causal learning, along with traditional experiments, is necessary. Attention mechanisms can be a reasonable addition [10].

References

1. Al-Absi, H.R., Refaee, M.A., Rehman, A.U., Islam, M.T., Belhaouari, S.B., Alam, T.: Risk factors and comorbidities associated to cardiovascular disease in Qatar: a machine learning based case-control study. IEEE Access **9**, 29929–29941 (2021)
2. Baek, M., et al.: Accurate prediction of protein structures and interactions using a three-track neural network. Science **373**(6557), 871–876 (2021)
3. Chen, R., Liu, X., Jin, S., Lin, J., Liu, J.: Machine learning for drug-target interaction prediction. Molecules **23**(9), 2208 (2018)

4. Cui, F., Zhang, Z., Zou, Q.: Sequence representation approaches for sequence-based protein prediction tasks that use deep learning. Brief. Funct. Genomics **20**(1), 61–73 (2021)
5. Eslami Manoochehri, H., Nourani, M.: Drug-target interaction prediction using semi-bipartite graph model and deep learning. BMC Bioinform. **21**, 1–16 (2020)
6. Ezzat, A., Wu, M., Li, X.L., Kwoh, C.K.: Drug-target interaction prediction via class imbalance-aware ensemble learning. BMC Bioinform. **17**(19), 267–276 (2016)
7. Faulon, J.L., Misra, M., Martin, S., Sale, K., Sapra, R.: Genome scale enzyme-metabolite and drug-target interaction predictions using the signature molecular descriptor. Bioinformatics **24**(2), 225–233 (2008)
8. Fu, G., Ding, Y., Seal, A., Chen, B., Sun, Y., Bolton, E.: Predicting drug target interactions using meta-path-based semantic network analysis. BMC Bioinform. **17**(1), 1–10 (2016)
9. He, T., Heidemeyer, M., Ban, F., Cherkasov, A., Ester, M.: SimBoost: a read-across approach for predicting drug-target binding affinities using gradient boosting machines. J. Cheminform. **9**(1), 1–14 (2017)
10. Hua, Y., Song, X., Feng, Z., Wu, X.: MFR-DTA: a multi-functional and robust model for predicting drug-target binding affinity and region. Bioinformatics **39**(2), btad056 (2023)
11. Jiang, M., et al.: Drug-target affinity prediction using graph neural network and contact maps. RSC Adv. **10**(35), 20701–20712 (2020)
12. Jiménez, J., Skalic, M., Martinez-Rosell, G., De Fabritiis, G.: K deep: protein-ligand absolute binding affinity prediction via 3D-convolutional neural networks. J. Chem. Inf. Model. **58**(2), 287–296 (2018)
13. Lee, H., Kim, W.: Comparison of target features for predicting drug-target inter-actions by deep neural network based on large-scale drug-induced transcriptome data. Pharmaceutics **11**(8), 377 (2019)
14. Li, J., Zheng, S., Chen, B., Butte, A.J., Swamidass, S.J., Lu, Z.: A survey of current trends in computational drug repositioning. Brief. Bioinform. **17**(1), 2–12 (2016)
15. Lim, J., Ryu, S., Park, K., Choe, Y.J., Ham, J., Kim, W.Y.: Predicting drug-target interaction using a novel graph neural network with 3D structure-embedded graph representation. J. Chem. Inf. Model. **59**(9), 3981–3988 (2019)
16. Mousavian, Z., Masoudi-Nejad, A.: Drug-target interaction prediction via chemoge-nomic space: learning-based methods. Expert Opin. Drug Metab. Toxicol. **10**(9), 1273–1287 (2014)
17. Mukherjee, S., Ghosh, M., Basuchowdhuri, P.: DeepGLSTM: deep graph convo-lutional network and LSTM based approach for predicting drug-target binding affinity. In: Proceedings of the 2022 SIAM International Conference on Data Mining (SDM), pp. 729–737. SIAM (2022)
18. Nguyen, T., Le, H., Quinn, T.P., Nguyen, T., Le, T.D., Venkatesh, S.: GraphDTA: predicting drug-target binding affinity with graph neural networks. Bioinformatics **37**(8), 1140–1147 (2021)
19. Öztürk, H., Özgür, A., Ozkirimli, E.: DeepDTA: deep drug-target binding affinity prediction. Bioinformatics **34**(17), i821–i829 (2018)
20. Pahikkala, T., et al.: Toward more realistic drug-target interaction predictions. Brief. Bioinform. **16**(2), 325–337 (2015)
21. Pan, L., et al.: MFDNN: multi-channel feature deep neural network algorithm to identify covid19 chest X-ray images. Health Inf. Sci. Syst. **10**(1), 4 (2022)
22. Peng, J., Li, J., Shang, X.: A learning-based method for drug-target interaction prediction based on feature representation learning and deep neural network. BMC Bioinform. **21**(13), 1–13 (2020)

23. Peng, J., et al.: An end-to-end heterogeneous graph representation learning-based framework for drug-target interaction prediction. Briefings Bioinform. **22**(5), bbaa430 (2021)
24. Perlman, L., Gottlieb, A., Atias, N., Ruppin, E., Sharan, R.: Combining drug and gene similarity measures for drug-target elucidation. J. Comput. Biol. **18**(2), 133–145 (2011)
25. Samara, K.A., Al Aghbari, Z., Abusafia, A.: Glimpse: a glioblastoma prognostication model using ensemble learning—a surveillance, epidemiology, and end results study. Health Inf. Sci. Syst. **9**, 1–13 (2021)
26. da Silva Rocha, S.F., Olanda, C.G., Fokoue, H.H., Sant'Anna, C.M.: Virtual screening techniques in drug discovery: review and recent applications. Curr. Top. Med. Chem. **19**(19), 1751–1767 (2019)
27. Stärk, H., Ganea, O., Pattanaik, L., Barzilay, R., Jaakkola, T.: EquiBind: geometric deep learning for drug binding structure prediction. In: International Conference on Machine Learning, pp. 20503–20521. PMLR (2022)
28. Stokes, J.M., et al.: A deep learning approach to antibiotic discovery. Cell **180**(4), 688–702 (2020)
29. Thafar, M.A., et al.: DTi2Vec: drug-target interaction prediction using network embedding and ensemble learning. J. Cheminform. **13**(1), 1–18 (2021)
30. Tunyasuvunakool, K., et al.: Highly accurate protein structure prediction for the human proteome. Nature **596**(7873), 590–596 (2021)
31. Van Laarhoven, T., Nabuurs, S.B., Marchiori, E.: Gaussian interaction profile kernels for predicting drug-target interaction. Bioinformatics **27**(21), 3036–3043 (2011)
32. Vázquez, J., López, M., Gibert, E., Herrero, E., Luque, F.J.: Merging ligand-based and structure-based methods in drug discovery: an overview of combined virtual screening approaches. Molecules **25**(20), 4723 (2020)
33. Wang, M., Li, P., Qiao, P., et al.: The virtual screening of the drug protein with a few crystal structures based on the adaboost-SVM. Comput. Math. Methods Med. **2016** (2016)
34. Wang, P., et al.: Structure-aware multimodal deep learning for drug-protein interaction prediction. J. Chem. Inf. Model. **62**(5), 1308–1317 (2022)
35. Wang, S., Du, Z., Ding, M., Rodriguez-Paton, A., Song, T.: KG-DTI: a knowledge graph based deep learning method for drug-target interaction predictions and Alzheimer's disease drug repositions. Appl. Intell. **52**(1), 846–857 (2022)
36. Wang, Y.B., You, Z.H., Yang, S., Yi, H.C., Chen, Z.H., Zheng, K.: A deep learning-based method for drug-target interaction prediction based on long short-term memory neural network. BMC Med. Inform. Decis. Mak. **20**(2), 1–9 (2020)
37. Wang, Y., Zeng, J.: Predicting drug-target interactions using restricted Boltzmann machines. Bioinformatics **29**(13), i126–i134 (2013)
38. Wu, J., Lv, X., Jiang, S.: BSageIMC: drug repositioning based on bipartite graph convolutional networks and transcriptomics data. In: Li, X. (ed.) IASC 2021. LNDECT, vol. 80, pp. 376–383. Springer, Cham (2022). https://doi.org/10.1007/978-3-030-81007-8_42
39. Xia, Z., Wu, L.Y., Zhou, X., Wong, S.T.: Semi-supervised drug-protein interaction prediction from heterogeneous biological spaces. In: BMC Systems Biology, vol. 4, pp. 1–16. BioMed Central (2010)
40. Yang, F., Xue, F., Zhang, Y., Karypis, G.: Kernelized multitask learning method for personalized signaling adverse drug reactions. IEEE Trans. Knowl. Data Eng. (2021)

41. Yang, Z., Zhong, W., Zhao, L., Chen, C.Y.C.: MGraphDTA: deep multiscale graph neural network for explainable drug-target binding affinity prediction. Chem. Sci. **13**(3), 816–833 (2022)

42. Yin, X.X., et al.: Automatic breast tissue segmentation in MRIs with morphology snake and deep denoiser training via extended stein's unbiased risk estimator. Health Inf. Sci. Syst. **9**, 1–21 (2021)

43. Yuan, Y., et al.: A novel strategy for prediction of human plasma protein binding using machine learning techniques. Chemom. Intell. Lab. Syst. **199**, 103962 (2020)

44. Zhang, J., Liu, B.: A review on the recent developments of sequence-based protein feature extraction methods. Curr. Bioinform. **14**(3), 190–199 (2019)

45. Zhang, W., Lin, W., Zhang, D., Wang, S., Shi, J., Niu, Y.: Recent advances in the machine learning-based drug-target interaction prediction. Curr. Drug Metab. **20**(3), 194–202 (2019)

46. Zhang, Y.F., et al.: SPVec: a word2vec-inspired feature representation method for drug-target interaction prediction. Front. Chem. **7**, 895 (2020)

47. Zhao, Z., Bourne, P.E.: Harnessing systematic protein-ligand interaction fingerprints for drug discovery. Drug Discovery Today (2022)

KNN-Based Patient Network and Ensemble Machine Learning for Disease Prediction

Haohui Lu[ID] and Shahadat Uddin[✉][ID]

School of Project Management, Faculty of Engineering, The University of Sydney,
Level 2, 21 Ross St, Forest Lodge, NSW 2037, Australia
{haohui.lu,shahadat.uddin}@sydney.edu.au

Abstract. Machine learning has the ability to predict outcomes and identify features that contribute to chronic disease prediction, enabling the classification of patients based on features. The aim of this study is to enhance the accuracy of chronic disease prediction using network analytics and machine learning, and to identify the features that contribute to this prediction. For our case study, we utilise administrative claim data, which includes patients with and without specific chronic diseases. The KNN network constructor is employed and compared to uncover hidden patient relationships. Subsequently, five network features (i.e., degree centrality, eigenvector centrality, closeness centrality, betweenness centrality, and clustering coefficient) are extracted from the network to train ensemble machine learning models along with demographic and behavioral features. The performance of various ensemble machine learning methods was analysed to determine prediction accuracy. The boosting technique exhibited exceptional accuracy for chronic disease prediction. Moreover, age, gender, and the clustering coefficient were identified as features contributing to the prediction. This research can assist healthcare practitioners in making more informed decisions from their data. Stakeholders stand to gain multiple benefits, including enhanced patient care and improved diagnostic efficiency.

Keywords: Disease prediction · Machine learning · Network analytics · Patient network

1 Introduction

Chronic diseases and conditions have become a public health and economic burden in many nations around the world [23]. For instance, diabetes is a significant health concern that can lead to various long-term health problems, including cardiovascular and renal issues. Many of these problems can result in elevated healthcare costs. According to an annual report for 2017 to 2018, health spending in Australia exceeded $150 billion and averaged over $7,000 per person [3]. The most common type of diabetes is Type 2 diabetes (T2D), which can often

© The Author(s), under exclusive license to Springer Nature Singapore Pte Ltd. 2023
Y. Li et al. (Eds.): HIS 2023, LNCS 14305, pp. 296–305, 2023.
https://doi.org/10.1007/978-981-99-7108-4_25

be prevented through a healthy lifestyle [4]. Since T2D is a progressive condition with variable early symptoms, it is frequently preventable with early detection, especially for those aware of the associated risks. Thus, predicting the risk of T2D is vital not only for individuals but also for public health stakeholders and insurance companies.

Numerous studies have investigated T2D risk prediction using machine learning [21]. Anderson et al. [1] developed a model from electronic health records achieving an AUC of 0.76. Deberneh and Kim [11] predicted T2D risk annually, finding ensemble models superior. Islam et al. [17] utilised various machine learning methods, including logistic regression and random forest, to assess T2D risk. Lama et al. [25] identified T2D risks using machine learning, emphasising features like body mass index and diabetes heredity.

While many studies have concentrated on specific diseases, chronic diseases don't occur in isolation. They often share risk factors influenced by genetic, environmental, and behavioral variables [5]. Recently, Social Network Analysis (SNA) has gained popularity in addressing this, with techniques applied to healthcare data to form disease networks [22]. Lu et al. [28] introduced a patient network for predicting chronic diseases, but these works primarily utilise traditional machine learning without comparing various ensemble methods.

This study uses a network analytics approach to uncover hidden patient relationships, followed by ensemble methods for T2D risk prediction. Ensemble learning combines multiple model predictions to improve accuracy [12]. While models are categorised as 'black-box' or 'white-box', the health sector often prefers interpretable 'white-box' models [15]. Our research uniquely integrates a patient network and transparent ensemble models to predict T2D risks.

2   Material and Methods

This research aims to predict T2D risk using administrative data from Australia's CHBS. We first extracted relevant data, formed a patient network for chronic conditions, then proceeded with data pre-processing and feature selection. The selected ensemble methods are elaborated upon, followed by discussions on model evaluation and validation.

2.1   Study Setting and Population

The administrative dataset of this study encompasses patients under the CHBS fund hospitalised from 1995–2018, containing medical histories of about 1.24 million anonymised patients. Each record includes details like patient ID, demographics, medical service data, and specific disease codes using the ICD-9-AM and ICD-10-AM versions. These codes represent the medical issues faced by patients during their hospital stay.

2.2 Data Extraction and Inclusion

Given the over 20,000 distinct ICD codes in administrative data [34], it's impractical to use them all for predicting T2D risk. We focused on chronic diseases,
excluding unrelated disease codes. The Elixhauser index, designed primarily
for evaluating comorbidity in administrative data, was our basis due to its
widespread use [13]. After applying filtering criteria like selecting T2D patients
and episodes with relevant Elixhauser ICD codes, adapted from Quan et al.
[31], we identified 4,363 diabetic patients. From these, we randomly chose 4,000,
and an equivalent number from the 119,164 non-diabetic ones. Consequently, we
had a balanced dataset of 4,000 each of diabetic and non-diabetic for evaluating
ensemble machine learning methods.

2.3 Patient Network

The experimental findings of the network model suggest that considering label
information on neighbors may enhance prediction tasks [33]. Moreover, our previous studies also confirmed that features from the patient network (PN) or
using graph neural networks could improve prediction performance [26, 27].

In the PN, nodes represent the patient. If patients are diagnosed with the
same chronic disease, there is an edge between them. Otherwise, there is no
edge between the two patients. According to the literature, research suggests
that individuals with the same chronic diseases share risk factors such as a
history of smoking, obesity, and insufficient physical activity [2]. As a result,
we employ the PN to uncover hidden associations among patients, and we will
use features from the PN to predict the risk of T2D. In this study, we used the
KNN constructor to create the PN. KNN Constructor employs the k-Nearest
Neighbors technique [10]. The distance between each instance of the dataset is
measured using Euclidean distance metrics. The distance is the edge between
nodes. Afterwards, the k closest examples are selected, and edges are formed
between them for each instance. Figure 1 demonstrates the KNN constructor.
We select $k = 3$. Given the reference node, the k closest points are connected.

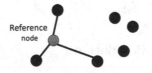

Fig. 1. KNN constructor

2.4 Feature Selection

We derive two types of features from the dataset and PN: network features and
patient features. These two feature vectors are concatenated to predict the risk
of T2D in patients with chronic diseases. Feature engineering will be explained
in the subsequent subsections.

Network Features. To achieve high prediction accuracy, effective features must be extracted from the PN. Consequently, we extract five types of features from the PN: Eigenvector centrality, Katz centrality, Closeness centrality, Betweenness centrality, and Clustering coefficient. Each feature will be detailed subsequently. Table 1 summarises the network features.

Table 1. Features Extracted from the PN with their Formulas and Notations

Feature	Description	Formula & Notation
Eigenvector Centrality	Measure of a node's influence [6]	$x_v = \frac{1}{\lambda} \sum_{t \in G}^{n} A_{vt} x_t$ Where λ is a positive coefficient, A_{vt} is the adjacency matrix
Katz Centrality	Centrality depending on neighbours [19]	$x_v = \alpha \sum_{t \in G}^{n} A_{vt} x_t + \beta$ Where α and β are coefficients, A_{vt} is the adjacency matrix
Closeness Centrality	Nodes disseminating information [14]	$C_{closeness}(u) = \frac{1}{\sum_{y \in N} d(u,v)}$ Where N is the set of nodes, $d(u,v)$ is the shortest path between u and v
Betweenness Centrality	Node's effect on information flow [32]	$C_{betweenness}(u) = \sum_{s \neq v \neq t} \frac{\sigma_{st}(u)}{\sigma_{st}}$ Where $\sigma_{st}(u)$ is the number of paths between s and t containing u, and σ_{st} is the path between s and t
Clustering Coefficient	Node network clustering [16]	$C_u = \frac{2T(u)}{\deg(u)(\deg(u)-1)}$ Where $T(u)$ is the number of triangles and $\deg(u)$ is the degree of node u

Patient Features. According to the literature, age, gender, and behaviour are risk factors for chronic diseases [9]. Therefore, in addition to the network features, gender, age, and smoking behaviour are used as patient features. Age is normalised (i.e., rescaled from 0 to 1). Gender is categorised with a score of 0 for female patients and 1 for male patients. The score for smoking behaviour is a discrete number, and we utilise ICD codes to determine whether a patient is a smoker. If at least one ICD code matches, the patient's behavioural risk score is 1. Otherwise, it is 0.

2.5   Machine Learning Ensemble Methods

The performance of machine learning ensemble models can vary across datasets depending on the features. As a result, several models and methodologies were reviewed and compared in this study to identify the one that offers the best performance for our dataset. Five machine learning ensemble methods will be explored in this research: Averaging, Max voting, Stacking, Bagging, and Boosting. Table 2 presents a summary of the methods.

Table 2. Ensemble Techniques and Descriptions

Technique	Description	Reference
Averaging	A modelling averaging ensemble mixes the predictions from each model equally. This procedure takes the average of all the predictions for the final outcome. In regression issues, averaging is used	[12]
Max Voting	An ensemble method integrating the predictions of numerous models. Each model's predictions are treated as votes, with the majority serving as the final prediction. A single model is built on several models, predicting output based on the majority of votes	[36]
Stacking	Learns how to aggregate predictions from multiple algorithms using a meta-learning technique. Models in a stack sequence predict a portion of the training data, with a meta learner generalising features for the final prediction	[39]
Bagging	Multiple instances of an estimator are built on subsets of the training set, with their predictions aggregated. Bagging introduces randomisation in its construction process to minimise the variance of a base estimator	[12]
Boosting	A sequential technique that reduces error, turning a weak learner into a strong one. It involves weighting data samples, with wrongly predicted points having increased weights in iterations for better accuracy in subsequent iterations	[12]

2.6   Model Evaluation

This study employed the confusion matrix for model evaluation, which summarised the classifier's performance on the test data. Subsequently, we used performance metrics, including accuracy, recall, precision, and F1 score, to compare the performances of different ensemble methods.

3   Results

In this study, we utilised an administrative claim dataset to construct the prediction model. Three patient features were considered: age, gender, and smoking. In addition to these patient features, five network features were employed. The dataset contains 8,000 patient records. We used an equal number of T2D and non-T2D patients to address the class imbalance issue. To construct prediction models, we randomly divided the dataset into training and test sets at a 0.90:0.10 ratio. The subsequent subsections detail the performance evaluation, feature importance, and evaluation of network features.

3.1 Performance Evaluation

For T2D risk prediction, six ensemble machine learning techniques (Averaging, Max voting, Bagging, Boosting, Stacking, and Blending) were used. We also employed random forest [7] as a baseline for performance comparison. Concurrently, the hyperparameters for the models were optimised to achieve optimal prediction accuracy. We utilised Python, the Sknet [35], and the Scikit-learn (sklearn) module [29] to train the machine learning models. For the averaging method, three model learning classifiers (i.e., Logistic Regression, Random Forest, and Support Vector Machine) were used to average the results. The same models were employed for max voting, stacking, and blending to ensure a fair comparison. Additionally, we used eXtreme Gradient Boosting (XGBoost) [8] for the boosting model and random forest as the base estimator for the bagging classifier. Table 3 displays the accuracy and performance measures of the models using KNN constructors. The default value was utilised for the network constructor [35].

Table 3. Performance of ensemble models using KNN Constructor

Models	Accuracy	Precision	Recall	F1-score
Random forest	0.8300	0.8667	0.7800	0.8211
Averaging	0.7975	0.8240	0.7650	0.7916
Max voting	0.8250	0.8439	**0.7975**	0.8201
Bagging	0.8325	0.8778	0.7725	0.8218
Boosting	**0.8405**	**0.9053**	0.7650	**0.8293**
Stacking	0.8337	0.8719	0.7825	0.8248
Blending	0.8350	0.8807	0.7750	0.8245

For the KNN constructor, according to Table 3, Boosting had the highest accuracy, precision, and F1-score. Thus, Boosting is seen to outperform other models. Among the various risk prediction algorithms based on healthcare data [11,18,24,37], XGBoost has shown the highest accuracy. XGBoost uses the second-order Taylor series to approximate the loss function's value, and regularisation helps in reducing the chance of overfitting.

3.2 Feature Importance

The boosting model performed best among the six ensemble models. Therefore, we applied feature importance in the XGBoost model to evaluate the significance of the chosen network and patient features. Figure 2 depicts the feature importance as determined by XGBoost. Age, gender, and the clustering coefficient, with feature importance values over 0.05, had a notable influence on model performance. The clustering coefficient for a patient measures how closely its neighbors are connected in the network. Patients with higher scores often cluster together, affecting how they are classified. Such patients might have distinct underlying characteristics. Therefore, network features are essential. However, age is a dominant factor in our top-performing model. Clinically, adults aged 45 and over constitute a significant portion of T2D patients [30]. There's also increasing evidence of significant sex and gender differences, with the rising prevalence of T2D and related comorbidities [20]. These observations align with the results of our XGBoost model.

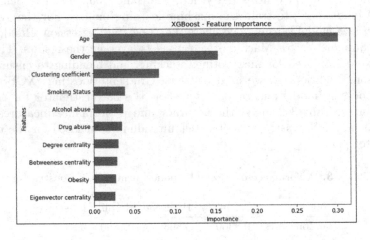

Fig. 2. Feature importance for XGBoost model

4   Discussion

T2D is one of the primary noncommunicable chronic diseases that has been escalating at an alarming rate worldwide. The overall number of diabetics is expected to rise from 171 million in 2000 to 366 million by 2030 [38]. This study aimed to predict the risk of T2D using network analysis and ensemble machine learning approaches. Four patient features, namely age, gender, smoking, and drinking, and five network features (degree centrality, eigenvector centrality, closeness centrality, betweenness centrality, and clustering coefficient) were employed for the models. Models incorporating network analysis exhibited remarkable performance, with accuracies ranging from 0.7975 to 0.8405. Our models integrate additional network features beyond the risk variables identified in earlier research. The results suggest that age, gender, and the clustering coefficient are pivotal, aligning with previous studies [11, 23]. Our approach addressed the limitations of earlier research, which largely depended on patient characteristics, and consequently produced models with notably high accuracies.

Furthermore, we highlighted our data engineering method that extracts patient similarity and incorporates it as new variables into administrative claim data.

The integration of AI technology in the medical realm has paved the way to address various medical challenges. In the context of ensemble methods, the commendable prediction capability of the boosting model underscores the potential in curating health plans for patients. Patients identified as high-risk for type 2 diabetes using the ensemble methods discussed in this study might benefit from specific regimens. Such patients could be advised to modify their lifestyle, curbing detrimental habits like smoking and drinking, which can either prevent or reduce the risk of T2D. Furthermore, timely intervention and treatment for high-risk patients can mitigate the progression of their condition.

Nonetheless, this study has its limitations. We solely relied on administrative claim data, and integrating other data sources could enhance the generalisability of our findings. Moreover, this study omits certain underlying medical conditions not covered in the Elixhauser index, such as stroke and ischemic heart disease. Concerning behavioral risk factors, our research didn't account for drugs as a risk factor, as we didn't analyse pharmaceutical data. Future studies might encompass diverse datasets and juxtapose the insights with our current findings.

5   Conclusion

This research devised a unique framework to predict the risk for T2D patients, utilising network methods and ensemble machine learning techniques. A patient network was constructed from the Australian administrative claim data, from which features were subsequently extracted. These features then informed six ensemble machine learning prediction models, aiming to pinpoint at-risk T2D patients. The boosting models, leveraging the KNN Constructor, demonstrated remarkable predictive accuracy. The results affirm that the fusion of network analytics with ensemble machine learning methods can be aptly applied for chronic disease risk prediction. Consequently, this research can empower healthcare professionals to make informed decisions based on their data. The potential benefits are manifold, spanning enhanced patient care to increased diagnostic efficiency.

References

1. Anderson, J.P., et al.: Reverse engineering and evaluation of prediction models for progression to type 2 diabetes: an application of machine learning using electronic health records. J. Diab. Sci. Technol. **10**(1), 6–18 (2016)
2. Australian Institute of Health and Welfare: Evidence for chronic disease risk factors (2016). https://www.aihw.gov.au/reports/chronic-disease/evidence-for-chronic-disease-risk-factors/contents/summary. Accessed 26 Mar 2023
3. Australian Institute of Health and Welfare: Chronic disease (2023). https://www.aihw.gov.au/reports-data/health-conditions-disability-deaths/chronic-disease/overview. Accessed 26 Mar 2023

4. Australian Institute of Health and Welfare: Diabetes (2023). https://www.aihw.gov.au/reports-data/health-conditions-disability-deaths/diabetes/overview. Accessed 26 Mar 2023
5. Barabási, A.L.: Network medicine-from obesity to the "diseasome" (2007)
6. Bonacich, P.: Factoring and weighting approaches to status scores and clique identification. J. Math. Sociol. **2**(1), 113–120 (1972)
7. Breiman, L.: Random forests. Mach. Learn. **45**, 5–32 (2001)
8. Chen, T., Guestrin, C.: XGBoost: a scalable tree boosting system. In: Proceedings of the 22nd ACM SIGKDD International Conference on Knowledge Discovery and Data Mining, pp. 785–794 (2016)
9. Comino, E.J., et al.: Impact of diabetes on hospital admission and length of stay among a general population aged 45 year or more: a record linkage study. BMC Health Serv. Res. **15**, 1–13 (2015)
10. Cover, T., Hart, P.: Nearest neighbor pattern classification. IEEE Trans. Inf. Theory **13**(1), 21–27 (1967)
11. Deberneh, H.M., Kim, I.: Prediction of type 2 diabetes based on machine learning algorithm. Int. J. Environ. Res. Public Health **18**(6), 3317 (2021)
12. Dietterich, T.G.: Ensemble methods in machine learning. In: Kittler, J., Roli, F. (eds.) MCS 2000. LNCS, vol. 1857, pp. 1–15. Springer, Heidelberg (2000). https://doi.org/10.1007/3-540-45014-9_1
13. Elixhauser, A., Steiner, C., Harris, D.R., Coffey, R.M.: Comorbidity measures for use with administrative data. Med. Care **36**, 8–27 (1998)
14. Freeman, L.C., et al.: Centrality in social networks: conceptual clarification. Soc. Netw. Crit. Concepts Sociol. **1**, 238–263. Routledge, Londres (2002)
15. Gong, H., Wang, M., Zhang, H., Elahe, M.F., Jin, M.: An explainable AI approach for the rapid diagnosis of COVID-19 using ensemble learning algorithms. Front. Public Health **10**, 874455 (2022)
16. Holland, P.W., Leinhardt, S.: Transitivity in structural models of small groups. Comp. Group Stud. **2**(2), 107–124 (1971)
17. Islam, M.M., et al.: Identification of the risk factors of type 2 diabetes and its prediction using machine learning techniques. Health Syst. **12**, 1–12 (2022)
18. Jha, M., Gupta, R., Saxena, R.: Cervical cancer risk prediction using XGBoost classifier. In: 2021 7th International Conference on Signal Processing and Communication (ICSC), pp. 133–136. IEEE (2021)
19. Katz, L.: A new status index derived from sociometric analysis. Psychometrika **18**(1), 39–43 (1953)
20. Kautzky-Willer, A., Harreiter, J., Pacini, G.: Sex and gender differences in risk, pathophysiology and complications of type 2 diabetes mellitus. Endocr. Rev. **37**(3), 278–316 (2016)
21. Kavakiotis, I., Tsave, O., Salifoglou, A., Maglaveras, N., Vlahavas, I., Chouvarda, I.: Machine learning and data mining methods in diabetes research. Comput. Struct. Biotechnol. J. **15**, 104–116 (2017)
22. Khan, A., Uddin, S., Srinivasan, U.: Comorbidity network for chronic disease: a novel approach to understand type 2 diabetes progression. Int. J. Med. Inform. **115**, 1–9 (2018)
23. Khan, A., Uddin, S., Srinivasan, U.: Chronic disease prediction using administrative data and graph theory: the case of type 2 diabetes. Expert Syst. Appl. **136**, 230–241 (2019)
24. Kwon, Y., et al.: Remission of type 2 diabetes after gastrectomy for gastric cancer: diabetes prediction score. Gastric Cancer **25**, 265–274 (2022)

25. Lama, L., et al.: Machine learning for prediction of diabetes risk in middle-aged Swedish people. Heliyon **7**(7), e07419 (2021)
26. Lu, H., Uddin, S.: A weighted patient network-based framework for predicting chronic diseases using graph neural networks. Sci. Rep. **11**(1), 22607 (2021)
27. Lu, H., Uddin, S., Hajati, F., Khushi, M., Moni, M.A.: Predictive risk modelling in mental health issues using machine learning on graphs. In: Australasian Computer Science Week 2022, pp. 168–175. Association for Computing Machinery (2022)
28. Lu, H., Uddin, S., Hajati, F., Moni, M.A., Khushi, M.: A patient network-based machine learning model for disease prediction: the case of type 2 diabetes mellitus. Appl. Intell. **52**(3), 2411–2422 (2022)
29. Pedregosa, F., et al.: Scikit-learn: machine learning in python. J. Mach. Learn. Res. **12**, 2825–2830 (2011)
30. Pippitt, K., Li, M., Gurgle, H.E.: Diabetes mellitus: screening and diagnosis. Am. Fam. Phys. **93**(2), 103–109 (2016)
31. Quan, H., et al.: Coding algorithms for defining comorbidities in ICD-9-CM and ICD-10 administrative data. Med. Care **43**, 1130–1139 (2005)
32. Shaw, M.E.: Group structure and the behavior of individuals in small groups. J. Psychol. **38**(1), 139–149 (1954)
33. Shi, Y., Huang, Z., Feng, S., Zhong, H., Wang, W., Sun, Y.: Masked label prediction: Unified message passing model for semi-supervised classification. arXiv preprint arXiv:2009.03509 (2020)
34. The Australian Classification of Health Interventions: ICD-10-AM (2020). https://www.accd.net.au/icd-10-am-achi-acs/. Accessed 26 Mar 2023
35. Toledo, T.: sknet: a python framework for machine learning in complex networks. J. Open Source Softw. **6**(68), 3864 (2021)
36. Tsoumakas, G., Partalas, I., Vlahavas, I.: A taxonomy and short review of ensemble selection. In: Workshop on Supervised and Unsupervised Ensemble Methods and Their Applications, pp. 1–6 (2008)
37. Uddin, S., Wang, S., Lu, H., Khan, A., Hajati, F., Khushi, M.: Comorbidity and multimorbidity prediction of major chronic diseases using machine learning and network analytics. Expert Syst. Appl. **205**, 117761 (2022)
38. Wild, S., Roglic, G., Green, A., Sicree, R., King, H.: Global prevalence of diabetes: estimates for the year 2000 and projections for 2030. Diab. Care **27**(5), 1047–1053 (2004)
39. Wolpert, D.H.: Stacked generalization. Neural Netw. **5**(2), 241–259 (1992)

Medical Imaging and Dataset Exploration

Optimizing the Size of Peritumoral Region for Assessing Non-Small Cell Lung Cancer Heterogeneity Using Radiomics

Xingping Zhang[1,4,5], Guijuan Zhang[3], Xingting Qiu[b], Jiao Yin[4], Wenjun Tan[7], Xiaoxia Yin[1], Hong Yang[1(✉)], Kun Wang[4], and Yanchun Zhang[2,4,5(✉)]

[1] Cyberspace Institute of Advanced Technology, Guangzhou University, Guangzhou 510006, China
hyang@gzhu.edu.cn
[2] School of Computer Science and Technology, Zhejiang Normal University, Jinhua 321000, China
[3] Department of Respiratory and Critical Care, First Affiliated Hospital of Gannan Medical University, Ganzhou 341000, China
[4] Institute for Sustainable Industries and Liveable Cities, Victoria University, Melbourne 3011, Australia
{xingping.zhang,yanchun.zhang}@vu.edu.au
[5] Department of New Networks, Peng Cheng Laboratory, Shenzhen 518000, China
[6] Department of Radiology, First Affiliated Hospital of Gannan Medical University, Ganzhou 341000, China
[7] Key Laboratory of Intelligent Computing in Medical Image, Ministry of Education, Northeastern University, Shenyang 110189, China

Abstract. Objectives: Radiomics has a novel value in accurately and noninvasively characterizing non-small cell lung cancer (NSCLC), but the role of peritumoral features has not been discussed in depth. This work aims to systematically assess the additional value of peritumoral features by exploring the impact of peritumoral region size. **Materials and methods:** A total of 370 NSCLC patients who underwent preoperative contrast-enhanced CT scans between October 2017 and September 2021 were retrospectively analyzed. The study was carefully designed with a radiomics pipeline to predict lymphovascular invasion, pleural invasion, and T4 staging. To assess the impact of peritumoral features, tumor regions of interest (ROIs) annotated by two medical experts were automatically expanded to produce peritumoral ROIs of different regional sizes, with edge thicknesses of 1 mm, 3 mm, 5 mm, and 7 mm. In a custom pipeline, prediction models were constructed using peritumoral features with different margin thicknesses and intratumoral features of the primary tumor. **Results:** Radiomics features combining intratumoral and peritumoral regions were created based on the best features of each ROI. Models incorporating peritumoral features yielded varying degrees of improvement in AUCs compared to models using only intratumoral features. The choice of peritumoral size may impact the

---

X. Zhang, G. Zhang, X. Qiu, J. Yin, W. Tan, X. Yin, H. Yang, K. Wang, Y. Zhang—All authors contribute equally to this work.

Y. Li et al. (Eds.): HIS 2023, LNCS 14305, pp. 309–320, 2023.
https://doi.org/10.1007/978-981-99-7108-4_26

degree of improvement in radiomics analysis. **Conclusions:** The integration of peritumoral features has shown potential for improving the predictive value of radiomics. However, selecting an appropriate peritumoral region size is constrained by various factors such as clinical issues, imaging modalities, and ROI annotations. Therefore, future radiomics studies should consider these factors and optimize peritumoral features to cater to specific applications.

Keywords: Radiomics · NSCLC · Tumor heterogeneity · Quantitative imaging · Peritumoral region

1   Introduction

Lung cancer stands as a pervasive malignancy. The subset of non-small cell lung cancer (NSCLC) encompasses a substantial proportion of the overall diagnosed cases, ranging from 80% to 90% [4]. The survival and recurrence of NSCLC patients can benefit from the accurate prediction of tumor aggressiveness, lymph node metastasis (LNM), lymphovascular invasion (LVI), and pleural invasion (PI), which enables individualized treatment [6,35]. Proper preoperative assessment of these factors, closely related to prognosis, is crucial in selecting the appropriate treatment strategy for NSCLC patients [35]. Traditional preoperative evaluation based on low-dose multidetector computed tomography (CT) is the conventional method [10,22,30,37], but its accuracy is low, and misdiagnosis may occur.

Medical imaging methods have been applied in various fields including knowledge graph, privacy protection and security [34,41–43]. With the application of AI techniques in medical imaging [1,18,25,27], radiomics has proven to be a promising approach that is receiving increasing attention [7,31,46]. It can extract many quantitative features and provide insights through statistical analysis of radiological features, revealing details of the tumor microenvironment. This approach is cost-effective, non-invasive, and allows the naked eye to uncover heterogeneous biomarkers of undetectable tumors [8,23,24]. Many radiomics-based studies have demonstrated successful assessment and predictive capabilities in cancer identification, LNM, LVI, and survival and treatment response [3,9,47]. Song et al. [29] found that CT radiomics features can be used to differentiate adenocarcinoma and squamous cell carcinoma. Li et al. [19] and Wang et al. [36] demonstrated that radiomics features could predict PI and provide survival risk stratification in NSCLC.

While previous radiomics studies have primarily focused on the intratumoral region [5,12,15,33,38], evidence suggests that the peritumoral region can also provide potentially critical information [2,17,36]. Recent advances in NSCLC research indicate that subtle structural changes in the peritumoral region may serve as biomarkers for various key outcomes, including LVI and overall survival [3], acquired drug-resistant T790M mutations [11], and excessive progression during immunotherapy [32]. Notably, several recent publications have highlighted the role of peritumoral features in pancreatic cancer [39], glioblastoma

[20], breast cancer [40], and hepatocellular carcinoma [44], underscoring the valuable yet easily overlooked tumor information within the peritumoral regions. In our previous study, we incorporated features extracted from the marginal areas surrounding lung cancer lesions, with a thickness of 3 mm on CT images, to enhance the performance in assessing tumor heterogeneity. Zhang et al. [45] and Hu et al. [14] reported that combining intratumoral and peritumoral features from pretreatment CT scans could more accurately predict prognostic risk stratification in lung adenocarcinoma and response to neoadjuvant chemotherapy in patients with esophageal cancer. In their studies, the peritumoral region was defined by a 5-mm and 10-mm radius ring around the tumor and an area manually delineated by medical experts.

However, the optimal size of the peritumoral region has not been discussed in depth. This study further investigated the impact of peritumoral region size on predicting LVI, PI, and T-stage in NSCLC to examine the role of peritumoral features in radiomics analysis.

2   Material and Methods

2.1   Patients

Ethical approval for this study was obtained from the Institutional Review Board of the First Affiliated Hospital of Gannan Medical University, and the requirement for informed consent was waived. The details of the inclusion and exclusion criteria for patient recruitment are described in our previous study. A total of 370 patients with histologically confirmed diagnoses of NSCLC were enrolled, and the collected data included preoperative enhanced CT images and complete clinicopathological information such as age, sex, and smoking status. The dataset was randomly divided into training and validation cohorts in a 7:3 ratio. The demographic and clinical characteristics of all patients are presented in Table 1.

2.2   ROI Segmentation and Pre-processing

Patients underwent CT examinations using GE Revolution (256 channels) and Somatom Definition (64 channels) scanners [13, 26]. Two medical experts manually outlined the tumor region of interest (ROI) on CT images in DICOM format using 3D Slicer (version 4.11.2020.09.30). An initial annotation was done by a physician with five years of experience, followed by review and refinement by a physician with ten years of experience. A consensus was reached for the final results. Peritumoral ROIs were obtained by automatically expanding the intratumoral ROIs by 1 mm, 3 mm, 5 mm, and 7 mm using an in-house algorithm, excluding areas outside the expanded lung. Figure 1 illustrates a representative CT image and its corresponding intratumoral and peritumoral ROIs.

To account for the anisotropic voxel spacing in the selected CT images and ensure the reliability of radiological features, we performed resampling to achieve an isotropic voxel space. All images were resampled using the B-spline interpolation algorithm, adjusting the voxel spacing of the ROIs to $1.0\,mm^3$. This voxel spacing was chosen to minimize any potential information distortion from the operation.

Table 1. Clinical and demographic characteristics.

Characteristic	LVI (n=370)		PI (n=370)		T Staging (n=370)	
	Yes (n=145)	No (n=225)	Yes (n=281)	No (n=89)	T4 (n=120)	Other (n=250)
Age (y)		0.196_p		$< 0.05^*$		0.588_p
Mean	63.5±10.2	62.0±10.9	63.2±10.8	60.5±9.7	63.2±9.9	62.2±11.0
Gender		0.249_p		0.602_p		0.868_p
Male	95 (65.5)	134 (59.6)	176 (62.6)	53 (59.6)	75 (62.5)	154 (61.6)
Female	50 (34.5)	91 (40.4)	105 (37.4)	36 (40.4)	45 (37.5)	96 (38.4)
Smoking status		0.184_p		0.353_p		0.066_p
Smoker	76 (52.4)	102 (45.3)	139 (49.5)	39 (43.8)	66 (55.0)	112 (44.8)
Nonsmoker	69 (47.6)	123 (54.7)	142 (50.5)	50 (56.2)	54 (45.0)	138 (55.2)
Tumor location		0.779_p		0.020_p		0.629_p
RUL	34 (23.4)	76 (33.8)	71 (25.3)	39 (43.8)	32 (26.7)	78 (31.2)
RML	17 (11.7)	17 (7.6)	27 (9.6)	7 (7.9)	16 (13.3)	18 (7.2)
RLL	37 (25.5)	31 (13.8)	58 (20.6)	10 (11.2)	24 (0.0)	44 (17.6)
LUL	41 (28.3)	69 (30.7)	88 (31.3)	22 (24.7)	37 (30.8)	73 (29.2)
LLL	16 (11.0)	32 (14.2)	37 (13.2)	11 (12.4)	11 (9.2)	37 (14.8)

Unless otherwise mentioned, the meaning of the data is n (%). The subscript p on the right side represents the p-value. RUL=right upper lobe, RML=right middle lobe, RLL=right lower lobe, LUL=left upper lobe, LLL=left lower lobe.

2.3   Feature Extraction

Two sets of radiomics features, namely the original and filtered feature sets, were extracted from the intratumoral and peritumoral ROIs using PyRadiomics. The original feature set was obtained directly from the original images, while the filtered feature set was derived after applying wavelet transform (8 types) to the original images. The original feature set includes seven types of features (first-order statistical, shape, GLCM, GLRLM, GLSZM, NGTDM, and GLDM), totaling 867 features for each ROI. Shape features are not computed in the filtered feature set. More detailed information can be found in [46].

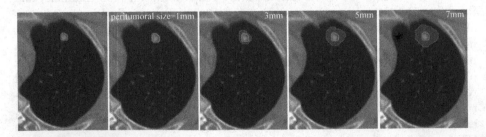

Fig. 1. A representative set of enhanced CT images of the intratumoral region and different peritumoral region sizes of the ROIs.

2.4 Selection of the Best Features

To mitigate overfitting, we performed feature selection and modeling in a separate training cohort, using a validation cohort solely for evaluating the prediction model. Before feature selection, two preprocessing steps were implemented: z-score normalization for all features to improve stability and a synthetic minority oversampling technique algorithm to address category imbalance. These steps aimed to enhance training efficiency and address data challenges.

For feature selection, we employed the following methods to eliminate uncorrelated and redundant features: (1) Univariate selection: The Mann-Whitney U test and Pearson linear correlation coefficient were utilized to retain features with p-values < 0.05 and correlation coefficients between categories < 0.75. (2) Minimum Redundancy Maximum Relevance (mRMR) algorithm: Features with the highest discriminative power, exhibiting the highest correlation with the predicted category but the lowest correlation with other features, were identified. (3) Least Absolute Shrinkage and Selection Operator algorithm (LASSO): The remaining features were inputted into LASSO, and features with non-zero coefficients were considered the most important predictors. These methods collectively enabled us to select relevant and informative features for the analysis.

We applied the feature selection method described for each ROI and prediction category. For the combined features in the intratumoral and peritumoral regions, their best features were combined and further selected using LASSO to identify the most important predictors. To prevent overfitting, up to 10 features were retained for each model.

2.5 Model Building and Performance Evaluation

The eligible features were utilized to develop a multivariate logistic regression model. Parameter optimization was performed in the training cohort using a grid search method with 5-fold cross-validation. To ensure unbiased estimation, 10-fold cross-validation was applied to the training and validation cohorts. Performance evaluation of the models included calculating the receiver operating characteristic (ROC) curve, the area under the curve (AUC), accuracy, sensitivity, and specificity.

To examine the impact of peritumoral region size, we finally constructed the radiomics model, combined model (1 mm), combined model (3 mm), combined model (5 mm), and combined model (7 mm) in each prediction category.

3 Results

In the prediction model of LVI, the number of features selected from the intratumoral region was 9. Additionally, when considering different peritumoral region sizes, the number of features selected was 10 for 1 mm, 10 for 3 mm, 10 for 5 mm, and 10 for 7 mm. For the other two prediction tasks, the number of features selected from the intratumoral region, peritumoral region (1 mm), peritumoral region (3 mm), peritumoral region (5 mm), and peritumoral region (7 mm) were 10, 10, 10, 10, and 9 in PI. Similarly, for T-staging, the number of selected features was 10, 10, 7, 10, and 10. These results indicate that the optimal features chosen by the prediction model differ in the number of peritumoral features when combining intratumoral and peritumoral features for the three tasks.

Figure 2 displays the ROC curves illustrating the performance of the best features obtained for predicting LVI, PI, and T staging using both the intratumoral ROI and combined ROI in the validation cohort. Meanwhile, Table 2 summarizes the detailed performance metrics for each model and task in the training and validation cohorts. These results demonstrate that including peritumoral features in the combined models has led to improvements in prediction performance to varying extents compared to models that solely utilize intratumoral features. Specifically, for LVI, the AUC increased by −0.003–0.025; for PI, the AUC increased by 0.04–0.065; and for T-stage, the AUC also increased by 0.012–0.052. These findings highlight the significant contribution of peritumoral features to the predictive capabilities of the radiomics models.

Table 2. Predictive performance of radiomics models based on intratumoral ROI and ROIs with different peritumoral region sizes in training and validation cohorts.

Task	Model	Training cohort			Validation cohort		
		AUC	95%CI	ACC	AUC	95%CI	ACC
LVI	Radiomics	0.740	[0.722–0.756]	0.664	0.706	[0.693–0.721]	0.669
	Combined (1mm)	0.772	[0.748–0.781]	0.694	0.711	[0.698–0.724]	0.656
	Combined (3mm)	0.779	[0.755–0.788]	0.696	0.703	[0.689–0.717]	0.661
	Combined (5mm)	**0.781**	[0.765–0.797]	0.713	**0.731**	[0.719–0.745]	0.688
	Combined (7mm)	0.747	[0.724–0.758]	0.668	0.717	[0.703–0.730]	0.686
PI	Radiomics	0.900	[0.886–0.905]	0.818	0.768	[0.755–0.784]	0.781
	Combined (1mm)	0.907	[0.896–0.915]	0.830	0.808	[0.795–0.820]	0.820
	Combined (3mm)	**0.915**	[0.903–0.921]	0.838	**0.833**	[0.821–0.846]	0.804
	Combined (5mm)	0.912	[0.901–0.919]	0.805	0.826	[0.812–0.839]	0.798
	Combined (7mm)	0.908	[0.897–0.916]	0.815	0.813	[0.799–0.824]	0.782
T Staging	Radiomics	0.808	[0.793–0.822]	0.729	0.775	[0.761–0.788]	0.788
	Combined (1mm)	**0.821**	[0.807–0.835]	0.742	**0.827**	[0.815–0.839]	0.758
	Combined (3mm)	0.810	[0.796–0.824]	0.719	0.799	[0.786–0.812]	0.737
	Combined (5mm)	0.813	[0.799–0.827]	0.724	0.825	[0.813–0.837]	0.751
	Combined (7mm)	0.817	[0.783–0.831]	0.732	0.787	[0.774–0.800]	0.713

AUC=area under the curve, CI=confidence interval, ACC=accuracy.

The prediction of LVI showed the best performance in the validation cohort when including a 5 mm-thick peritumoral region feature. On the other hand, peritumoral region sizes of 3 mm and 1 mm yielded superior predictive model performance for the identification of PI and T staging. These findings indicate that the optimal size of the most informative peritumoral region may not be

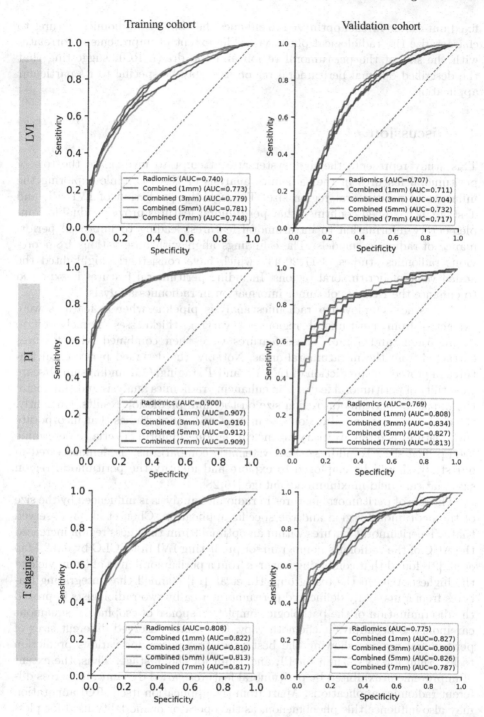

Fig. 2. ROC curves of prediction models based on intratumoral region and different peritumoral region sizes were generated for various tasks.

fixed but can be further optimized to enhance the ability of radiomics features to characterize the radiological phenotype. The extent of improvement correlates with the size of the peritumoral region and the drawn ROI, suggesting that the described optimal peritumoral region size may be specific to its particular application.

4 Discussion

This study represents the first systematic attempt to investigate the role of peritumoral features in the radiomics analysis of NSCLC while exploring the influence of peritumoral region size. Through the prediction of LVI, PI, and T-stage, it has been confirmed that peritumoral features provide valuable complementary information to intratumoral features, leading to improved performance of radiomics models. These findings align with observations from previous radiomics studies [3,17,20,44], which have consistently highlighted the added value of peritumoral regions. Including peritumoral features is expected to enhance the richness of tumor information in radiomics analysis.

This study employed a radiomics analysis pipeline wherein features were extracted from peritumoral regions of varying thicknesses, namely 1 mm, 3 mm, 5 mm, and 7 mm. These features were then combined with features extracted from the intratumoral areas. Notably, the designed peritumoral features improved the prediction of LVI, PI, and T staging. Our findings underscore the utility of peritumoral features in enhancing radiomics analysis and emphasize the impact of peritumoral region size on the final prediction results. Currently, the choice of peritumoral region size in most radiomics studies that incorporate such features is often arbitrary or unclear, lacking uniform criteria to determine the optimal size. To address this, systematic comparisons, as demonstrated in our study, should be employed to explore and identify the peritumoral region size that can yield maximum advantage [16,28].

The role of peritumoral features in radiomics analysis is influenced by the size of the peritumoral region and the specific application. Chen et al. [3] observed that CT peritumoral features within an optimal 9 mm thickness region increased the AUC of the radiomics nomogram for predicting LVI in NSCLC by 0.07. Mao et al. [21] found that combining features from a peritumoral area of 5 mm yielded the highest AUC in the test group. Hu et al. [14] claimed that integrating features from a manually delineated peritumoral area by two radiologists improved the discrimination of the pathologic complete response of esophageal squamous carcinoma to neoadjuvant chemotherapy. Our study observed different sizes of peritumoral regions showing the best predictive power for various prediction tasks: 5 mm for LVI, 3 mm for PI, and 1 mm for the T stage. Thus, the extent of improvement exhibited by peritumoral features varied dynamically across different radiomics applications. Apart from the application itself, ROI annotation may also influence this phenomenon, as the operator or modality used for plotting ROI can vary across applications. These influences should be considered when designing future radiomics studies.

5   Conclusion

This study provides preliminary evidence that the peritumoral region has critical but easily overlooked additional information about the tumor. Including peritumoral features can help improve the potential for applying radiomics analysis and should be considered in future radiomics studies. In addition, different characteristics of peritumoral size can impact the final performance of prediction models, and the optimal peritumoral size may be inconsistent across applications. Therefore, optimization of peritumoral features should be considered when integrating peritumoral regions.

Acknowledgements. This work was supported by the Overseas Joint Training Program and the Innovative Research Grant Program (Grant No. 2022GDJC-D20) for Postgraduates of Guangzhou University, as well as by the National Natural Science Foundation of China (Grant No. 61971118) and the Natural Science Foundation of Guangdong (Grant No. 2022A1515010102).

References

1. Alvi, A.M., Siuly, S., Wang, H.: A long short-term memory based framework for early detection of mild cognitive impairment from EEG signals. IEEE Trans. Emerg. Top. Comput. Intell. **7**, 375–388 (2023). https://api.semanticscholar.org/CorpusID:250397486
2. Braman, N., et al.: Association of peritumoral radiomics with tumor biology and pathologic response to preoperative targeted therapy for HER2 (ERBB2)-positive breast cancer. JAMA Netw. Open **2**(4), e192561–e192561 (2019)
3. Chen, Q.L., et al.: Intratumoral and peritumoral radiomics nomograms for the preoperative prediction of lymphovascular invasion and overall survival in non-small cell lung cancer. Eur. Radiol. **33**(2), 947–958 (2023)
4. Chetan, M.R., Gleeson, F.V.: Radiomics in predicting treatment response in non-small-cell lung cancer: current status, challenges and future perspectives. Eur. Radiol. **31**(2), 1049–1058 (2021)
5. Chong, H.H., et al.: Multi-scale and multi-parametric radiomics of gadoxetate disodium-enhanced MRI predicts microvascular invasion and outcome in patients with solitary hepatocellular carcinoma <= 5 cm. Eur. Radiol. **31**(7), 4824–4838 (2021)
6. Cong, M.D., et al.: Development of a predictive radiomics model for lymph node metastases in pre-surgical CT-based stage IA non-small cell lung cancer. Lung Cancer **139**, 73–79 (2020)
7. Cortiula, F., et al.: Immunotherapy in unresectable stage iii non-small-cell lung cancer: state of the art and novel therapeutic approaches. Ann. Oncol. **33**(9), 893–908 (2022)
8. Deniz, E., Sobahi, N., Omar, N., Şengur, A., Acharya, U.R.: Automated robust human emotion classification system using hybrid EEG features with ICBrainDB dataset. Health Inf. Sci. Syst. **10**, 1–14 (2022). https://api.semanticscholar.org/CorpusID:253422345
9. Dercle, L., et al.: Identification of non-small cell lung cancer sensitive to systemic cancer therapies using radiomics. Clin. Cancer Res. **26**(9), 2151–2162 (2020)

10. Du, J., Michalska, S., Subramani, S., Wang, H., Zhang, Y.: Neural attention with character embeddings for hay fever detection from Twitter. Health Inf. Sci. Syst. **7**, 1–7 (2019). https://api.semanticscholar.org/CorpusID:204456482

11. Fan, Y., et al.: Preoperative MRI-based radiomics of brain metastasis to assess T790M resistance mutation after EGFR-TKI treatment in NSCLC. J. Magn. Reson. Imaging **57**, 1778–1787 (2022)

12. Forouzannezhad, P., et al.: Multitask learning radiomics on longitudinal imaging to predict survival outcomes following risk-adaptive chemoradiation for non-small cell lung cancer. Cancers **14**(5), 1228 (2022)

13. Hu, H., Li, J., Wang, H., Daggard, G., Shi, M.: A maximally diversified multiple decision tree algorithm for microarray data classification (2006). https://api.semanticscholar.org/CorpusID:12168114

14. Hu, Y.H., et al.: Assessment of intratumoral and peritumoral computed tomography radiomics for predicting pathological complete response to neoadjuvant chemoradiation in patients with esophageal squamous cell carcinoma. JAMA Netw. Open **3**(9), e2015927–e2015927 (2020)

15. Huang, Y., et al.: Preoperative prediction of mediastinal lymph node metastasis in non-small cell lung cancer based on 18F-FDG PET/CT radiomics. Clin. Radiol. **78**(1), 8–17 (2023)

16. Jiang, H., Zhou, R., Zhang, L., Wang, H., Zhang, Y.: Sentence level topic models for associated topics extraction. World Wide Web **22**, 1–16 (2018). https://api.semanticscholar.org/CorpusID:53085050

17. Jiang, L., et al.: Radiogenomic analysis reveals tumor heterogeneity of triple-negative breast cancer. Cell Rep. Med. **3**(7) (2022)

18. Lee, J., Park, J.S., Wang, K., Feng, B., Tennant, M., Kruger, E.: The use of telehealth during the coronavirus (COVID-19) pandemic in oral and maxillofacial surgery - a qualitative analysis. EAI Endorsed Trans. Scalable Inf. Syst. **9**, 2 (2021). https://api.semanticscholar.org/CorpusID:244846117

19. Li, J.Q., et al.: ITHscore: comprehensive quantification of intra-tumor heterogeneity in NSCLC by multi-scale radiomic features. Eur. Radiol. **33**(2), 893–903 (2023)

20. Liu, D., et al.: Radiogenomics to characterize the immune-related prognostic signature associated with biological functions in glioblastoma. Eur. Radiol. **33**(1), 209–220 (2023)

21. Mao, N., et al.: Intratumoral and peritumoral radiomics for preoperative prediction of neoadjuvant chemotherapy effect in breast cancer based on contrast-enhanced spectral mammography. Eur. Radiol. **32**(5), 3207–3219 (2022)

22. Ninatti, G., Kirienko, M., Neri, E., Sollini, M., Chiti, A.: Imaging-based prediction of molecular therapy targets in NSCLC by radiogenomics and AI approaches: a systematic review. Diagnostics **10**(6), 359 (2020)

23. Pandey, D., Wang, H., Yin, X., Wang, K.N., Zhang, Y., Shen, J.: Automatic breast lesion segmentation in phase preserved DCE-MRIS. Health Inf. Sci. Syst. **10**, 9 (2022). https://api.semanticscholar.org/CorpusID:248924735

24. Pang, X., Ge, Y.F., Wang, K.N., Traina, A.J.M., Wang, H.: Patient assignment optimization in cloud healthcare systems: a distributed genetic algorithm. Health Inf. Sci. Syst. **11**, 30 (2023). https://api.semanticscholar.org/CorpusID:259277247

25. Rehman, O.M.H., Al-Busaidi, A.M., Ahmed, S., Ahsan, K.: Ubiquitous healthcare system: architecture, prototype design and experimental evaluations. EAI Endorsed Trans. Scalable Inf. Syst. **9**, 6 (2018). https://api.semanticscholar.org/CorpusID:245777204

26. Sarki, R., Ahmed, K., Wang, H., Zhang, Y., Wang, K.N.: Convolutional neural network for multi-class classification of diabetic eye disease. EAI Endorsed Trans. Scalable Inf. Syst. **9**, 5 (2018). https://api.semanticscholar.org/CorpusID:245295045

27. Siddiqui, S.A., Fatima, N., Ahmad, A.: Chest X-ray and CT scan classification using ensemble learning through transfer learning. EAI Endorsed Trans. Scalable Inf. Syst. **9**, e8 (2022). https://api.semanticscholar.org/CorpusID:249557133

28. Singh, R., et al.: Antisocial behavior identification from twitter feeds using traditional machine learning algorithms and deep learning. ICST Trans. Scalable Inf. Syst. (2023). https://api.semanticscholar.org/CorpusID:258671645

29. Song, F., et al.: Radiomics feature analysis and model research for predicting histopathological subtypes of non-small cell lung cancer on CT images: a multidataset study. Med. Phys. **50**, 4351–4365 (2023)

30. Sun, Y., Li, J., Xu, Z., Liu, Y., Hou, L., Huang, Z.Z.: Exploring relationship between emotion and probiotics with knowledge graphs. Health Inf. Sci. Syst. **10**, 1–11 (2022). https://api.semanticscholar.org/CorpusID:252182735

31. Tomaszewski, M.R., Gillies, R.J.: The biological meaning of radiomic features. Radiology **298**(3), 505–516 (2021)

32. Vaidya, P., et al.: Novel, non-invasive imaging approach to identify patients with advanced non-small cell lung cancer at risk of hyperprogressive disease with immune checkpoint blockade. J. Immunother. Cancer **8**(2), 11 (2020)

33. Vicini, S., et al.: A narrative review on current imaging applications of artificial intelligence and radiomics in oncology: focus on the three most common cancers. Radiol. Med. **127**(8), 819–836 (2022)

34. Vimalachandran, P., Liu, H., Lin, Y., Ji, K., Wang, H., Zhang, Y.: Improving accessibility of the Australian my health records while preserving privacy and security of the system. Health Inf. Sci. Syst. **8**, 1–9 (2020). https://api.semanticscholar.org/CorpusID:222233812

35. Wang, M.N., Herbst, R.S., Boshoff, C.: Toward personalized treatment approaches for non-small-cell lung cancer. Nat. Med. **27**(8), 1345–1356 (2021)

36. Wang, T.T., et al.: Radiomics for survival risk stratification of clinical and pathologic stage IA pure-solid non-small cell lung cancer. Radiology **302**(2), 425–434 (2022)

37. Wu, L.Y., Lou, X.J., Kong, N., Xu, M.S., Gao, C.: Can quantitative peritumoral CT radiomics features predict the prognosis of patients with non-small cell lung cancer? A systematic review. Eur. Radiol. **33**(3), 2105–2117 (2023)

38. Wu, Y.J., Wu, F.Z., Yang, S.C., Tang, E.K., Liang, C.H.: Radiomics in early lung cancer diagnosis: from diagnosis to clinical decision support and education. Diagnostics **12**(5), 1064 (2022)

39. Xie, N., et al.: Peritumoral and intratumoral texture features based on multiparametric MRI and multiple machine learning methods to preoperatively evaluate the pathological outcomes of pancreatic cancer. J. Magn. Reson. Imaging **58**(2), 379–391 (2022)

40. Xu, H., et al.: Intratumoral and peritumoral radiomics based on dynamic contrast-enhanced MRI for preoperative prediction of intraductal component in invasive breast cancer. Eur. Radiol. **32**(7), 4845–4856 (2022)

41. Yin, J., Tang, M., Cao, J., Wang, H., You, M., Lin, Y.: Vulnerability exploitation time prediction: an integrated framework for dynamic imbalanced learning. World Wide Web **25**, 401–423 (2021). https://api.semanticscholar.org/CorpusID:237746297

42. You, M., Yin, J., Wang, H., Cao, J., Miao, Y.: A minority class boosted framework for adaptive access control decision-making. In: WISE (2021). https://api.semanticscholar.org/CorpusID:244852711
43. You, M., et al.: A knowledge graph empowered online learning framework for access control decision-making. World Wide Web **26**, 827–848 (2022). https://api.semanticscholar.org/CorpusID:250007362
44. Yu, Y.X., et al.: GD-EOB-DTPA-enhanced MRI radiomics to predict vessels encapsulating tumor clusters (VETC) and patient prognosis in hepatocellular carcinoma. Eur. Radiol. **32**(2), 959–970 (2022)
45. Zhang, X.B., et al.: Prognostic analysis and risk stratification of lung adenocarcinoma undergoing EGFR-TKI therapy with time-serial CT-based radiomics signature. Eur. Radiol. **33**(2), 825–835 (2023)
46. Zhang, X.P., et al.: Deep learning with radiomics for disease diagnosis and treatment: challenges and potential. Front. Oncol. **12**, 773840 (2022)
47. Zhang, X.P., et al.: Prospective clinical research of radiomics and deep learning in oncology: a translational review. Crit. Rev. Oncol. Hematol. **179**, 103823 (2022)

Multi-dimensional Complex Query Optimization for Disease-Specific Data Exploration Based on Data Lake

Zhentao Hu[1], Kaige Wang[1(✉)], Weifan Wang[1(✉)], Wenkui Zheng[2],
Yong Zhang[3], Xin Li[4], Gao Fei[5], Wenyao Li[2], and Luoxi Wang[6]

[1] School of Artificial Intelligence, Henan University, Zhengzhou 450046, China
{hzt,wkg}@henu.edu.cn, 1838030030@vip.henu.edu.cn
[2] School of Software, Henan University, Kaifeng 475004, China
[3] BNRist, DCST, RIIT, Tsinghua University, Beijing 100084, China
zhangyong05@tsinghua.edu.cn
[4] Beijing Tsinghua Changgung Hospital, School of Clinical Medicine, Tsinghua University, Beijing 100084, China
Horsebackdancing@sina.com
[5] Henan Justice Police Vocational College, Zhengzhou 450018, China
[6] The Experimental High School Attached To Beijing Normal University, Beijing 100032, China

Abstract. In the medical field, huge amounts of multi-modal medical data are generated daily from various smart devices. Besides EMRs, medical data include a large amount of unstructured data such as MRI scans, CT scans, and X-rays. These massive, heterogeneous multi-modal data bring the big challenge to explore medical data. While traditional databases and data warehouses can identify valuable datasets for medical researchers through complex multi-dimensional queries on structured medical data, they face limitations in terms of query efficiency and the ability to explore multi-modal data. Therefore, in order to solve these problems, we propose the implementation of multi-dimensional complex query optimization for multi-modal medical data based on data lake. Firstly, we design an efficient data layout optimization strategy that aggregates data meeting the conditions of queries, thereby reducing the data throughput of the system during the query process. Secondly, leveraging the benefits of data layout optimization, we establish high-dimensional indexes for multi-modal medical data to improve the efficiency of multi-dimensional query.

Keywords: Data Lake · Multi-modal medical data · Data layout optimization · High-dimensional index

1 Introduction

With the rapid advancement of information technology and various digital medical devices, tremendous amounts of multi-modal medical data are recorded.

Y. Li et al. (Eds.): HIS 2023, LNCS 14305, pp. 321–330, 2023.
https://doi.org/10.1007/978-981-99-7108-4_27

These complex and diverse medical data include structured data, such as EMR and EHR, as well as unstructured data [1], including MRI scans, CT scans, and X-rays etc. Using data exploration techniques to extract valuable information from these data can effectively assist medical professionals in making treatment decisions [2–4]. Among various approaches to data exploration, complex queries are commonly employed in medical data exploration, involving intricate condition filtering, association operations, and frequent access to data. The multi-dimensional query has a high frequency and is severely time-consuming among the subqueries of the complex query by analyzing the complex query process.

The database technology is early adopted within the medical field to handle multi-dimensional complex queries on structured medical data and provide data support for treatment decisions [5]. It can meet the need for quick data queries in the case of less medical data. However, when it comes to analysis tasks involving a large amount of data, the database technology may encounter limitations. To solve this issue, the data warehouse technology is applied to manage large-scale structured medical data and leverage the arithmetic power of distributed clusters to improve data query efficiency [6]. The data warehouse technology offers improved performance for handling extensive datasets. In recent years, data warehouse systems have faced challenges in analyzing multi-modal medical data due to the increasing demand for efficient data querying, as well as the exponential growth of unstructured data in the healthcare domain, among other factors.

In order to solve the problems of database and data warehouse in healthcare data exploration, researchers began to apply data lake technology to healthcare data exploration. The data storage systems based on data lake have better data aggregation capabilities to handle larger data sizes. However, the current data exploration frameworks in medical domain based on data lake technology faces two challenges as follows:

1. Workload. In many frameworks, querying data stored according to the original distribution requires scanning a large amount of irrelevant data, which can create unnecessary workload.
2. Efficiency. In the real scene, medical workers frequently need to obtain real-time results. However, existing frameworks suffer from inefficient multi-dimensional queries, which hinder medical workers' ability to perform real-time analysis of diseases.

The main contributions are summarized as follows:

1. We implemented data layout optimization based on data lake. The data that meets the query criteria are aggregated together so that a large amount of irrelevant data is skipped in the query process, effectively reducing the system throughput.
2. We design an optimization method for multi-dimensional queries of medical data based on data layout optimization. High-dimensional indexes are created for selected multi-dimensional query columns during data clustering to further improve the efficiency of multi-dimensional queries.

The rest of this paper is organized as follows. Section 2 introduces the related work. Section 3 gives the system architecture. Section 4 introduces query optimization techniques and data layout optimization methods for multi-dimensional queries. Section 5 presents a performance comparison experimental analysis. Section 6 summarizes the paper and points out future research direction.

2 Related Work

At present, the data warehouse is an important tool for storing and analyzing structured data. However, due to the lack of management of unstructured data within the medical field, the data lake technology is used to solve the problem of multi-modal data storage in data warehouses. The existing data storage system based on data lake can store data in any format and solve the data management problem of multi-modal medical data, but there are still limitations in querying multi-modal data. As shown in Table 1, 1–4 are related studies of data warehouses, and 5–9 are related work of data lakes.

Table 1. Comparison of related researches.

	Related research	Multi-sources heterogeneous data acquisition	Multi-sources heterogeneous data storage	Multi-sources heterogeneous data management	Multi-modal data fusion	Multi-dimensional query optimization	Data layout optimization	Visual exploration
1	Ali et al. [7]	O	O	O	O	O	O	●
2	Helmut et al. [8]	O	O	O	O	O	O	●
3	Mohammad et al. [9]	O	O	O	O	O	O	●
4	Ding et al. [10]	O	O	O	O	O	O	●
5	Joseph et al. [11]	●	●	●	O	O	O	●
6	Iran A et al. [12]	●	●	●	●	O	O	●
7	Ren et al. [13]	●	●	●	●	O	O	●
8	Bian et al. [14]	O	O	O	O	O	●	●
9	Zhang et al. [15]	●	●	●	●	O	O	●
10	**Ours et al.**	●	●	●	●	●	●	●

Note: ● indicates that the tables feature is supported, and O is not

There are also researches about data layout optimization. Bian et al. [14] implemented data storage layout optimization in the open source storage system Pixels, adding the missing I/O scheduling policy in S3 column storage to solve the high latency problem in cloud object storage. Qiao et al. [16] proposed a new heterogeneous copy construction algorithm and adaptive routing policy based on NoSQL database, which can generate optimal layout of heterogeneous replicas to achieve the optimal query throughput for a specific workload. The above proposed methods reduce the workload of the system, but cannot be applied to medical scenarios with large data volumes and complex queries of high-dimensional medical data.

The multi-dimensional query is one of the leading causes of slow data queries. Wang et al. [17] combined Hilbert space-filling curves and clustering indexes and proposed a Hilbert curve-based clustering index structure to implement multi-dimensional queries for the NoSQL database HBASE. Yang et al. [18] proposed a secure and efficient multi-dimensional range query algorithm MMRQ for TMWSN to guarantee the privacy of sensor data, query primitives, and query results and improve the multi-dimensional query efficiency of data. Although such optimization algorithms have been proposed, there is a dearth of research in constructing high-dimensional indexes for unstructured data.

3   Architecture Design

Our architecture is established on a heterogeneous medical data fusion framework(HMDFF) supporting multi-modal query [15], utilizing Apache Hudi as data lake platform and Apache Spark as computational engine. We implement the layout optimization strategy of multi-modal data based on Apache Hudi, and we further manage multi-modal data by constructing a high-dimensional index. In this section, we present the key design of our architecture.

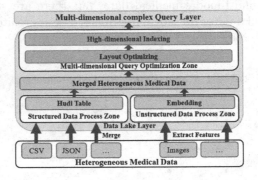

Fig. 1. System architecture overview

3.1   Architecture Overview

The architecture of our framework is presented in Fig. 1. It consists of five main modules: data lake layer, structured data process zone, unstructured data process zone, multi-dimensional query optimization zone, and multi-dimensional complex query layer. Data lake layer loads and merges multi-modal medical data through Apache Spark, and transforms data in different formats into a unified DataFrame data structure, which can be accessed through the rich APIs provided by the SparkSQL platform. Structured data process zone writes the merged structured data into Hudi table for persistent storage. Unstructured data process zone extracts feature vectors from unstructured data, such as medical images, by employing pre-trained deep learning models. These feature vectors are then transformed into columns within DataFrame. Multi-dimensional query optimization zone optimizes data layout and constructs high-dimensional index according to the data exploration needs and data characteristics. Multi-dimensional complex query layer queries transformed multi-modal data using specific query statements efficiently.

From the implementation point of view, our framework uses application programming interfaces (APIs) provided by Apache Hudi for the optimization of multi-modal data, constructing high-dimensional index. For the DataFrame transformed by data merging or feature extracting, we initially develop a suitable clustering plan, such that nearby data in the high-dimensional space are close to each other, thereby achieving data layout optimization. On this basis, high-indexes are constructed for multi-dimensional datasets, to address multi-dimensional query problems in the field of multi-modal medical complex query.

4   Multi-dimensional Complex Query Optimization

Due to the data characteristics of complex query scenarios in healthcare, we propose to take the advantages of Spark cluster in terms of data structure and computing efficiency, optimizing data layout and constructing high-dimensional indexes on data lake platform, Apache Hudi.

4.1   The Optimization of Data Layout

Traditional medical storage systems store data in an order that is not available to query engines. If the data is stored in the order of the condition columns in the query statement, the data throughput during the query process can be greatly reduced. Figure 2 shows two ways of data layout for the same dataset, Data Layout 1 is a data table formed after storing the data in its original order, and Data Layout 2 is a data table created after aggregating the data. The amount of data read is different when the same query statement is executed on two tables. For example, to find the data of red, 9 data reads are required on Data layout 1, while only 3 data reads are required on Data layout 2.

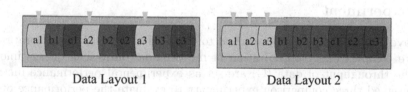

Data Layout 1   Data Layout 2

Fig. 2. Layouts of same dataset

Therefore, we choose the parquet-based Hudi table as the physical table for high-dimensional data storage, utilizing Clustering function provided by Apache Hudi to develop inline clustering plan for the data. The frequency of data clustering can be controlled by adjusting the parameters of the specified APIs. For better result, we set the clustering frequency to the highest. This means that it will re-order each batch of data written to the Hudi table by the selected columns, and store data with similar values in the selected feature columns in the same parquet file, which makes a large amount of irrelevant data to be skipped during the data query.

4.2   The Construction of High-Dimensional Index

In medical data exploration, multi-modal data are high-dimensional, such as patient's age, gender, disease type, etc. Furthermore, medical image data such as X-rays have multi-dimensional features including background, foreground, grayscale, pixels and edges. Due to data from each dimension to be traversed and compared in the traditional high-dimensional query, it makes query times for high-dimensional datasets to increase rapidly. In our framework, we address the problem by creating high-dimensional indexes for each column in accordance with the conditions of high-dimensional queries.

Before indexing the high-dimensional multi-modal healthcare dataset, we need to fuse the heterogeneous data. To be more specific, the structured and semi-structured data (including CSV, JSON, SQL files) is transformed into a unified DataFrame by SparkSQL, which subsequently acts as a loading container for the multi-modal data to be fused. For unstructured data (MRI, CT scans, X-rays), we first use pre-trained deep learning models to extract the corresponding feature vectors for the different features of data and transform them into different feature columns in the DataFrame.

Eventually, we further optimize the data clustering parameters, and enable the construction of high-dimensional index for the fused multi-modal medical data during the data writing process. We specify the feature columns that need to be indexed, so that the data is reordered according to the selected columns, and an index file is generated as it is written to the Hudi table. When performing a multi-criteria query on a Hudi table, the query engine will generate the appropriate data filters based on the index file to find the data that matches the query criteria quickly, improving the efficiency of multi-dimensional queries on medical structured data.

5   Experiment

We have applied the proposed method to the field of sepsis data exploration to achieve complex query optimization of multi-modal data. The query time (s) and the throughput of data (G) are set as experimental performance metrics. We designed three comparison experiments to evaluate the performance of the proposed method in this paper.

5.1   Experimental Environment and Datesets

We maintain consistent hardware and software configurations throughout experiments to ensure accurate and meaningful comparisons between the data lake framework and the distributed PostgreSQL database. They are deployed in clusters with three nodes, each including an 11th Gen Intel 16-core processor, 16GB of operating memory, and the 64-bit version 18.04.6 of the Ubuntu operating system.

We choose to use structured data from the MIMIC-IV database and X-ray images as the experimental validation dataset through research and analysis of datasets in the field of sepsis. The structured data includes the inputevents table, labevents table, and chartevents table, which are essential for conducting multi-dimensional queries in the sepsis field. They contain 42.9G of structured data and 37,110 X-ray images, with the largest dataset containing 329,499,789 pieces of data.

5.2   Performance Evaluation

The query statement in the performance evaluation scheme is executed three times and the average result is taken as the experimental result. The data in Fig. 3 clearly illustrates the benefits of our method. Our method effectively minimizes the throughput of data access during the query process to aggregate similar data together. However, the distributed PostgreSQL approach to perform multi-dimensional queries requires scanning the entire table, and the data throughput of the system is often the size of the entire dataset. On the other hand, the default method of Apache Hudi creates a large number of small files in the process of writing to the Hudi table, which in turn increases the throughput of data access in the query operation.

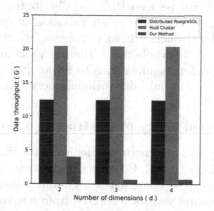

Fig. 3. Data throughput comparison of different dimensions

As shown in Fig. 4(a). Our method consistently delivers exceptional query efficiency, regardless of the increasing data volume, when subjected to the same multi-dimensional query conditions. This advantage becomes more pronounced in comparison to the other two methods, particularly when dealing with large volumes of data. Through the creation of high-dimensional indexes for each data entry during the data aggregation process, we enable rapid and precise data retrieval, resulting in accelerated query performance. In contrast, the distributed PostgreSQL method and the default Hudi method exhibit lower efficiency due to the requirement of comparing each data entry during multi-dimensional queries. This limitation becomes particularly evident when dealing with large data volumes.

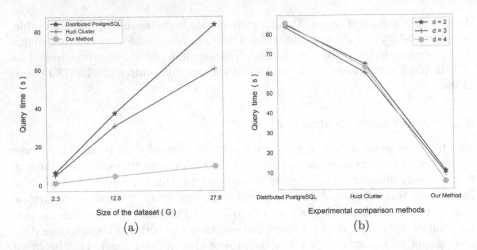

Fig. 4. Time-consuming comparison of different dataset sizes and dimensions

The data in Fig. 4(b) highlight the advantages of our method in multi-dimensional queries. It can be seen that the distributed PostgreSQL method and the Hudi method do not show much variation in query time when performing multi-dimensional queries from the figure, which indicates that they need to scan the data of the whole table. However, our method enables multi-dimensional queries of different dimensions to be completed quickly by building high-dimensional indexes for multi-dimensional query columns.

5.3   Multi-dimensional Query of Unstructured Data

In some medical scenarios, unstructured medical data is needed to assist doctors in their work, including EMR, CT scans, X-rays, etc. To accurately retrieve patients' medical records, we construct a high-dimensional index for unstructured data based on feature vectors generated from unstructured data.

Suppose a doctor needs to retrieve similar X-ray images from three features: grayscale, edge, and foreground, to diagnose the disease of sepsis for a patient. Based on our framework, this problem can be settled according to the following steps: First, the corresponding X-ray image dataset is uploaded to the data lake for persistence. Next, the pre-trained deep learning model is used to extract the feature vectors for different features of the image. Then, a high-dimensional index is built for the extracted multiple feature quantities. Finally, similar images are queried and query results are returned based on the X-ray images selected by the physician and the query features. We implemented the query process for this scene using a dataset of 37,110 X-ray images. The multi-dimensional query of unstructured data is implemented in terms of functionality.

6   Conclusion and Future Work

We implement a multi-dimensional complex query optimization method of multimodal medical data using APIs provided by Apache Hudi. In the data writing process, a data layout optimization strategy is developed. This strategy clusters the data that meets the query criteria, thereby reducing the amount of data that the system needs to access during the query process. In the data clustering process, high-dimensional indexes are created for selected feature columns of multi-model medical data to speed up the execution of multi-dimensional queries and solve the multi-dimensional query problem for unstructured data. In the future, we will apply clustering algorithms in the query process of multi-source heterogeneous data, and model various types of query statements to enhance intelligence and efficiency of data exploration.

Acknowledgements. This work was supported by National Key R&D Program of China (No.2020AAA0109603), National Natural Science Foundation of China (No.62202332), Diversified Investment Foundation of Tianjin (No.21JCQNJC009 80) and key funding from National Natural Science Foundation of China (No.9206 7206)

References

1. Li, T.: Enabling Precision Medicine by Integrating Multi-modal Biomedical Data. Georgia Institute of Technology, Atlanta, GA, USA (2021)
2. Pan, L., et al.: MFDNN: multi-channel feature deep neural network algorithm to identify covid19 chest x-ray images. Health Inf. Sci. Syst. **10**(1), 4 (2022)
3. Pandey, D., Wang, H., Yin, X., Wang, K., Zhang, Y., Shen, J.: Automatic breast lesion segmentation in phase preserved DCE-MRIS. Health Inf. Sci. Syst. **10**(1), 9 (2022)
4. Tawhid, M.N.A., Siuly, S., Wang, K., Wang, H.: Automatic and efficient framework for identifying multiple neurological disorders from EEG signals. IEEE Trans. Technol. Soc. **4**(1), 76–86 (2023). https://doi.org/10.1109/TTS.2023.3239526
5. Mohamad, B., Orazio, L., Gruenwald, L.: Towards a hybrid row-column database for a cloud based medical data management system. In: 1st International Workshop on Cloud Intelligence, pp. 1–4. ACM, New York (2012)
6. Sebaa, A., et al.: Medical big data warehouse: architecture and system design, a case study: improving healthcare resources distribution. J. Med. Syst. **42**, 59 (2018)
7. Neamah, A.F.: Flexible data warehouse: towards building an integrated electronic health record architecture. In: 2020 International Conference on Smart Electronics and Communication (ICOSEC), pp. 1038–1042. IEEE (2020)
8. Spengler, H., Gatz, I., Kohlmayer, F., Kuhn, K.A., Prasser, F.: Improving data quality in medical research: a monitoring architecture for clinical and translational data warehouses. In: 2020 IEEE 33rd International Symposium on Computer Based Medical Systems (CBMS), pp. 415–420. IEEE (2020)
9. Khan, M.Z., Kidwai, M.S., Ahamad, F., Khan, M.U.: Hadoop based EMH framework: a big data approach. In: 2021 International Conference on Advance Computing and Innovative Technologies in Engineering (ICACITE), pp. 1068–1070. IEEE (2021)

10. Ding, S., Mao, C., Zheng, W., Xiao, Q., Wu, Y.: Data exploration optimization for medical big data. In: Traina, A., Wang, H., Zhang, Y., Siuly, S., Zhou, R., Chen, L. (eds.) Health Information Science, HIS 2022. Lecture Notes in Computer Science, vol. 13705, pp. 145–156. Springer, Cham (2022). https://doi.org/10.1007/978-3-031-20627-6_14

11. Mesterhazy, J., Olson, G., Datta, S.: High performance on-demand de-identification of a petabyte-scale medical imaging data lake. arXiv preprint arXiv:2008.01827 (2020)

12. Melchor-Uceda, I.A., Olivares-Rojas, J.C., Gutiérrez-Gnecchi, J.A., García-Ramírez, M.C., Reyes-Archundia, E., Téllez-Anguiano, A.C.: Data ingestion system for interoperability and integration of hospital data online and in real time. In: 2021 Mexican International Conference on Computer Science (ENC), pp. 1–5. IEEE (2021)

13. Ren, P., et al.: MHDP: an efficient data lake platform for medical multi-source heterogeneous data. In: Xing, C., Fu, X., Zhang, Y., Zhang, G., Borjigin, C. (eds.) WISA 2021. LNCS, vol. 12999, pp. 727–738. Springer, Cham (2021). https://doi.org/10.1007/978-3-030-87571-8_63

14. Bian, H., Ailamaki, A.: Pixels: an efficient column store for cloud data lakes. In: 2022 IEEE 38th International Conference on Data Engineering (ICDE), pp. 3078–3090. IEEE (2022)

15. Zhang, Y., et al.: A heterogeneous multi-modal medical data fusion framework supporting hybrid data exploration. Health Inf. Sci. Syst. **10**(1), 22 (2022)

16. Qiao, J., et al.: Heterogeneous replicas for multi-dimensional data management. In: Nah, Y., Cui, B., Lee, S.-W., Yu, J.X., Moon, Y.-S., Whang, S.E. (eds.) DASFAA 2020, Part I. LNCS, vol. 12112, pp. 20–36. Springer, Cham (2020). https://doi.org/10.1007/978-3-030-59410-7_2

17. Wang, X., Sun, Y., Sun, Q., Lin, W., Wang, J.Z., Li, W.: HCIndex: a Hilbert-Curve based clustering index for efficient multi-dimensional queries for cloud storage systems. Clust. Comput. **26**(3), 2011–2025 (2023)

18. Yang, W., Liu, L., Liu, Y., Fan, L., Lu, W.: Secure and efficient multi-dimensional range query algorithm over TMWSNs. Ad Hoc Netw. **130**, 102820 (2022)

Analyzing Health Risks Resulting from Unplanned Land Use Plan and Structure: A Case Study in Historic Old Dhaka

Nishat Tasnim Manami$^{(\boxtimes)}$, Ashik Mostafa Alvi⊙, and Siuly Siuly⊙

Victoria University, Melbourne, VIC, Australia

{nishat.manami,ashik.alvi,siuly.siuly}@vu.edu.au

Abstract. Dhaka, the capital and largest city of Bangladesh, is the economic and historical core of the country. The old part of it, is known as Old Dhaka which holds great importance in the country of Bangladesh, as it serves as a vibrant hub of cultural heritage and valuable resources. It raises concerns due to its high population density and unplanned urban planning. The present situation is impacting the physical and mental health of the people living here. The presence of air and water pollution in Old Dhaka contributes to various health issues, while the unplanned structure of the area adds to a sense of insecurity among its residents. Moreover, the lack of community resilience further exposes the locality to vulnerabilities. There is a lot of research that has been done on Old Dhaka regarding specific words, community resilience, built structures, and so on. These studies have elaborated on the existing situation but are hardly related to the situation regarding health concerns. To comprehend the effect of the unplanned design on the health of the residents, the author of this paper conducted interviews with 120 individuals, along with observation, photographic analysis, and a cause-and-effect diagram. It facilitated comprehending how people's health is being impacted and what possible place-based solutions are available for addressing this. This research will assist future researchers as well as government or private agencies in prioritizing health in Old Dhaka.

Keywords: Old Dhaka · Placed-based approach · Health · Social Resilience

1 Introduction

Old Dhaka, the capital of Bangladesh, holds significant economic importance, as it encompasses a rich history showcased through its old buildings and long-established local enterprises that have been passed down through generations [8]. However, with a substantial increase in population and rapid urbanization, Old Dhaka has become a notable example of uncontrolled development. Estimates suggest that a severe earthquake could occur soon [12]. Old Dhaka, with its numerous mixed-use buildings and chemical industries, is particularly vulnerable to both Earthquake and fire incidents.

Daisy, Naznin Sultana, et al. have attempted to determine the extant problem in Old Dhaka by analyzing Ward 30 using a place-based approach [9]. Using Pairwise ranking and a Venn diagram, they ranked the problems and investigated the relationships between various resources [11]. Using pairwise matrices and cause and effect diagrams, Tokey, Ahmad Ilderim, et al. presented redevelopment strategies for Ward 30 [10]. It mentioned health hazards contemplating the scenario, but these two papers did not specify how the unplanned urban design impacts physical and mental health [13]. However, this was a broad study that lacked the in-depth analysis required for place-based approaches.

In this paper, the author seeks to explain why old Dhaka needs improvement, how it is influencing the health of its residents, and what options are available to make it a better place. Following a place-based approach, the objective will be to identify the factors that contribute to the area's unfavorable living conditions and to identify options, including community participation that can make the area livable for its residents. This study will contribute to –

- Students and researchers will be able to obtain an in-depth analysis of health issues in old Dhaka, which will aid them in conducting further research on this topic.
- The government and health sector will have a clearer understanding of why Old Dhaka is a top priority in terms of health concerns.
- The study will concentrate on the physical and mental health of Old Dhaka residents, as opposed to the current study's emphasis on structures.

2 Methodology

In Old Dhaka, there are six distinct wards. Figure 1 shows six wards of Old Dhaka and Old Central Jail area with boundary specifications.

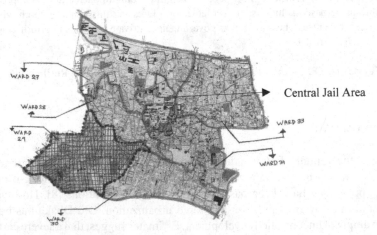

Fig. 1. Six wards of Old Dhaka including Old central jail area and the study area, ward 29.

With the polluted river Buriganga, high population density, and accessibility to amenities taken into consideration, the author has specifically chosen ward 29 for further investigation into the health and safety of its inhabitants [7]. Through a seven-day period of observation and photographic analysis, the author has determined that Ward 29 is a focal point for exploring the health and safety concerns of the residents.

To gain a comprehensive understanding of the correlation between the roads and the surrounding buildings, the author conducted on-site visits to closely observe and analyze the buildings near these roads [16]. The author has attempted to establish some maps that will aid in understanding the accessibility of the roads, accessibility to medical facilities, accessibility to fields and open spaces for the impact on mental health, and population density of the area to understand the health safety of the locals [14]. Table 1 shows a brief overview of the study area.

Table 1. A brief overview of the study area (Ward 29).

Location	• Ward 29 is located in South-West portion of Old Dhaka and is connected to the river Buriganga
Area	• Approximately 60,000 hectare
Population	• Around 70,599
Fire-stations	• Lalbagh and Palashi fire station
Major Roads	• Islambagh, Shayesta Khan Road, Goni Miar Haat, and Hazi Kali Road
Parks	• No available parks
Open spaces	• Three available open spaces

A total of 120 respondents were taken for interviews for this study. Since there were few resources and results, the author used a purposive selection method to choose respondents as a sample. A set of criteria was used in the purposive sampling method to ensure uniformity across all respondents. The criteria for this selection were-

1. Respondents have been involved with business in this area or have been living here for more than one year.
2. Respondents have some knowledge of this area and are active in community participation.

3   Result and Discussion

The study identified four main issues affecting the physical and mental health of the residents of Ward 29. The cause-and-effect diagram in Table 2, will provide a detailed understanding of this result.

Table 2. Cause and Effect diagram considering the physical and mental health of the residents of Ward 29, Old Dhaka.

Issue 1				
Effect	Water diseases	Affecting flor-fauna cycle	Blocking the road during rainy season	Unhealthy space for bad smell of water
Issue Water pollution				
Cause	Polluter river-Buriganga	Chemicals, Plastic materials	Medical and household waste	Poor drainage system
Issue 2				
Effect	Breathing issue	Cold and cough	Limiting the interest to go outside	Affecting social interaction
Issue	Air pollution			
Cause	Polluter river-Buriganga	Factory wastage	Overcrowded area and vehicles	Plastic burning
Issue 3				
Effect	Safety of people	Physical vulnerability	Social vulnerability	Mental health
Issue Unplanned built structure				
Cause	Lack of guidance	Population Density	Lack of proper maintenance	Lack of application of strict laws
Issue 4				
Effect	Vulnerable to any disaster	Physical and mental health	Affecting social connectivity	
Issue Lack of community resilience				
Cause	Lack of training	Lack of awareness	Lack of resources	

3.1 Health Determinants

The ward border line is adjacent to the Central Jail area and the Buriganga River. Due to its high population density and significant industrial and commercial activities, the people who reside and work in this area are constantly exposed to risks [20]. It is important to note that most of the buildings close to Buriganga are commercial and mixed-use ones. There are numerous factories in the area involved in the production of chemicals, plastics, and electrical products, which pose a significant fire hazard risk.

The majority of the buildings have inhabitants in the upper floors and mixed-use industries at the lower level [5]. The air pollution caused by the chemical and plastic manufacturers is harming the locals. People who suffer from asthma and other respiratory illnesses are caused by the poor air quality brought on by pollution [6].

60% of the respondents said they had trouble breathing in this area, 12% said they didn't, and the remaining respondents were not sure (Fig. 2). In addition, 25% of them stated having asthma, 49% of them noted having a cough, a runny nose, or burning eyes, and the other people said they don't have any health issues (Fig. 3).

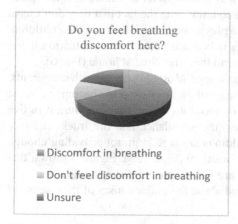

Do you feel breathing discomfort here?

- Discomfort in breathing
- Don't feel discomfort in breathing
- Unsure

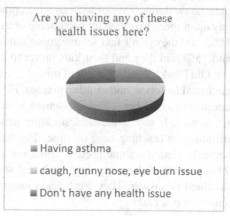

Are you having any of these health issues here?

- Having asthma
- caugh, runny nose, eye burn issue
- Don't have any health issue

Fig.2. A pie chart showing breathing discomfort percentage among the respondents.

Fig. 3. A pie chart showing health issue percentage among the residents.

The few roads are wide enough to allow a fire brigade to reach the area quickly, according to surveys. Figure 4 shows that few roads exist between 3 and 9 m, with the majority being less than 3 m. Figure 5 shows the road width with a pie chart that defines the condition of the road of Ward 29.

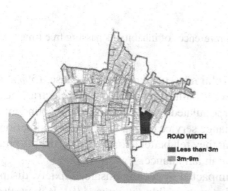

ROAD WIDTH
- Less than 3m
- 3m-9m

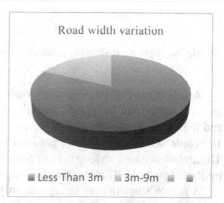

Road width variation

- Less Than 3m   - 3m-9m

Fig. 4. Different Road variations in ward 29.

Fig. 5. A pie chart showing the percentage of road width variation.

3.2 Built Environments and Health

A significant proportion of respondents said they get good communication with their neighbors in terms of neighborhood relations. They exhibited mental health and a sense of community with them. This positive relationship helps them to reach out for support that highlights a favorable outcome concerning mental health within the community [15].

On the other hand, the lack of open areas and pedestrians is having an impact on the local young people. When asked to women, why people prefer to remain at home rather than go outdoors, 75% of women have come to terms with the fact that they don't have any open space to utilize for socializing or as a playground for the kids and their children. 10% said they don't feel secure going outdoors because of the dense population there, and 15% said they and their kids prefer to spend their free time at home (Fig. 6).

Old Dhaka Ward 29 is full of mixed-use buildings. Most of them are with restaurants, chemical factories, and printing presses. Fire hazard for this reason has become the most common hazard here. The unplanned wire connections make the place unsafe to live in as well. If any vulnerable situation arises, the ambulance and fire truck will face difficulty in reaching here on time. The buildings are here built not providing enough setback. Here are some present scenarios of ward 29 (Figs. 7, 8). Figure 9 shows, that 75% percent of them say they don't feel secure living here, 15% dispute this, and 10% declined to answer. They were again inquired about the major causes of their sense of safety in this place.

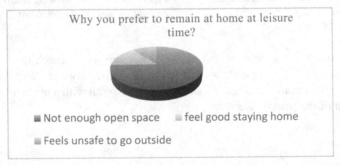

Fig. 6. A pie chart showing percentages of preferences of inhabitants passing free time.

According to Fig. 10, 35% of respondents claimed a fire danger as the cause, 15% told an unplanned urban design, 20% mentioned weak built structure, 18% cited electric lines, and the remaining respondents cited an overpopulated region. Among the respondents, 10 people agreed they couldn't get an ambulance service during their extreme situation. The ambulance took so long time to come that they felt better about reaching the hospital by Rickshaw or CNG rather than waiting for an ambulance.

A person's health may be significantly impacted by feeling unsafe. Anxiety, disappointment, and post-traumatic stress disorder are possible outcomes [19]. It may also worsen illnesses linked to stress, such as cardiovascular disease or hypertension. Additionally, it may restrict their social interactions and lead to social isolation. So, ensuring safety should be the priority for any place to live in.

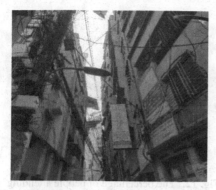

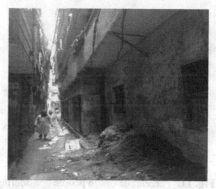

Fig. 7. Unplanned wire connection in ward 29, which is vulnerable to fire and earthquakes.

Fig. 8. Building without maintenance setbacks and blockage in the drainage system

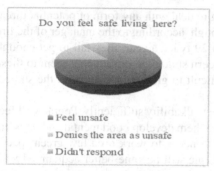

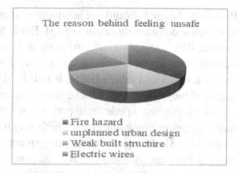

Fig. 9. A pie chart showing the percentage of people with safety concerns.

Fig. 10. A pie chart showing the percentage of the reasons behind feeling unsafe.

3.3 Community Resilience

It has already been shown via several studies and research that it is risky and hazardous to live in Old Dhaka due to fire and earthquake hazards. Mixed-use structures, plastic industries, and vulnerable buildings were all characteristics that made this neighborhood dangerous to live in [4].

Most attendees are those who come here to work every day. On a regular basis, students conduct observations while passing through the roadways, analyzing the surrounding environment where businesspeople and service providers operate. This practice allows them to evaluate any possible risks or hazards that may exist. Figures 11 and 12 show the basic knowledge of the interviewers to face any vulnerable situation. The ability to deal with stress and trauma to their highest degree makes individuals stronger against developing mental health disorders. Additionally, developing resilience has a big impact on public health. Social cohesiveness, participation in the community, and the availability of support networks are all factors that enhance health outcomes, and they are all directly related to community resilience.

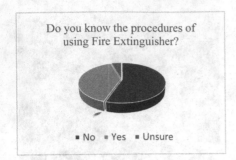

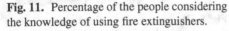

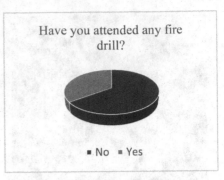

Fig. 11. Percentage of the people considering the knowledge of using fire extinguishers.

Fig. 12. The percentage of people attending fire drills.

4 Place-Based Approaches Focusing Health in Old Dhaka

People in the area should get adequate training to deal with any form of potential threat to increase community resilience [3]. Even though, according to the manager of the fire station, they attempt to offer training in Ward 29 twice a year, they fail to get enough participation from residents. The primary concern should be introducing them to these vulnerabilities and their effects. It will be difficult to grab their interest in the subject matter if they don't comprehend the situation.

There must be a pedestrian path to improve walkability sufficiently. People will feel more confident being outdoors, which may help them develop good mental and physical wellness [18]. Along with this, the government needs to work on a few green spaces and public areas in Ward 29. By doing so, people will become better acquainted with the open areas, which would boost public gatherings and help improve local youngsters and women's mental health. The local population's mental and physical health may be favorably impacted by the change [2]. Increased social interaction, stress relief, and community involvement are all expected to ensue from it.

After careful examination, we may conclude that in Fig. 14, four key highways are those that can remain open in the most dangerous circumstances. The road beside the river is already 5 m wide, making it possible to link two open areas and create a decent path for pedestrians.

The other three roads may also be utilized as a major road, connecting most of this ward while also serving as an emergency route for the fire department and ambulance. It is important to mark the dead end so that hospitals and fire stations may utilize a different route to get there.

The location of the plastic and chemical plants should be changed to reduce air pollution and fire hazards [1]. Once again, the mixed-use buildings that are mostly situated along the waterworks road need to be reorganized. For Burigange, the government has to take steps to ensure adequate water recycling, which will aid in reducing environmental hazards. In this situation, community engagement in efforts to clean the water, remove trash from the river's surroundings, and create a healthy environment might be an effective strategy [16]. Additionally, more trees will aid in air purification as well (Fig. 13).

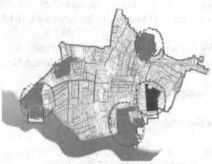

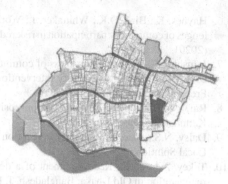

Fig. 13. Available open spaces in ward 29. **Fig. 14.** Proposed connection to the open spaces and emergency road identification.

5 Conclusion

The Buriganga River and the area's many historic structures are its major assets. It is essential to reorganize the neighborhood to guarantee its safety and security if the government is to capitalize on the power of the populace. Adequate training should be provided to the locals so they can manage unanticipated events and implement the appropriate safety measures. The public has to be made aware of the risks posed by chemical and plastic manufacturers as well as possible fire threats and natural disasters by both public and private organizations.

The locals or people often are not aware of these unique construction regulations, legislation, and safety issues. The place-based approach will aid in boosting community resilience and involvement. A resilient community promotes the surroundings necessary for families, people, and individuals to achieve personal resilience. Resilient communities recognize the importance of mental health and establish support systems to address and promote mental well-being. The required support networks are designed to be available to people through building social relationships, encouraging community involvement, and providing mental health services. This may aid in lowering stress, preventing mental health issues, and enhancing psychological resilience in general. Applying a place-based framework may help make old Dhaka a healthier environment for its inhabitants.

References

1. Bangladesh Bureau of Statistics (BBS), Household Population and density by residence and communication table C.01
2. Cutter, Susan L., et al.: A place-based model for understanding community resilience to natural disasters. Glob. Environ. Change **18**(4), 598–606 (2008)
3. Field Survey, 2017, 2022, 2023
4. Fresque-Baxter, J.A., Armitage, D.: Place identity and climate change adaptation: a synthesis and framework for understanding. Wiley Interdisc. Rev.: Clim. Change **3**(3), 251–266 (2012)
5. Guillaumont, P.: Vulnerability and resilience: a conceptual framework applied to three Asian countries—Bhutan, Maldives, and Nepal (2017)

6. Haynes, K., Bird, D.K., Whittaker, J.: Working outside 'the rules': opportunities and challenges of community participation in risk reduction. Int. J. Disaster Risk Reduction **44**, 101396 (2020)

7. Jamshidi, E., et al.: Effectiveness of community participation in earthquake preparedness: a community-based participatory intervention study of Tehran. Disaster Med. Public Health Preparedness **10**(2), 211–218 (2016)

8. Rai, N., Bikash, T.: A study on purposive sampling method in research. Kathmandu: Kathmandu School Law **5** (2015)

9. Daisy, N.S., et al.: Community Perception on the Redevelopment of Old Dhaka Based on Local Solutions

10. Tokey, A.I., et al.: Redevelopment of a dense area: a participatory planning approach for regeneration in Old Dhaka, Bangladesh. J. Reg. City Plan. **31**(3), 217–236 (2020)

11. c. Assessing social vulnerability to earthquake hazard in Old Dhaka, Bangladesh. Asian J. Environ. Disaster Manag. **3**(3), 285–300 (2011)

12. Chisty, M.A., Md Mizanur, R.: Coping capacity assessment of urban fire disaster: an exploratory study on ward no: 30 of Old Dhaka area. Int. J. Disaster Risk Reduction **51**, 101878 (2020)

13. Alvi, A.M., et al.: A study to find the impacts of strikes on students and local shopkeepers in Bangladesh. In: World Congress on Sustainable Technologies (WCST-2019) (2019)

14. Alvi, A.M., et al.: Impacts of blockades and strikes in Dhaka: a survey. Int. J. Innov. Bus. Strat. **6**(1), 369–377 (2020)

15. Paul, S., Alvi, A.M., Rahman, R.M.: An analysis of the most accident prone regions within the Dhaka Metropolitan Region using clustering. Int. J. Adv. Intell. Paradigms **18**(3), 294–315 (2021)

16. Alvi, A.M., et al.: An adaptive image smoothing technique based on localization. In: Developments of Artificial Intelligence Technologies in Computation and Robotics: Proceedings of the 14th International FLINS Conference (FLINS 2020) (2020)

17. Paul, S., et al.: Analyzing accident prone regions by clustering. Adv. Top. Intell. Inf. Database Syst. **9**, 3–13 (2017)

18. Pang, X., et al.: Patient assignment optimization in cloud healthcare systems: a distributed genetic algorithm. Health Inf. Sci. Syst. **11**(1), 30 (2023)

19. Sarki, R., et al.: Automated detection of mild and multi-class diabetic eye diseases using deep learning. Health Inf. Sci. Syst. **8**(1), 32 (2020)

20. Sarki, R., et al.: Convolutional neural network for multi-class classification of diabetic eye disease. EAI Endorsed Trans. on Scalable Inf. Syst. **9**(4), e5 (2022)

Elderly Care and Knowledge Systems

Home Self-medication Question-Answering System for the Elderly Based on Seq2Seq Model and Knowledge Graph Technology

Baoxin Wang[1], Shaofu Lin[1(⊠)], Zhisheng Huang[2,3,4], and Chaohui Guo[1]

[1] Faculty of Information Technology, Beijing University of Technology, Beijing 100124, China
linshaofu@bjut.edu.cn
[2] Department Computer Science, Vrije University Amsterdam, Amsterdam, Netherlands
[3] Clinical Research Center for Mental Disorders, Shanghai Pudong New Area Mental Health Center, Tongji University School of Medicine, Shanghai, China
[4] Deep Blue Technology Group, Shanghai, China

Abstract. With the deepening of aging, chronic diseases of the elderly are the main burden of disease in most countries in the world. The prevalence of chronic diseases in urban areas in China is as high as 75%. Many elderly people use multiple drugs for a long time. Home self-medication problems occur frequently. In order to alleviate this problem to a certain extent, knowledge graph technology and a deep learning model are used to design a home self-medication question-answering system for the elderly and their caregivers. Explore a feasible way of providing automated online consultation intelligent services. In this paper, we have collected medication as well as professional Q&A (question and answer) data in the field of aging health, and constructed a knowledge graph that meets the characteristics of medication use in the elderly. Based on the matching rules in the question judging module, the problems entered by users are classified. For professional knowledge related to diseases and medications of the elderly, the question-answering system uses the knowledge graph to search for answers. For other basic knowledge related to elderly health, the system uses the BERT model to vectorize its users' questions, then matches the questions by calculating cosine similarity, thus finding the corresponding answers. The system adds the Seq2Seq model as a supplement to the answer retrieval method of the knowledge graph. The testing results shows that the system provides online consultation services more accurately and efficiently for home self-medication for the elderly and their caregivers.

Keywords: Elderly health · Home Self-medication · Knowledge Graph · Template Matching · Seq2Seq Model

1 Introduction

Along with the deepening of aging and the increasing number of elderly people, the disease spectrum of the population in China is also undergoing significant changes, starting to shift from a pattern of mainly infectious diseases to a pattern of mainly chronic

© The Author(s), under exclusive license to Springer Nature Singapore Pte Ltd. 2023
Y. Li et al. (Eds.): HIS 2023, LNCS 14305, pp. 343–353, 2023.
https://doi.org/10.1007/978-981-99-7108-4_29

diseases. According to the latest data released by the National Health Commission, as of the end of 2018, the number of elderly people with chronic diseases in China has exceeded 180 million, accounting for up to 75% [1]. With the deepening of public hospital reform, the average length of stay has been reduced, forcing elderly people who have entered a stable period after the acute phase of chronic diseases to return to their communities and families for long-term care and treatment. Due to the lack of medical knowledge, effective medication guidance and medication consultation, many elderly people with chronic diseases at home in communities are prone to mistaking and missing medication, delaying the process of disease treatment [2].MIRA J J et al. [3] showed that the incidence of medication errors in elderly people is as high as 75%, and the most common types of errors are taking inaccurate dosage, missing medication, mixing drugs, taking expired or improperly stored medications. Medication errors can deepen the adverse effects of drugs. With the rapid development of social informatization, people have become more and more dependent on online consultation and use it as the first choice for daily diagnosis and treatment. But there are still some problems with online consultation. For instance, most of the online consultations are answered by doctors in their spare time, and the real-time answer is not guaranteed [4]. Thus the knowledge graph-based Q&A system in the medical field can somewhat alleviate this situation. The knowledge graph is represented in the structure of < entity, relation, entity >, which has very obvious advantages in knowledge representation and retrieval compared with the traditional relational model [5]. As one of the important applications of the knowledge graph, the Q&A system can accept questions from users in the form of natural language [6]. The system recognizes the question through template matching and finds the answer to the question in the knowledge graph, then returns the answer in natural language to the user [7]. Compared with traditional search engines, Q&A system can provide users with reliable information more accurately and efficiently [8].

At present, a considerable number of scholars have applied knowledge graph-based Q&A system to medical and health fields. Y Zhang et al. [9] proposed a highly efficient data fusion framework supporting data exploration for heterogeneous multi-modal medical data based on data lake. Xie Y [10] constructed a Chinese traditional medical pathology knowledge graph, combined with the KNN algorithm to answer medical questions. Zhang Chongyu [11] proposed a solution for knowledge graph construction and knowledge graph automatic Q&A system, and completed the design and implementation of a medical-assisted Q&A service platform. Huang Wei et al. [12] enabled users to get answers to medical questions online in real time, thus improving the user experience. Zhang Minglei [13] realized a Q&A system based on the knowledge graph of medical treatment through the integration of medical open-source data and took the Web end as an interactive platform to help patients query relevant disease information. Cheng Zijia et al. [14] designed and implemented an automatic Q&A model based on knowledge graph to address the problems of insufficient comprehending ability and recall ratio of the Q&A system, optimizing and improving the query rate. Xing Z et al. [15] combined medical background information with the Seq2Seq model, selected an independent recurrent neural network (RNN) as the encoder and decoder of the model, and established an automatic question-answering system for the medical guidance station. All the above mentioned scholars have well integrated the Q&A system with the medical and healthcare domain and have their own application areas. However, there are relatively few Q&A systems that combine deep learning models with knowledge graph technology for providing information related to home medication for the elderly.

To address the above issues, we construct a knowledge graph and deep learning technology-based home medication Q&A system for the elderly. Four types of datasets are collected and processed in this paper, including the expertise dataset of medication for elderly patients, the expertise dataset of diseases of elderly people, the basic Q&A dataset about elderly patients and the basic chat dataset between doctors and patients. Based on the four types of datasets, the corresponding Q&A strategies are designed in this paper. The elderly patients' medication expertise dataset and elderly disease expertise dataset are used to construct the elderly disease medication expertise semantic data, and the specialized answers in the knowledge graph are obtained by keyword extraction and template matching. The basic Q&A dataset about elderly patients is used to construct the basic Q&A semantic data of elderly patients, and the best answers are matched using the sentence vector similarity algorithm. In this paper, the Seq2Seq model is trained using the patient-doctor chat dataset as a complement to the above two Q&A strategies. Combining the above Q&A strategies, this system can provide online consultation service for home medication for the elderly population and their companions, as well as answers to non-specialized questions.

2 Models and Algorithms

2.1 BERT Models

The BERT (Bidirectional Encoder Representation from Transformers) model [16] based on the Transformer model of bidirectional encoder representation has achieved impressive results in natural language processing. The BERT model is a pre-trained language model that transforms words in a text that cannot be computed directly into vectors or matrices that can be used for computation, reflects the meaning of words in the text by such vectorized numbers. Previous language models would correspond one word to one vector, which results in the misrepresentation of polysemous words. The BERT model successfully breaks through this problem.

In this paper, the BERT model is fine-tuned using the base Q&A dataset about elderly patients. The BERT model uses the encoder of the Transformer model. By inputting the format of the underlying Q&A dataset, the BERT model outputs the training results of a black-box model consisting of multiple Transformers. This enables the fine-tuned BERT model to synthesize contextual Q&A pairs. The fine-tuned BERT model is used to vectorize the questions in the basic Q&A dataset about elderly patients. The sentence vectors are then deposited into the existing basic Q&A semantic data about elderly patients and stored in the knowledge graph in order to find the best answer by the method of Q&A vector matching.

2.2 Seq2Seq Model

In addition to the specialized and basic forms of Q&A, the daily Q&A for elderly patients also includes non-specialized forms of Q&A. Knowledge graphs are good at storing limited, fixed expertise, but are difficult to adapt flexibly to non-specialized Q&A formats. To solve the above problem, the Seq2Seq (Sequence to sequence) model [17] is introduced, which is a variant of recurrent neural network. The model structure consists of two parts, an encoder and a decoder, where it accepts input in the form of a sequence of words and its output is also a sequence of words. In encoder, the sequence is converted into a fixed-length vector, and then the vector is converted into the desired sequence output by decoder. In this paper, we use the LSTM (Long Short-Term Memory) model in both the encoder and decoder.

The simple seq2seq model is superior for short sentences. In this paper, Seq2Seq model is trained using physician-patient conversation data. The encoder part of the model encodes all the input sequences into a uniform semantic vector, which is then decoded by the decoder. Since the semantic vectors for doctor-patient dialogs contain all the information in the original sequence, its limited length causes the degradation of the model's accuracy. Besides, if the encoder is implemented in the above way, only the last hidden layer state of the encoder will be used and the information utilization would be low. To solve this problem, this paper adds attention mechanism, which is a mechanism that allows the encoder to compile vectors and dynamically adjust them in real time based on the current decoding content of the decoder. The semantic vectors are no longer fixed, but the weights are adjusted to input different semantic vectors at each moment in time. This can enhance the memory capacity of the neural network and complete a learning task on semantic data from physician-patient conversations.

2.3 Cosine Similarity Algorithm

In this paper, the cosine similarity algorithm [18] is used to compare the similarity between two questions. The algorithm uses the cosine of the angle between two vectors in a vector space as a measure of the magnitude of the difference between two questions. The closer the cosine degree is to 1, i.e., the closer the angle is to 0 degrees, the more similar the two question vectors are; conversely, the closer the cosine degree is to 0, i.e., the closer the angle is to 90 degrees, the less similar the two question vectors are. Therefore, by calculating the cosine distance between the question vectors, the similarity between the questions can be obtained. The user input question is vectorized and then the cosine similarity is computed with the question vectors in the knowledge graph. If the result is greater than the similarity threshold, the answer is based on the answer corresponding to the question vector in the knowledge graph.

Suppose A and B are two n-dimensional vectors, A is [A1, A2,..., An], and B is [B1, B2,..., Bn], the cosine of the angle θ between A and B is shown in Eq. (1):

$$\cos\theta = \frac{\sum_{i=1}^{m}(A_i \times B_i)}{\sqrt{\sum_{i=1}^{n}(A_i)^2} \times \sqrt{\sum_{i=1}^{n}(B_i)^2}} \tag{1}$$

3   Construction of Dataset and Knowledge Graph

3.1   Dataset

The importance of datasets in Q&A system cannot be underestimated. As the basis for model training, datasets provide rich samples that enable models to learn the semantics, context, and syntax of questions to generate accurate answers.

The data sources of this paper are diversified and come from the authoritative medical websites on the Internet, which are Doctor Seeker (www.xywy.com), Dingxiang Doctor (www.dxy.com) and Family Doctor (www.familydoctor.com.cn). The data have been obtained by means of web crawlers, and the required data have been crawled from the above websites. The expertise data set of medications for elderly patients has been obtained from the medication and disease data of elderly people on the Family Doctor Online website. The expertise dataset of medications for elderly patients has been obtained from the general knowledge of diseases on the Doctor Seeker and the disease data related to the geriatric section on the Family Doctor. The data set of basic questions and answers about elderly patients has been obtained from the consultation window for elderly people on the website of Dr. Dingxiang for the general public. The specific data types are shown in Table 1.

Table 1. Dataset of the home self-medication question answering system for the elderly

Dataset Name	Dataset Properties
Elderly patients Drug Dataset	Name, Indication, Usage_dosage, Ingredients, Characteristics, Adverse_reactions, Contraindications, Precautions, Drug_interactions, Pharmacological_action, Storage, Approval_number, Manufacturer
Elderly Disease dataset	Name, Other_name, Parts, People, Departments, Symptoms, Drug, Check, Producers, Cause, Symptoms_desc, Diagnosis, Treatment, Food, Health, Infect, Inheritance
Basic question and answer dataset about elderly patients	Problem sentence vector, Question, Answer
Basic doctor-patient chat dataset	Question, Answer

3.2   Construction of Knowledge Graph

A large amount of fixed and specialized domain knowledge can be stored in the knowledge graph, ensuring the accuracy of the content from the root. The answers for the queries are derived from these accurate data, which ensures the authority of the answers. The use of knowledge graph technology can also improve the intelligence of the Q&A system. Knowledge graphs describe things in the form of a triple consisting of two entities and the relationship between them. Such a feature of the knowledge graph makes it possible to link different entities through relationships in the process of matching queries, enabling intelligent queries.

In order to increase the diversity of information in the knowledge graph, and thus increase the flexibility of the Q&A system, this system integrates "semantic data of professional knowledge of medication for diseases of the elderly" and "semantic data of basic questions and answers about elderly patients". In the first part of the data, the system extracts entities, relationships, and attributes from the data, and carries an neo4j server to combine the data with Cypher statements to create entities, entity relationship edges, and entity association edges in the knowledge graph. In the second part of the data, the system first vectorizes the questions through the BERT model, and then stores the corresponding answers as attributes of the vectorized questions in the knowledge graph. The knowledge graph can be divided into two categories, which are professional knowledge of medication for the elderly and basic Q&A knowledge about elderly patients. The above two semantic data were merged to construct the knowledge graph used in this system. The knowledge graph is shown in Fig. 1:

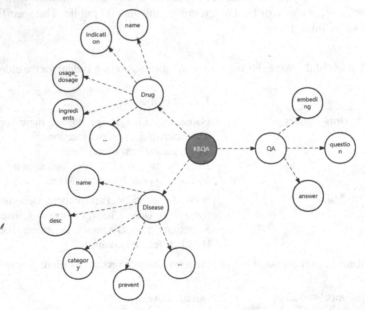

Fig. 1. Knowledge graph of the home self-medication question-answering system for the elderly

4 Question Judgment and Answer Generation Method

4.1 Users and Problem Types

Traditional search engines retrieve web resources to find the most valuable information for users after they make a request. In contrast, domain-specific knowledge Q&A system uses artificial intelligence technology to analyze questions in real time and determine exactly what knowledge the user needs, thus reducing the cost of judgments and attempts the user needs to make. The system is designed for three main groups of people: partially healthy elderly people, escorts, and other members of the public. Most of the questions from the elderly are about their own conditions, such as whether they are suffering from diseases, how to treat their diseases, and what causes their health conditions. Most of the questions from the escorts are about the professional problems of the elderly patients, such as how to take care of them when they are sick, what is the manufacturer of the medication they need, and what equipment they need. Other questions from the public were mostly basic questions about home medication, such as what medication should be taken for pneumonia in the elderly, how to take Pulmonary tablets, and what are the contraindications after taking Pulmonary tablets medication, etc.

4.2 Overall Architecture Design of the Question and Answer System

The home self-medication question-answering system for the elderly crawls public disease and drug data related to the elderly online. When asking questions to the system, the system can identify the entities in the question, and use template matching technology to answer questions related to medication for elderly diseases. At the same time, it also crawls the answer data of online physicians. When the elderly have similar questions, they can provide advice from online physicians, or the system can also chat with them. To some extent, this can serve as a supplement to the Q&A strategy.

This prototype system is designed and divided into modules, mainly including user interaction module, question judgment module and answer generation module. The user interaction module serves as the interface between the system and the user, and is mainly responsible for the input of questions and the output of answers. The question judgment module is one of the core modules of this prototype system. Its main function is to receive the question text input from the user interaction module and derive the question type through dictionary query, template text and similarity calculation. The answer generation module receives the question text information from the user interaction module, combines it with the question types derived from the question judgment module, and uses the knowledge graph inference technique and text generation technology to derive the final answers. The overall architecture of this Q&A system is shown in Fig. 2.

Users input the question they want to ask and get the question type through the question judgment module. If the question is related to the semantic data of specialized knowledge on medication for elderly patients, the question is queried in the Knowledge Graph of Elderly Home Medication through knowledge graph inference, and the answer is generated. If the question is judged by the question judgment module to be basic Q&A semantic data about elderly patients, the answer is matched in the Knowledge Graph of Elderly Home Medication through sentence vector similarity matching. If the similarity between the most similar question and the question asked by the user is less than a threshold value, the answer is generated through the question query based on the seq2seq model for display. After verification, a similarity threshold of 0.95 achieved better results.

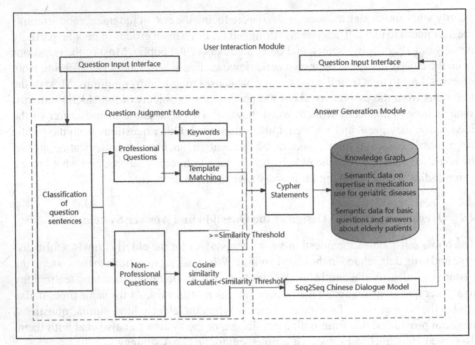

Fig. 2. General framework of the home self-medication question-answering system for the elderly

4.3 Question Judgment and Answer Generation

The question judgment module builds a dictionary of words matching entity types based on feature words. By constructing actree and filtering the problem using Ahocorasick algorithm [19], the feature words in the problem are extracted and then the problem is categorized based on the specific feature words. Finally returns the classification result of the question and the extracted key entities and types. In this paper, keywords such as drug names and disease names in the knowledge graph are extracted and integrated to form a drug dictionary, disease dictionary, symptom dictionary, food dictionary, department dictionary and drug manufacturer dictionary, as shown in Table 2.

The above dictionary combined with the question type template enables the determination of the question type. If the question involves expertise in medication for geriatric diseases, the keywords are combined with Cypher statements to query the best answer in the knowledge graph. The questions that do not involve professional knowledge are transformed into sentence vectors using the BERT model, and the similarity between the question text and the existing questions in the knowledge graph is calculated using the cosine similarity algorithm. The question sentence vectors with similarity thresholds are combined with Cypher statements to query the answers of questions similar to them in the knowledge graph, and the question texts with less than similarity thresholds are input into the trained Seq2Seq model to generate the answer texts. The similarity threshold for this experiment is derived by calculating the similarity of 10 pairs of question texts by the BERT model combined with the similarity algorithm, and the threshold is set to 0.95 by manual checking.

Table 2. Dictionary of the home self-medication question-answering system for the elderly

Question	Answer
Disease Dictionary	Aspiration pneumonia in the elderly, acute left heart failure in the elderly, ventricular tachycardia in the elderly, prostate hyperplasia in the elderly
Drug Dictionary	Pulaoan Tablet, Kidney Bone Dispersion, Kidney Bone Capsules, Nicergoline Capsules
Symptom Dictionary	Reverse cervical arch, positive hepatic-jugular venous reflux sign, sprain, walking with a large gait, coughing up yellow sputum
Food Dictionary	Tea egg, white fruit and chicken soup, sea shrimp and tofu, stir-fried tender cucumber, carp and sand nut soup
Department Dictionary	Otolaryngology, Traditional Chinese Medicine, Urology, Rehabilitation, Neurosurgery
Producer Dictionary	Guangdong Pidi Colloidal Pectin Bismuth Capsules, Liyi Menthylase for Injection, Shandong Luoxin Thiopronin for Injection, Guangxi Wuzhou Mao Dongqing Injection, Taiji Mianyang Pharmaceutical Qiju Dihuang Wan

4.4 Functional Testing and Application Verification

In this paper, the test dataset is divided into three parts for the three groups of people targeted by the system. The first part of the test data is composed of questions raised by professional geriatric doctors related to medication for elderly patients' diseases. The second part of the test data is for questions about geriatric diseases raised by the elderly and their caregivers. The final part of the test is for random questions and answers from the general public. Select 10 questions for each section for testing, and the test results are shown in Table 3.

For the first two parts of the test data, the Q&A system was accurate and answered quickly, however, for the randomized Q&A for the general public, the system will match the similarity based on the questions and the overall effectiveness of the system is average and needs to be improved. After entering the test data, part of the running picture is shown in Fig. 3.

Table 3. Test results of the home self-medication question-answering system for the elderly

Category	Number of tests	Correct quantity
Questions related to drug treatment of diseases in elderly patients raised by professional geriatric doctors	10	9
Questions raised by elderly people and their caregivers regarding elderly diseases	10	8
Public random Q&A	10	6

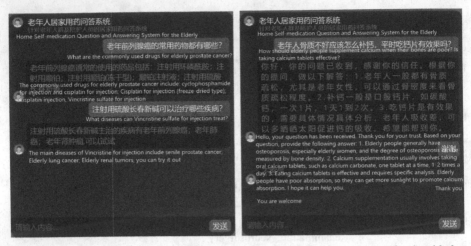

Fig. 3. Test interface of the home self-medication question-answering system for the elderly

5 Conclusion

The home self-medication question-answering system for the elderly combines the logical reasoning language of the knowledge graph with the probability calculation technology of deep learning, and provides flexible answers for the elderly and their caregivers. The combination of knowledge graph technology and deep learning models extends the types of questions that can be answered while ensuring professionalism. Professional questions from users can be answered with accurate and reliable knowledge from the knowledge graph. The text generation technology of deep learning models is used as a supplement to the knowledge graph to answer non-specialized questions in the form of daily chats. However, the system still has flaws. We will address the following issues in our next work: 1) Comparing multiple text similarity calculation methods; 2) Improving the quality of the training set of the Seq2Seq model; 3) Expand professional data in the medical field, improve the system question matching mode, and further improve the accuracy of the question answering system.

References

1. Wang, X.: Vulnerability evaluation and characteristics of elderly population with chronic diseases in China. J. Northeast Univ. (Soc. Sci. Ed.) **25**(1), 96–105 (2023). https://doi.org/10.15936/j.cnki.1008-3758.2023.01.011
2. Yao, L., et al.: Analysis and suggestions on medication safety for elderly people with chronic diseases at home in the context of the "Healthy China" strategy. China Primary Health Care **32**(10), 44–46 (2018)
3. Mira, J.J., Lorenzo, S., Guilabert, M., et al.: A systematic view of patient medication error on self-administering medication at home. Expert Opin. Drug Saf. **14**(6), 815–838 (2015)
4. Cai, Y., Wang, J., Douglas, J.: Design, and algorithm parallelization of medical Question answering based on Knowledge graph. Technol. Innov. **05**, 22–24 (2023)

5. Wang, Q., Mao, Z., Wang, B., et al.: Knowledge graph embedding: a survey of approaches and applications.IEEE Trans. Knowl. Data Eng. **29**(12), 2724–2743 (2017)
6. Dimitrakis, E., Sgontzos, K., Tzitzikas, Y.: A survey on question answering systems over linked data and documents. J. Intell. Inf. Syst. **55**(2), 233–259 (2020)
7. Singh, R., Subramani, S., Du, J., et al.: Antisocial behavior identification from Twitter feeds using traditional machine learning algorithms and deep learning. EAI Endorsed Trans. Scalable Inf. Syst. **10**(4), e17–e17 (2023)
8. Yang, M., Zhong, J., Hu, P., et al.: AI-driven question-answer service matching. In: 2017 Second International Conference on Mechanical, Control and Computer Engineering (ICMCCE). IEEE, 141–145 (2017)
9. Zhang, Y., Sheng, M., Liu, X., et al.: A heterogeneous multi-modal medical data fusion framework supporting hybrid data exploration. Health Inf. Sci. Syst. **10**(1), 22 (2022)
10. Xie, Y.: A TCM question and answer system based on medical records knowledge graph. In: 2020 International Conference on Computing and Data Science (CDS). IEEE, pp. 373–376 (2020)
11. Chongyu, Z.: Application Research and Implementation of Automatic Question Answering Based on Knowledge Graph. Beijing University of Posts and Telecommunications, Beijing (2019)
12. Wei, H., Li, L., Pengna, X.: Analysis and research on automatic Question answering of medical Knowledge graph. Fujian Comput. **37**(11), 100–103 (2021)
13. Zhang, M.: Research on automatic question-answering technology based on Knowledge graph of medical diseases. Beijing: Beijing University of Posts and Telecommunications (2021)
14. Zijia, C., Chong, C.: User question understanding and answer content organization for epidemic disease popularization. Data Anal. Knowl. Discov. **6**(S1), 202–211 (2022)
15. Xing, Z., Jingyi, D.: Seq2seq automatic question answering system of medical guide station based on background information. In: 2021 IEEE 5th Advanced Information Technology, Electronic and Automation Control Conference (IAEAC). IEEE, vol. 5, pp. 507–511 (2021)
16. Devlin, J., Chang, M.W., Lee, K., et al.: Bert: pre-training of deep bidirectional transformers
17. Ghazvininejad, M., Brockett, C., Chang, M.W., et al.: A knowledge grounded neural conversation model. In: Proceedings of the AAAI Conference on Artificial Intelligence, vol. 32, no. 1 (2018)
18. Gunawan, D., Sembiring, C.A., Budiman, M.A.: The implementation of cosine similarity to calculate text relevance between two documents. In: Journal of Physics: Conference Series. IOP Publishing, vol. 978, p. 012120 (2018)
19. Song, Y., Long, J., Li, F., et al.: A new adaptive multi string matching algorithm. Comput. Eng. Appl. **45** (6), 98–100123 (2009). https://doi.org/10.3778/j.issn.1002-8331.2009.06.028

Constructing Multi-constrained Cognitive Diagnostic Tests: An Improved Ant Colony Optimization Algorithm

Xi Cao[1], Yong-Feng Ge[2], and Ying Lin[3(✉)]

[1] Department of Computer Science and Information Technology,
La Trobe University, Melbourne 3086, Australia
[2] Institute for Sustainable Industries and Liveable Cities,
Victoria University, Melbourne 3011, Australia
[3] Department of Psychology,
Sun Yat-sen University, Guangzhou 510006, China
linying23@mail.sysu.edu.cn

Abstract. Most application scenarios of cognitive diagnostic tests (CDTs) are confronted with multiple constraints. Some existing well-developed algorithms for constructing CDTs transforms the test-construction problem into an optimization problem to improve the statistical performance of tests. However, tackling optimization problems with multiple constraints, particularly nonlinear ones, through previous optimization methods may not yield satisfactory outcomes. To address the multi-constrained CDT construction with greater efficiency, this paper introduces a method based on ant colony optimization (ACO-mTC). The method uses pheromone and heuristic information to guide the test-construction optimization. Pheromone signifies past construction experiences, while heuristic information integrates item discrimination indices and test constraint information. To facilitate the search to approximate feasible optima, each construction iteration is evaluated by item discrimination indices and test constraint information collectively. The effectiveness of the proposed method is demonstrated through a series of simulation experiments under various conditions. Comparative analysis with the random algorithm illustrates that ACO-mTC is more proficient in producing feasible tests with increased speed and enhanced statistical performance.

Keywords: Ant colony optimization · Cognitive diagnosis model · Multiple constraints · Test construction

1 Introduction

Cognitive diagnosis models (CDMs) stand as a significant theoretical advancement within psychometrics, emphasizing latent variables at the attribute level rather than encompassing the entire subject. With the development of CDMs, greater attention has been directed toward achieving more efficient and higher-quality cognitive diagnostic test (CDT) construction [4,11,14]. An effective strategy involves transforming the test construction into an optimization problem and employing optimization algorithms, such as the greedy algorithm [11], 0–1 programming [5], and evolutionary algorithms [4,14], to improve optimization efficiency and statistical performance.

Additionally, in real-world applications, CDT construction is often subject to multiple constraints. These constraints are related to either psychometric or non-psychometric characteristics [20]. Typically, psychometric constraints are requirements for test diagnostic capability, which can be characterized by the psychometric criteria such as validity [1] and target test information functions [15] within classical test theory and item response theory, respectively. In the context of CDMs, item discrimination indices can serve as the indicator of psychometric constraints. The range of non-psychometric constraints is more extensive. These constraints involve prerequisites for item selection that do not directly determine test diagnostic capability, such as item content and item type. Conventional optimization methods demonstrate limitations in effectively addressing problems characterized by multiple non-psychometric constraints. The optimization of CDT construction within the context of multiple constraints remains a challenging problem, holding significance for the practical implementation of cognitive diagnosis theory.

Drawing on a comprehensive view of prior literature and real-world scenarios, this study establishes a framework that delineates five constraints potentially emerging within CDTs. Targeting this framework, the current study introduces an ant colony optimization (ACO) algorithm for test construction. ACO, an optimization method proposed by Dorigo [3] and inspired by the foraging behavior of ants, enables both global and local searches, demonstrating robustness in addressing complex solution constructions. This study utilizes and adapts the ACO algorithm to effectively tackle the multi-constrained CDT construction problem.

The paper is organized into five sections. Section 2 provides an overview of the related work concerning CDT construction. Section 3 elaborates on the proposed ACO-mTC algorithm. Section 4 introduces the experimental design and presents the simulation results. The last section concludes the study and discusses potential directions for future research.

2 Related Work

Item discrimination indices are a series of indicators that quantify the diagnostic capability of CDTs and are extensively used in the construction of CDTs. In previous studies, two discrimination indices have been mainly employed: cognitive diagnosis information (CDI) [11] and attribute-level discrimination indices (ADI) [12]. The concept of utilizing the item selection method based on the item discrimination index for automated CDT construction was first introduced by Henson and Douglas [11]. In their method, the algorithm initially identifies and selects the item with the highest CDI and subsequently assesses whether the involvement of the remaining items aligns with predefined constraints. The algorithm then selects the item with the maximum CDI from the subset of items that satisfy the constraints. By iteratively evaluating and selecting items, the algorithm systematically assembles CDTs with high diagnostic validity.

To further enhance test quality, optimization algorithms have been employed for test assembly. Finkelman et al. [4] utilized the genetic algorithm (GA) [6,7,9] for this purpose. GA is a meta-heuristic algorithm that simulates the evolutionary process [8,17], driving solutions to evolve into the optimal state. The algorithm first applies Henson et al.'s CDI-based approach to generate the initial test population. Subsequently, it replaces items within individual tests to generate offspring tests and evaluates their performance through simulation. The algorithm then keeps the best-performing tests into the next iteration. Through iterative processes of mutation, evaluation, and selection, the test population evolves toward optimal test performance. While the GA approach enhances both test quality and adaptability, the computational process is complicated and time-consuming. Hence, to further improve the construction efficiency and test quality, Lin et al. [14] introduced a test-construction method based on ACO, referred to as ACO-TC. In their algorithm, an adaptive strategy is designed to determine the composition of item discrimination indices that are used as heuristic information in ACO-TC. The algorithm constructs tests based on heuristic information and measures tests according to heuristic information and pheromones that are based on the optimization history. ACO-TC optimizes the test population by repeating adaptation, selection, and update procedures. In comparison with the GA method, ACO-TC achieves higher computational speed and test quality.

CDT construction involves numerous constraints [11], such as attribute balance and maintaining equilibrium in multiple-choice answers. As the utilization of CDTs expands across diverse fields, addressing scenarios with multiple constraints becomes a pivotal consideration in refining the CDT construction methodology. In the context of tackling the single-constraint problem involving attribute balance, Lin et al. [14] conducted a comparative analysis among the CDI, GA, and ACO-TC algorithms. The results demonstrated that both the ACO-TC algorithm and GA method outperformed the CDI-based approach across most cases, with the ACO-TC algorithm exhibiting superiority over the GA method. However, limited attention has been directed toward the context of multiple constraints. Finkelman et al. [4] studied a double-constraint scenario involving attribute balance and answer distribution. They compared their method with the CDI-based approach and found that the GA algorithm produces significantly better results than the CDI method. To the best of our knowledge, no research has been done regarding CDT construction involving more than two constraints. In light of this gap, this study aims to develop a multi-constrained CDT construction algorithm, enhancing the efficacy and applicability of CDTs applied in complex real-world scenarios.

3 Method

3.1 Problem Definition

In this study, the CDT construction is converted into an optimization problem, wherein the aim is to optimize the objective performance of the test while subject to multiple constraints. By delving into the requisites of cognitive test construction within practical testing contexts, five non-psychometric constraints are identified. These encompass 1) the minimum number of items measuring each attribute, 2) the number of items measuring specific numbers of attributes, 3) the number of items of specific question types, 4) item interrelationships, and 5) item repetition. These constraints collectively encapsulate the multifaceted considerations in CDT construction for real-world application. For clarification, the test constraints and the objective function are defined as follows.

Constraints. Firstly, a CDT measures multiple attributes. If very few items in a test measure an attribute, the diagnostic capability of the test on this attribute will be weak; thereby, the test may not correctly measure students' mastery level on this attribute. Hence, this study manages the minimum number of items on each attribute in the test.

Secondly, in CDT, each individual item serves the purpose of evaluating either a solitary attribute or multiple attributes. The calculation of ADI for a given attribute involves aggregating ADIs of all items within the test on that attribute. Theoretically, in the case where every item within the test measures all attributes, the ADI for each attribute is expected to achieve the highest level. However, this results in a trade-off, as while the overall ADI is enhanced, the test's ability to discern an examinee's mastery at the attribute level diminishes. Consequently, a careful equilibrium must be struck between elevating the collective ADI and ensuring the accurate measurement of each individual attribute. As a result, this study encompasses control over the number of items assessing specific numbers of attributes.

Thirdly, considering that cognitive tests generally include multiple question types, such as multiple choice, blank-filling, and short essay, this study also integrates a mechanism for managing the number of items corresponding to specific question types.

In addition, item-related situations can arise in a test. For instance, the solution to one item might be inferred from the content of another item. This situation can potentially provide examinees with information beyond their actual knowledge, thereby compromising the accurate measurement of their genuine abilities. Besides, including duplicated items within a test is undesirable. Hence, this study restricts both item-related situations and instances of item repetition, ensuring that no relevant or duplicated items are incorporated into the test.

Objective Function. The objective function of a test comprises two integral components: the constraint satisfaction and the diagnostic capability.

Set the minimum number of items on attribute $k = 1, 2, ..., K$ as I_k, the number of items measuring $n = 1, 2, ..., N$ attributes as I_n, and the number of item being the question type of $t = 1, 2, ..., T$ as I_t. The constraint satisfaction of test $v = 1, 2, ..., V$ is computed by

$$S_v = \sum_{k=1}^{K} \frac{\max(I_k - I_k', 0)}{I_k} + \sum_{n=1}^{N} \frac{\text{abs}(I_n - I_n')}{I_n} + \sum_{t=1}^{T} \frac{\text{abs}(I_t - I_t')}{I_t}, \qquad (1)$$

where I_k' denotes the present number of items measuring attribute k in the test, I_n' represents the present number of items measuring n attributes in the test, and I_t' is the present number of items being question type t in the test. A smaller value of S_v signifies a higher degree of constraint satisfaction for test v. $S_v = 0$ denotes complete satisfaction of constraints by the test.

Drawing upon the construction model presented by Finkelman et al. [4], the minimum sum of ADI across all attributes is used to assess the diagnostic capability of the test in this study. In test v, the sum of ADI of all items on attribute k is represented by $SADI_{vk}$. The test's overall ADI is set as the minimum attribute-level ADI, described as

$$AADI_v = \min(SADI_{vk}). \qquad (2)$$

Combining the two components, the objective function of test v can be denoted by

$$F = AADI_v, \qquad (3)$$

subject to

$$S_v = 0. \qquad (4)$$

A higher value of F with no violations of constraints corresponds to an improved individual test.

3.2   Algorithm Design

The overall procedure of the proposed ACO-mTC is depicted in Fig. 1. In the optimization, initial values for pheromone concentration and other parameters are established. In each iteration, the heuristic information of items is computed based on the present state. Item selection takes place by incorporating both the heuristic information and pheromone concentration, employing the pseudo-random proportional rule. Once a test is constructed, updates are made to the best test, as well as the local pheromone for each item. The global pheromone is updated at the end of each iteration. The two essential processes of population construction and pheromone management are described in detail below.

Population Construction

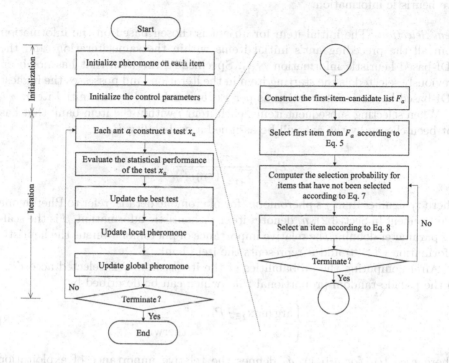

Fig. 1. Overall procedure of ACO-mTC.

Heuristic Information. ACO relies on heuristic information as a crucial guidance for optimization. In this study, the heuristic information includes both ADI and constraint satisfaction degrees. The ADI-based heuristic information is computed by

$$\eta_{(a)j} = \sum_{k=1}^{k} \alpha_{jk} \left(\frac{ADI_{jk} - mADI_k}{mADI_k} \right), \tag{5}$$

where α_{jk} is a binary variable denoting whether item j measures attribute k, ADI_{jk} represents item j's ADI on attribute k, and $mADI_k$ denotes the minimal ADI across all the items in the bank on attribute k.

The heuristic information associated with constraints is represented by $\eta_{(b)j}$, $\eta_{(c)j}$, $\eta_{(d)j}$, $\eta_{(e)j}$, and $\eta_{(f)j}$. Among these, the first three are determined by the extent of constraint violations corresponding to constraints 1 through 3, respectively. The remaining two are binary variables indicating the existence of constraints 4 and 5, respectively.

The comprehensive heuristic information for item j is an amalgamation of all the heuristic values mentioned earlier and is computed by

$$\eta_j = \frac{(\eta_{(a)j}^* + \eta_{(b)j}^* + \eta_{(c)j}^* + \eta_{(d)j}^*)\eta_{(e)j}\eta_{(f)j}}{4}, \tag{6}$$

where $\eta^*_{(a)j}$, $\eta^*_{(b)j}$, $\eta^*_{(c)j}$ and $\eta^*_{(d)j}$ symbolize the normalized forms of their respective heuristic information.

Item Selection. The initial item for an ant is chosen based on the information from all the preceding ant's initial items within the same iteration, and the ADI-based heuristic information $\eta_{(a)j}$. Specifically, the item that has not been previously selected as the starting item in the iteration, and possesses the highest ADI-based heuristic information as per Eq. 5, is selected as the initial item.

When selecting subsequent items, each item j within the item bank that has not been chosen by the ant will be assigned a probability P_j:

$$P_j = \frac{\tau_j \eta_j{}^\beta}{\sum_{j \in J}(\tau_j \eta_j{}^{\beta'})} \tag{7}$$

where τ_j signifies item j's pheromone (for pheromone details, refer to Pheromone Management in Sect. 3.2), η_j denotes item j's heuristic information, β is the scaling parameter defining the relative importance of pheromone versus the heuristic information ($\beta > 0$) and J represents the item bank.

After computing the probabilities of the items, item j is selected according to the pseudo-random proportional rule, which can be described by

$$j = \begin{cases} \arg\max_{j \in J} P_j, & \text{if } r \le q_0 \\ \widehat{j}, & \text{otherwise} \end{cases}, \tag{8}$$

where $r \sim Uniform(0,1)$, q_0 defines the relative importance of exploitation versus exploration ($q_0 \in (0,1)$), $\widehat{j}$ denotes the item selected based on item probabilities using roulette wheel selection. If r is smaller than q_0, the item j with the highest probability will be directly chosen; otherwise, a roulette wheel selection process is conducted.

Pheromone Management. In the ACO framework, every item within the bank is assigned a pheromone variable, initially set at τ_0. The value of τ_0 is computed based on a prior iteration preceding the optimization process.

The algorithm employs two pheromone-updating rules: the local updating rule and the global updating rule. Local updating takes place after each test construction. During this process, pheromone associated with items that have been selected in the tests within the iteration diminishes, thereby decreasing the likelihood of subsequent ants selecting these items. Specifically, the decay rule for item j is

$$\tau_j = (1 - \rho)\tau_j + \rho\tau_0, \tag{9}$$

where ρ is the pheromone decay parameter ($\rho \in (0,1)$). Following the completion of population construction, global updating is performed by adjusting pheromone associated with items within the present best test. The particular updating mechanism for item j is describes as follows:

$$\tau_j = (1 - \rho')\tau_j + \rho\Delta\tau_j, \tag{10}$$

where ρ' represents the pheromone updating parameter ($\rho' \in (0, 1)$), and $\Delta\tau_j$ is computed by

$$\Delta\tau_j = \begin{cases} \min(ADI_{jk}), & \text{if } j \in I_{\text{best}} \\ 0, & \text{otherwise} \end{cases}, \tag{11}$$

in which I_{best} denotes the current best individual in the population.

4 Simulation Experiments and Results

4.1 Experimental Design

In the simulation experiment, we generate a simulated item bank utilizing the reduced reparameterized unified model (r-RUM) [10], which is a widely used CDM. The simulated item bank comprises 300 items, measuring five attributes. According to the previous literature [11], the baseline probability is set in the range of [0.75, 0.95], while the penalty parameters range in [0.20, 0.95]. A detailed breakdown of the item bank composition is outlined in Table 1.

Table 1. Item bank composition.

Number of measuring	1 attribute	2 attributes	3 attributes
Multiple choice	50	60	10
Blank-filling	20	60	10
Short essay	10	20	60

Considering the test length varies across different application scenarios, this study investigates the algorithm performance at the test lengths of 20, 40, and 60. The experiment employs a population of 10 ants and is iterated 2,000 times. In terms of constraints, for each attribute, the minimum number of items measuring each attribute is designated as 1/4 of the test length. The numbers of items measuring 1, 2, and 3 attributes are set as 30%, 40%, and 50% of the test length, respectively. Additionally, the number of items classified as multiple choice, blank-filling, and short essay formats are set to 50%, 35%, and 15% of the test length, respectively. Other parameters are configured as follows: $\beta = 2$, $q_0 = 0.9$, and $\rho = \rho' = 0.1$.

4.2 Experiment Results

The results of the two algorithms under different test length scenarios are compared in Figs. 2 and 3. As the test length increases, the likelihood of the ACO-mTC algorithm generating feasible solutions stabilizes at 1. In contrast, the probability of the random algorithm achieving a feasible solution diminishes rapidly. In the case where the test length extends to 60 items, the probability of the random algorithm producing feasible solutions drops to 0 (refer to Fig. 2). In terms of feasible solutions, the average diagnostic capability of those generated by ACO-mTC substantially outperforms those produced by the random algorithm (p values approaching 0; refer to Fig. 3). Therefore, across various test length settings, ACO-mTC consistently generates feasible solutions with higher quality compared to the random algorithm.

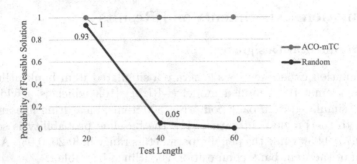

Fig. 2. Probability of generating feasible solutions for different test length settings.

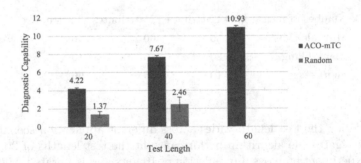

Fig. 3. Diagnostic capability for different test length settings.

There are overall 16 combinations of four constraints (the item repetition constraint is mandatorily restricted during the test construction process), as described in Table 2, where C1, C2, C3, and C4 respectively correspond constraint 1 through 4. The value "1" signifies the inclusion of the constraint, whereas "0" indicates its absence within the combination.

When the test length is set at 40 items, the evaluation of two algorithms under varying constraint combinations is illustrated in Figs. 4 and 5. Across different constraint scenarios, the likelihood of ACO-mTC algorithm producing feasible solutions stabilizes at 1. In most cases of the random algorithm, the probability remains at 1. However, a notable exception arises when two specific constraints coexist - namely, the minimum number of items for each attribute and the number of items being specific item types. In such cases, the probability of the random algorithm producing feasible solutions experiences a sharp reduction

Table 2. All combinations of four constraints.

Combination Number	C1	C2	C3	C4	Combination Number	C1	C2	C3	C4
1	0	0	0	0	9	1	0	0	1
2	1	0	0	0	10	1	0	1	0
3	0	1	0	0	11	1	1	0	0
4	0	0	1	0	12	1	1	1	0
5	0	0	0	1	13	1	1	0	1
6	0	0	1	1	14	1	0	1	1
7	0	1	0	1	15	0	1	1	1
8	0	1	1	0	16	1	1	1	1

to 0.1 (refer to Fig. 4). Moreover, a significant discrepancy is evident between the ACO-mTC algorithm and the random algorithm in terms of average diagnostic capability (p value approaching 0). ACO-mTC shows a higher level of robustness to the inclusion or exclusion of constraints, maintaining diagnostic capability consistently around 8. Conversely, the random algorithm displays instability, with diagnostic capability fluctuations ranging from 2 to 5.5 (refer to Fig. 5). Overall, ACO-mTC consistently assembles high-quality items that adhere to the specified constraints across diverse constraint combinations.

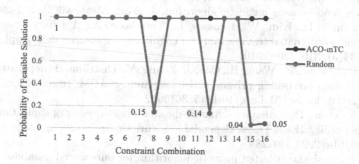

Fig. 4. Probability of feasible solutions for different constraint combinations.

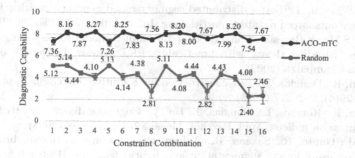

Fig. 5. Diagnostic capability for different constraint combinations.

5   Conclusion and Discussion

This paper addresses the multi-constrained CDT construction by utilizing the instrument of the ACO algorithm. Various constraints have been introduced to simulate the implementation of CDT in complex real-world scenarios. Simulation experiments verify the validity of the proposed algorithm. Results show that ACO-mTC has the capability to produce high-quality CDTs across different test length settings and diverse constraint combinations, significantly outperforming the random algorithm.

With the development of health information [13, 16, 23] and information technology [2, 18, 19, 21, 22], future research can further explore the application of automated test assembly in health-related domains.

References

1. Carmines, E.G., Zeller, R.A.: Reliability and Validity Assessment. Sage Publications, Thousand Oaks (1979)
2. Cheng, K., et al.: Secure k-NN query on encrypted cloud data with multiple keys. IEEE Trans. Big Data **7**(4), 689–702 (2017). https://doi.org/10.1109/TBDATA. 2017.2707552
3. Dorigo, M.: Optimization, learning and natural algorithms. Ph.D. thesis, Politecnico di Milano (1992)
4. Finkelman, M., Kim, W., Roussos, L.A.: Automated test assembly for cognitive diagnosis models using a genetic algorithm. J. Educ. Meas. **46**(3), 273–292 (2009)
5. Finkelman, M.D., Kim, W., Roussos, L., Verschoor, A.: A binary programming approach to automated test assembly for cognitive diagnosis models. Appl. Psychol. Meas. **34**(5), 310–326 (2010)
6. Ge, Y.F., Bertino, E., Wang, H., Cao, J., Zhang, Y.: Distributed cooperative coevolution of data publishing privacy and transparency. ACM Trans. Knowl. Discov. Data (2023). https://doi.org/10.1145/3613962
7. Ge, Y.F., et al.: Evolutionary dynamic database partitioning optimization for privacy and utility. IEEE Trans. Dependable Secure Comput. (2023). https://doi.org/10.1109/tdsc.2023.3302284
8. Ge, Y.F., et al.: Distributed memetic algorithm for outsourced database fragmentation. IEEE Trans. Cybernet. **51**(10), 4808–4821 (2021). https://doi.org/10.1109/tcyb.2020.3027962
9. Ge, Y.F., et al.: DSGA: a distributed segment-based genetic algorithm for multi-objective outsourced database partitioning. Inf. Sci. **612**, 864–886 (2022)
10. Hartz, S.M.: A Bayesian framework for the unified model for assessing cognitive abilities: Blending theory with practicality. Ph.D. thesis, University of Illinois, Urbana-Champaign (2002)
11. Henson, R., Douglas, J.: Test construction for cognitive diagnosis. Appl. Psychol. Meas. **29**(4), 262–277 (2005)
12. Henson, R., Roussos, L., Douglas, J., He, X.: Cognitive diagnostic attribute-level discrimination indices. Appl. Psychol. Meas. **32**(4), 275–288 (2008)
13. Jha, M., Gupta, R., Saxena, R.: A framework for in-vivo human brain tumor detection using image augmentation and hybrid features. Health Inf. Sci. Syst. **10**(1), 23 (2022). https://doi.org/10.1007/s13755-022-00193-9

14. Lin, Y., Gong, Y.J., Zhang, J.: An adaptive ant colony optimization algorithm for constructing cognitive diagnosis tests. Appl. Soft Comput. **52**, 1–13 (2017)
15. Lord, F.M.: Applications of Item Response Theory to Practical Testing Problems. Routledge, Milton Park (1980)
16. Pandey, D., Wang, H., Yin, X., Wang, K., Zhang, Y., Shen, J.: Automatic breast lesion segmentation in phase preserved DCE-MRIs. Health Inf. Sci. Syst. **10**(1), 9 (2022). https://doi.org/10.1007/s13755-022-00176-w
17. Pang, X., Ge, Y.F., Wang, K., Traina, A.J.M., Wang, H.: Patient assignment optimization in cloud healthcare systems: a distributed genetic algorithm. Health Inf. Sci. Syst. **11**(1), 30 (2023)
18. Patil, D.R., Pattewar, T.M.: Majority voting and feature selection based network intrusion detection system. EAI Endorsed Trans. Scalable Inf. Syst. **9**(6), e6–e6 (2022)
19. Singh, R., et al.: Antisocial behavior identification from twitter feeds using traditional machine learning algorithms and deep learning. EAI Endorsed Trans. Scalable Inf. Syst. **10**(4), e17–e17 (2023)
20. Swanson, L., Stocking, M.L.: A model and heuristic for solving very large item selection problems. Appl. Psychol. Meas. **17**(2), 151–166 (1993)
21. Wang, H., Yi, X., Bertino, E., Sun, L.: Protecting outsourced data in cloud computing through access management. Concurrency Comput. Pract. Experience **28**(3), 600–615 (2014). https://doi.org/10.1002/cpe.3286
22. You, M., et al.: A knowledge graph empowered online learning framework for access control decision-making. World Wide Web **26**(2), 827–848 (2022)
23. Zeng, Y., Liu, D., Wang, Y.: Identification of phosphorylation site using s-padding strategy based convolutional neural network. Health Inf. Sci. Syst. **10**(1), 29 (2022). https://doi.org/10.1007/s13755-022-00196-6

Health Informatics and Patient Safety in Pharmacotherapy

Antti Rissanen[1(✉)] and Marjo Rissanen[2]

[1] National Defence University, Helsinki, Finland
`antti.rissanen@mil.fi`
[2] Prime Multimedia Ltd, Helsinki, Finland

Abstract. Medication management is an essential part of patient safety. Problems related to prescribing, polypharmacy, and the interaction effects of drugs increase morbidity, mortality, and healthcare costs worldwide. Patients' knowledge of drug treatment could be improved in areas of the most common drug interactions and the general risks caused by drugs. The safety and effectiveness of medication for the elderly requires more effort especially in the area of high-risk medicines. Artificial intelligence–based decision support systems present new approaches for improving patient safety and medication management. However, before the full benefits of assistive technologies can be realized, these tools require proper validation.

Keywords: Pharmacotherapy · Patient Safety · Health Informatics

1 Introduction

Drug therapy is the most common medical intervention in healthcare [1]. Polypharmacy (PP), drug interactions, and other medicine-related adverse events mean a significant cause of morbidity and mortality worldwide [2, 3]. In the United States, approximately 8,000 people die yearly due to medication mistakes, and ordering errors account for nearly half of these errors [4]. System-related mistakes may be connected to ineffective processes, difficulties in communication and coordination, or technical malfunctions [5]. In England, around 237 million medication errors occur annually in the medication process chain [1]. Medication errors connected to transfers from one care unit to another form one priority area in WHO's safety scheme [6]. Pharmaceutical industry is growing rapidly. In 2020 global sales was more than $1,228.45 billion [7]. Adverse events in pharmacotherapy increase hospital admissions and prolong the length of hospital stays [8]. About 70% of adverse drug effects could be eliminated "if the right information about the right patient is available at the right time" [9].

In the management of pharmaceutical patient safety, key priority areas cover medication and device safety, information systems, professionals' competence, management, and appropriate reporting of adverse events. Information is needed on best practices and their effectiveness. Along with systematic data collection, meticulous analysis of damages and errors is necessary to improve process quality and reduce healthcare costs.

Y. Li et al. (Eds.): HIS 2023, LNCS 14305, pp. 366–374, 2023.
https://doi.org/10.1007/978-981-99-7108-4_31

[10–12] OECD survey (2018) shows that at least 25 countries routinely collect data on prescribed and dispensed medicines. In addition, they monitor medicine consumption and safety aspects for further analysis. This data can be linked with other information that relates to healthcare consumption. [13] Pharmacy-specific informatics evaluation should focus on interactions between environment, task, user, and tool. Such evaluation covers user, operational, and clinical outcomes, as well as up-to-date health informatics. [14] Stakeholders' interest in work safety, their continuous training, and clients' awareness and participation in safety matters are essential elements for advancements [15].

This study addresses two topics with the help of recent literature: 1) What kinds of issues in patient safety require more attention in the field of pharmacotherapy? 2) How health informatics and practices try to meet these challenges to improve patient safety? These challenges are examined in the light of the requirements of systemic coherence, in accordance with the research tradition of IT design science (DSR).

2 Pharmacotherapy and Patient Safety

Adverse drug events are common with antibiotics, antidiabetics, analgesics, and cardiovascular drugs [16]. Medication errors happen in all stages of process, such as during prescription, documentation, dosing, dispensing, or administration [17]. Effective mutual communication between service providers, customers, and professionals, as well as training practices, all need more attention [18, 19]. Underreporting of adverse drug reactions is one of the noticeable problems [20]. Pharmacovigilance (PV) provides verifiable information to the biopharmaceutical industry by regulating safety protocols in the field of pharmacotherapy [21].

The adverse effects of drugs increase with age and general frailty [22]. Age-related changes in liver and kidney function and in blood circulation affect drug kinetics and dynamics [23]. Psychosocial and psychological factors also have their effects [24]. The simultaneous use of several drugs by patients with multiple symptoms may increase adverse drug events despite appropriate medication policy [2]. However, inappropriate PP among the elderly requires attention [25]. PP risk may also increase due to difficulties with access to health services, chronic diseases, female gender, depression, and psychiatric diseases [26, 27]. Older patients do not necessarily get enough specific information about drugs. Especially anti-inflammatory medication for this group requires more attention [28]. Evaluations of PP in younger patients are sparse, but notable PP has been remarked upon in general practice among adult population [28].

Chronic disorders or continuous pain among the elderly may increase the necessity for intense pain medication, for which opioids can be prescribed [29]. Side effects vary between opioids. Insomnia and pain in the elderly can also increase dependence on benzodiazepines and opioids [30]. These drugs affect, for example, the central nervous system and can damage brain function in the elderly [31]. Individual variability for physiological effects increases with age, which means that consequences may also remain unclear [32]. Thus, careful use or even elimination of some medicines may come into question in pharmacotherapy for the elderly [32, 33]. The treatment intensity of the elderly population is low for several diseases [34]. This fact can lead to undertreatment of the main disease and excessive pain medication to compensate for it [35, 36].

3 Health Informatics and Drug Safety

3.1 Artificial Intelligence and Pharmacy Technology

Artificial intelligence (AI) is having a big impact in areas such as adverse drug events and diagnostic errors [37]. Pharmacy informatics helps in medication-specific data collection, analysis, storage, usage, distribution, and therapy management [38]. AI technologies serve several areas in the pharmaceutical industry like drug discovery, polypharmacology, hospital pharmacy, and dosage design [39].

AI and machine learning (ML) can decrease time in drug discovery and thereby decrease healthcare costs [40]. Toxicogenomics combines genetics and toxicological aspects of drugs and chemicals, thus giving it a crucial role in personalized medicine [41]. AI, novel ML, and deep learning approaches have transformed the field of PV in premarket drug safety and toxicity evaluation and in the assessment of biopharma industries but still require more research and validation [8, 21]. Premarketing clinical trials are often quick and may suffer from overly homogeneous test groups [42]. Despite available techniques, accurate prediction of drug-drug interactions (DDIs) remains a challenge [43]. Nowadays, social media may offer additional data for safety evaluation [42]. The need to obtain large amounts of high-quality data with accurate algorithmic interpretation and transparency means ongoing challenges [41].

3.2 Health Informatics in Patient Informing

Pharmacotherapy is the primary interventional strategy in healthcare [44]. Healthcare clients' general know-how in medication needs enhancement. In an adequate medication process, patients understand the basic information about and the functions and side effects of the prescribed drugs, and they are aware that their health and medication history can influence the medication and treatment decisions [45]. Healthcare professionals have an essential role in safe drug policy. Alongside that, support systems, applications, operating culture, and values have their place.

Customers can search for drug information on the Internet based on trade names or drug substance. In most countries, national drug information centers serve citizens' information needs. There are also independent mobile apps and platforms such as MyRx-Profile.com [46] that aid consumers in medication management and in preventing adverse drug reactions. There are even several disease-specific and also more general apps. Thus, digital pharmaceutical information is available on many medical specialty areas and sites [47]. However, clients find it demanding to find the most convenient, reliable and useful app with the best professional assistance [44]. Moreover, the apps' features do not always meet the needs of users for continuous use [48]. The need for assisting databases that guide clients in identifying high-quality mobile apps has been noted [49]. Simple medication alerts may help consumers in dosage and timing policy [50]. Likewise, medication follow-up tools exist for certain diagnoses [51]. Recently, ChatGPT has been used in many consumer-targeted health management apps to automate time-consuming tasks, like writing notes and reports [52]. The Smart and Healthy Aging through People Engaging in Supportive Systems (SHAPES) project aims to create an open European digital platform that assists older people in independent living as well in medication issues [53]. Still, in many countries, consumers' general knowledge about drug safety is unsatisfactory [20]. Urgent guidance is needed for both prescription and over-the counter medicines.

Better knowledge in pharmacotherapy can improve the vigilance of healthcare clients when sharing their medication history with their treating physician and healthcare professionals [34]. All approved medicine packages should contain information related to the medicine, and this is assumed to be the consumers' primary information about medicines, especially among elderly patients. Unfortunately, patients might not read the information. Spoken instructions or knowledge provided by pharmacy professionals are a good source of information, but due to automation (even medicines are delivered to pick-up boxes or home delivered by courier), the situation has changed. Therefore, access to professional informative pharmaceutical digital platforms seems important, also in self-medication [54].

Voice-based chatbots as reminders or instructors are seen as beneficial for older adults to improve medication-related adherence [55]. AI-based apps are considered promising in preventing the risk of opioid misuse in working population [56]. The accuracy of medicine related chatbots has been improved with the help of larger databases (e.g. Safedrugbot) [57, 58]. Chatbots can also decrease misinformation [59] in pharmacotherapy, and allow fast feedback, but unfortunately, the accuracy of answers cannot be guaranteed for demanding subquestions. Despite the utility values of ChatGPT, its use in public health still entails caution [60]. ChatGPT can partially predict and explain DDIs but may also provide incomplete information [61]. For better accuracy, significant barriers need to be removed, such as missing content and references, and reproducibility issues [62].

3.3 Health Informatics as Doctors' Aid

It is essential that doctors are aware of the harms and costs of adverse effects associated with drug treatment. Appropriate feedback systems and efficient consultation opportunities can enhance doctors' competence in pharmacotherapy. Computerized prescriber order entries and clinical decision support systems (CDSS) would prevent or at least reduce prescribing errors [3]. CDSS provide assistance in clinical practice (e.g., alerts, reminders, prescribing, image interpretation, and diagnostic aid). However, it is thought that they have not reached their full capacity due to hitches (e.g., low confidence, lack of relevance, low suitability to working flow) in user acceptance by physicians. [63] Properly applied AI-enabled CDSS can advance patient safety by improving error recognition in drug management but require validation [64].

DDIs and drug allergy alerts can lead to inappropriate alerts [63], requiring specificity and sensitivity enhancements for better serviceability. The development of a digital twin scheme in pharmacotherapy promises new perspectives for more personalized healthcare [65]. Digital therapeutics serve as complementary interventions (often as stand-alone solutions) for existing therapeutic strategies and are used, for example, in combination or as a replacement of other therapeutics (e.g., pharmacotherapy or psychotherapy) [66]. Their role in, for example, chronic pain and mental disorders may increase with technology development [66, 67]. These apps or solutions may be integrated with sensors and into wearables.

There are several promising examples regarding AI's positive effects in clinical practice. ML models have been successfully tested in the personalized pharmacotherapy of epilepsy [68]. AI can cut costs with a more exact identification of responders to specific asthma drugs [69]. Imprecisions in known and documented drug allergies in the EHRs are usual and can be organized better with the aid of AI [69]. AI-supported web applications have been used to detect interactions more quickly and to reduce the side effects of PP among elderly patients [70]. AI has also been used to find the best antidepressant and optimal dosage to evade undesirable side effects [71].

4 Discussion and Concluding Remarks

It is important that consumers receive pharmaceutical information that in its depth and accuracy suits their specific needs [72]. Adequate general knowledge about pharmacotherapy is also important among healthcare clients. This is an integral part of the professional intensity level of patient care. In healthcare the goal is a functioning systemic entity where different areas support each other. Medication related information is mainly in text form. For medicinal purposes, in most cases text-based material is not necessarily less informative than, for example, video material [73]. However, video clips or animations may clarify the basics of pharmacology (e.g. mechanisms of drug action, ways of giving medicine, absorption and biotransformation, physiological and environmental factors). Rigorous development, testing, validation, and reevaluations are necessary steps to avoid negative outcomes [74]. High-quality big data and AI are inseparable because AI systems are as good as connected training data [75]. AI development should align with people's values and interests, and related social and ethical aspects should be highlighted alongside technical aspects [52]. High-quality theoretical and empirical investigations are constantly needed to find the optimal ways of integrating AI into public healthcare [76].

The remarkable amount of adverse events in pharmacotherapy can be considered organizational wicked problems that mean additional costs but also lower image quality for the sector. Design science research (DSR) in information systems underlines synergy thinking, flexible manageability, and alignment between people, organization, and novel technical systems. This scheme requires creativity and understanding of the mutual coherence of interventions, as well as the ability to use human resources in a meaningful way as part of this process. Thus, the "cycles between design science and behavioral science" require attention when developing "best practices" for identified problems in the pharmaceutical area as well [77].

Emergent technologies and novel solutions for patient safety in pharmacotherapy comprise only one piece within the overall healthcare system. Thus, safety in pharmacotherapy is an area which requires effective efforts also at organizational levels. Alongside tutorial and educational interventions for professionals and clients, deeper investigations into system-related causes for erroneous procedures should also be given more attention. Such attention also means challenges for health informatics designers. In addition, rigorous assessment of the elements of prosperous health informatics entails more attention and resources [34]. Transparency related to adverse events in pharmacotherapy can enhance awareness of risky procedures and thereby finally improve image quality issues in organizations. Effective prevention of medication errors ultimately means better cost-effectiveness of healthcare.

References

1. Elliott, R.A., Camacho, E., Jankovic, D., Sculpher, M.J., Faria, R.: Economic analysis of the prevalence and clinical and economic burden of medication error in England. BMJ Qual. Saf. **30**, 96–105 (2021)
2. Chowdhary, R., Roshi, Tandon, V.: Role of free web based software in evaluating the profile of drug-drug interactions. J. Cardiovasc. Dis. **13**, 399–404 (2022)
3. Erstad, B.L., Romero, A.V., Barletta, J.F.: Weight and size descriptors for drug dosing: too many options and too many errors. Am. J. Health Syst. Pharm. **80**, 87–91 (2023)
4. Tariq, R.A., Vashisht, R., Sinha, A., Scherbak, Y.: Medication dispensing errors and prevention. StatPearls, Treasure Island, FL, USA (2020)
5. Rodziewicz, T.L., Hipskind, J.E.: Medical error prevention. StatPearls [Internet]. Treasure Island (FL), StatPearls Publishing (2020)
6. Elliott, R., Camacho, E.M., Gavan, S., Keers, R., Chuter, A.: Estimating the impact of enabling NHS information systems to share patients' medicines information digitally. University of Manchester (reports). (2023)
7. Hole, G., Hole, A.S., McFalone-Shaw, I.: Digitalization in pharmaceutical industry: what to focus on under the digital implementation process? Int. J. Pharm. X. **3**, 100095 (2021)
8. Basile, A.O., Yahi, A., Tatonetti, N.P.: Artificial intelligence for drug toxicity and safety. Trends Pharmacol. Sci. **40**, 624–635 (2019)
9. Kaelber, D.C., Bates, D.W.: Health information exchange and patient safety. J. Biomed. Inform. **40**, S40–S45 (2007)
10. Panagioti, M., et al.: Prevalence, severity, and nature of preventable patient harm across medical care settings: systematic review and meta-analysis. BMJ **366**, l4185 (2019)
11. Khalili, M., Mesgarpour, B., Sharifi, H., Daneshvar Dehnavi, S., Haghdoost, A.A.: Interventions to improve adverse drug reaction reporting: a scoping review. Pharmacoepidemiol. Drug Saf. **29**, 965–992 (2020)
12. Ikonen, T., Welling, M.: Parempaa potilasturvallisuutta. Lääkärilehti **75**, 1211–1219 (2020)
13. Organisation: using routinely collected data to inform pharmaceutical policies – OECD. https://www.oecd.org/health/health-systems/routinely-collected-data-to-inform-pharmaceutical-policies.htm. Accessed 09 June 2023
14. Ogundipe, A., Sim, T.F., Emmerton, L.: Development of an evaluation framework for health information communication technology in contemporary pharmacy practice. Exploratory Res. Clin. Soc. Pharm. **9**, 100252 (2023)
15. Mustonen, P., Ikonen, T., Rauhala, A., Leskelä, R.-L., Virkki, M.: Potilas- ja asiakasturvallisuudelle uusi kansallinen mittaristo **76**, 2892–3289 (2021)
16. Alqenae, F.A., Steinke, D., Keers, R.N.: Prevalence and nature of medication errors and medication-related harm following discharge from hospital to community settings: a systematic review. Drug Saf. **43**, 517–537 (2020)
17. Kopanz, J., et al.: Burden of risks in the analogue and digitally-supported medication use process and potential for solutions to increase patient safety in the hospital: a mixed method study (2022). https://doi.org/10.21203/rs.3.rs-1593296/v1
18. Burgener, A.M.: Enhancing communication to improve patient safety and to increase patient satisfaction. Health News **39**, 128–132 (2020)
19. Organization, W.H.: Ethics and governance of artificial intelligence for health: WHO guidance. (2021)

20. Leskur, D., et al.: Adverse drug reaction reporting via mobile applications: a narrative review. Int. J. Med. Inform. **168**, 104895 (2022)
21. Taylor, K., May, E., Powell, D., Ronte, H.: Deloitte insights, Intelligent post-launch patient support, Enhancing patient safety with AI. https://www2.deloitte.com/mt/en/pages/about-del oitte/topics/deloitte-insights.html. Accessed 07 June 2023
22. Hubbard, R.E., O'Mahony, M.S., Woodhouse, K.W.: Medication prescribing in frail older people. Eur. J. Clin. Pharmacol. **69**, 319–326 (2013)
23. Surale-Patil, A., Salve, P., Singh, L., Shah, A., Shinde, A.: Prevention of drug interaction in geriatric patients. Eur. Chem. Bulletin. **12**, 3355–3363 (2023)
24. Christopher, C., et al.: Medication use problems among older adults at a primary care: a narrative of literature review. Aging Med. **5**, 126–137 (2022)
25. Organization, W.H.: Medication safety in polypharmacy: Technical report. World Health Organization (2019)
26. Yaghi, G., Chahine, B.: Potentially inappropriate medications use in a psychiatric elderly care hospital: a cross-sectional study using beers criteria. Health Sci. Rep. **6**, e1247 (2023)
27. Ersoy, S., Engin, V.: Accessibility to healthcare and risk of polypharmacy on chronically ill patients. JCPSP-J. Coll. Phys. Surg. Pak. **29** (2019)
28. Rachamin, Y., et al.: Prescription rates, polypharmacy and prescriber variability in Swiss general practice—a cross-sectional database study. Front. Pharmacol. **13**, 832994 (2022)
29. Roberto, K.A., Teaster, P.B., Lindberg, B.W., Blancato, R.: A first (and disturbing) look at the relationship between the opioid epidemic and elder abuse: insights of human service professionals. J. Appl. Gerontol. **40**, 1231–1235 (2021)
30. Nieciecka, A., et al.: Addictions in the elderly–review article. J. Health Study Med. **22**, 43–67 (2022). https://doi.org/10.36145/JHSM2022.10
31. ELDesoky, E.S.: Pharmacokinetic-pharmacodynamic crisis in the elderly. Am. J .Ther. **14**, 488–498 (2007)
32. Wilder-Smith, O.H.: Opioid use in the elderly. Eur. J. Pain **9**, 137–140 (2005)
33. Pergolizzi, J., et al.: Opioids and the management of chronic severe pain in the elderly: consensus statement of an international expert panel. (Buprenorphine, fentanyl, hydromorphone, methadone, morphine, oxycodone). Pain Pract. **8**, 287–313 (2008)
34. Rissanen, M.: Comprehending translational design scenarios and implications in consumer health informatics. Doctoral Dissertation, Aalto University (2021)
35. Schofield, P.: The assessment of pain in older people: UK national guidelines. Age Ageing **47**, i1–i22 (2018)
36. Johansson, M.M., et al.: Pain characteristics and quality of life in older people at high risk of future hospitalization. Int. J. Env. Res. Public Health **18**, 958 (2021)
37. Bates, D.W., et al.: The potential of artificial intelligence to improve patient safety: a scoping review. NPJ Digit. Med. **4**, 54 (2021)
38. Jarab, A.S., Al-Qerem, W., Mukattash, T.L.: Information technology in pharmacy practice: barriers and utilization. J. Appl. Pharm. Sci. **13**, 150–155 (2023)
39. Raza, M.A., et al.: Artificial intelligence (AI) in pharmacy: an overview of innovations. Innov. Pharm. **13**, 13–13 (2022)
40. Bhagat, P.M.: Artificial Intelligence in Healthcare. IJSRET **7**, 796–800 (2021)
41. Singh, A.V., et al.: Integrative toxicogenomics: advancing precision medicine and toxicology through artificial intelligence and OMICs technology. Biomed. Pharmacother. **163**, 114784 (2023)
42. Liu, J., Wang, Y., Huang, L., Zhang, C., Zhao, S.: Identifying adverse drug reaction-related text from social media: a multi-view active learning approach with various document representations. Information **13**, 189 (2022)
43. KafiKang, M., Hendawi, A.: Drug-Drug interaction extraction from biomedical text using relation BioBERT with BLSTM. Mach. Learn. Knowl. Extr. **5**, 669–683 (2023)

44. Tabi, K., et al.: Mobile apps for medication management: review and analysis. JMIR Mhealth Uhealth **7**, e13608 (2019)
45. Ross, M.: What's the Importance of Medication Education for Patients? https://blog.cureatr. com/the-importance-of-medication-education-for-patients. Accessed 23 June 2023
46. MyRXprofile It Could Save Your Life (2023). https://www.myrxprofile.com/
47. Fauque, E.J.A.: Évaluation de l'information et du conseil pharmaceutique numérique existant en dermatologie. Analyse critique et proposition d'un nouvel outil (2020). https://dumas.ccsd. cnrs.fr/dumas-02970039
48. Vaghefi, I., Tulu, B.: The continued use of mobile health apps: insights from a longitudinal study. JMIR Mhealth Uhealth **7**(8), e12983 (2019)
49. Portenhauser, A.A., Terhorst, Y., Schultchen, D., Sander, L.B., Denkinger, M.D., Stach, M., et al.: Mobile apps for older adults: systematic search and evaluation within online stores. JMIR Aging **4**, e23313 (2021)
50. Fahamin, Ali, R., Lipi, I.A.: Medication Alert: A fore-and-aft Android-Based Hospitality Corps Sturdy for Progressive Repeated Medication Alert System. SSRN 4460501 (Elsevier) (2023). https://doi.org/10.2139/ssrn.4460501
51. Romero-Jimenez, R., et al.: Design and implementation of a mobile app for the pharmacotherapeutic follow-up of patients diagnosed with immune-mediated inflammatory diseases: eMidCare. Front. Immunol. **13**, 915578 (2022)
52. Al Kuwaiti, A., et al.: A review of the role of artificial intelligence in healthcare. J. Personal. Med. **13**, 951 (2023)
53. Spargo, M., et al.: Shaping the future of digitally enabled health and care. Pharmacy. **9**, 17 (2021)
54. Fainzang, S.: Managing medicinal risks in self-medication. Drug Saf. **37**, 333–342 (2014)
55. Gudala, M., Ross, M.E.T., Mogalla, S., Lyons, M., Ramaswamy, P., Roberts, K.: Benefits of, barriers to, and needs for an artificial intelligence–powered medication information voice chatbot for older adults: interview study with geriatrics experts. JMIR Aging **5**, e32169 (2022)
56. Islam, A.R., et al.: An artificial intelligence-based smartphone app for assessing the risk of opioid misuse in working populations using synthetic data: pilot development study. JMIR Formative Res. **7**, e45434 (2023)
57. Williams, L.: 11 Healthcare Chatbots Which Can Improve Patient Experience. https://get referralmd.com/2019/03/11-healthcare-chatbots-that-improve-patient-experience/. Accessed 09 June 2023
58. Lee, D.: AI-based healthcare chatbot. Int. Res. J. Eng. Technol. **10**, 563–568 (2023)
59. Parmar, P., Ryu, J., Pandya, S., Sedoc, J., Agarwal, S.: Health-focused conversational agents in person-centered care: a review of apps. NPJ Digit. Med. **5**, 21 (2022)
60. Zhang, Y., Pei, H., Zhen, S., Li, Q., Liang, F.: Chat Generative pre-trained transformer (Chat-GPT) usage in healthcare – science direct. Gastroenterol. Endosc. **1**, 139–143 (2023). https:// doi.org/10.1016/j.gande.2023.07.002
61. Juhi, A., et al.: The capability of ChatGPT in predicting and explaining common drug-drug interactions. Cureus. **15**, 1–7 (2023)
62. Morath, B., et al.: Performance and risks of ChatGPT used in drug information: an exploratory real-world analysis. Eur. J. Hosp. Pharm. (2023)
63. Khairat, S., Marc, D., Crosby, W., Al Sanousi, A.: Reasons for physicians not adopting clinical decision support systems: critical analysis. JMIR Med. Inform. **6**, e8912 (2018)
64. Choudhury, A., Asan, O.: Role of artificial intelligence in patient safety outcomes: systematic literature review. JMIR Med. Inform. **8**, e18599 (2020)
65. Kamel Boulos, M.N., Zhang, P.: Digital twins: From personalised medicine to precision public health. J. Personal. Med. **11**, 745 (2021)
66. Fürstenau, D., Gersch, M., Schreiter, S.: Digital therapeutics (DTx). Bus. Inf. Syst. Eng. **65**, 1–12 (2023)

67. Wang, C., Lee, C., Shin, H.: Digital therapeutics from bench to bedside. NPJ Digit. Med. **6**, 38 (2023)

68. Chiang, S., Rao, V.R.: Choosing the best antiseizure medication—can artificial intelligence help? JAMA Neurol. **79**, 970–972 (2022)

69. MacMath, D., Chen, M., Khoury, P.: Artificial intelligence: exploring the future of innovation in allergy immunology. Curr. Allergy Asthma Rep. **23**, 1–12 (2023)

70. Akyon, S.H., Akyon, F.C., Yılmaz, T.E.: Artificial intelligence-supported web application design and development for reducing polypharmacy side effects and supporting rational drug use in geriatric patients. Front. Med. **10**, 1029198 (2023)

71. Lisbona, N.: How artificial intelligence is matching drugs to patients - BBC News, https://www.bbc.com/news/business-65260592. Accessed 17 08 2023

72. Rissanen, M.: Ways for enhancing the substance in consumer-targeted eHealth. In: Wang, H., Siuly, S., Zhou, R., Martin-Sanchez, F., Zhang, Y., Huang, Z. (eds.) HIS 2019. LNCS, vol. 11837, pp. 306–317. Springer, Cham (2019). https://doi.org/10.1007/978-3-030-32962-4_28

73. Smith, I.P., et al.: The impact of video-based educational materials with voiceovers on preferences for glucose monitoring technology in patients with diabetes: a randomised study. Patient-Patient-Centered Outcomes Res. 1–15 (2023). https://doi.org/10.1007/s40271-022-00612-9

74. HealthITSecurity, S.: Leveraging Artificial Intelligence to Support Medication Adherence. https://healthitanalytics.com/features/leveraging-artificial-intelligence-to-support-medication-adherence. Accessed 17 Aug 2023

75. Merchant, S.: Stanford's AIMI is Revolutionizing Healthcare AI by Providing Free Big Data to Researchers – AIM. https://www.aimblog.io/2021/09/02/stanfords-aimi-is-revolutionizing-healthcare-ai-by-providing-free-big-data-to-researchers/. Accessed 17 Aug 2023

76. Alghadier, M., Kusuma, K., Manjunatha, D., Kabra, P., Zaleha, M.: A study of various applications of artificial intelligence (AI) and machine learning (ML) for healthcare services. Technology **5**(1), 87–94 (2023)

77. Hevner, A., Chatterjee, S.: Design science research in information systems. In: Design research in information systems. Integrated Series in Information Systems, vol. 22, pp. 9–22. Springer, Boston (2010). https://doi.org/10.1007/978-1-4419-5653-8_2

Author Index

A

Ahmed, Khandakar 91
Ahmed, Mohiuddin 65, 101
Alkhafaji, Sarmad K. D. 127
Alvi, Ashik Mostafa 331

B

Bai, Jinsheng 261

C

Cao, Xi 354
Chan, Ka Ching 17
Chen, Fazhan 40
Chen, Guozhu 283
Chen, Yanhua 135
Choosri, Noppon 235

D

Dart, Martin 65

F

Fang, Zhen 223
Fei, Gao 213, 321
Fu, Haojie 40
Fu, Yu 161

G

Ge, Yong-Feng 79, 354
Gomutbutra, Pattama 235
Gopalakrishnan, Abinaya 17
Grosser, Mark 187, 223
Guo, Chaogui 50
Guo, Chaohui 343
Guo, Kairui 223
Gururajan, Raj 17

H

Hai, Nan 213
Hao, Chenxiao 199

Hao, Rui 199
Haque, Umme Marzia 3
He, Beijia 50
Hong, Wei 175
Hong, Wenjuan 135
Hu, Chenping 135
Hu, Zhentao 321
Huang, Yi 261
Huang, Zhisheng 40, 50, 135, 161, 343

J

Jahan, Samsad 79
Jalal, Sarab 127
Jaworsky, Markian 115

K

Kabir, Enamul 3, 79
Khanam, Rasheda 3
Kittisares, Adisak 235

L

Lettrakarnon, Peerasak 235
Li, Chao 199
Li, Shuo 30
Li, Wenyao 199, 213, 321
Li, Xia 30
Li, Xin 213, 321
Li, Yan 247, 271
Lin, Hua 187, 223
Lin, Shaofu 50, 161, 343
Lin, Ying 354
Liu, Yanjun 149
Liu, Ying 30
Lu, Haohui 296
Lu, Jie 187, 223
Luo, Daizhong 149
Luo, Jinyuan 283

M
Ma, Xinqiang 261
Manami, Nishat Tasnim 331
Moonsamy, Avisen 101

N
Nowrozy, Raza 91

P
Pan, Lei 115
Peng, Dandan 283
Pokhrel, Shiva Raj 115

Q
Qin, Hongyun 135
Qiu, Xingting 309

R
Rissanen, Antti 366
Rissanen, Marjo 366

S
Sadiq, Muhammad Tariq 247
Sanguansri, Atigorn 235
Sheng, Ming 199
Shi, Wen 283
Siuly, Siuly 247, 331

T
Tan, Wenjun 309
Tao, Xiaohui 115

U
Uddin, Shahadat 296

V
Venkataraman, Revathi 17

W
Wang, Baoxin 343
Wang, Can 135

Wang, Hua 79
Wang, Kaige 321
Wang, Kate 149, 175
Wang, Kun 309
Wang, Luoxi 199, 321
Wang, Weifan 321
Wei, Shicheng 271
Wen, Paul 247
Wu, Mengjia 187
Wu, Qianqian 40

X
Xie, Linhai 283
Xu, Puti 175
Xu, Zhenkai 161

Y
Yang, Hong 283, 309
Yang, Wencheng 271
Yang, Yue 223
Yin, Jiao 149, 175, 309
Yin, Xiao-Xia 283
Yin, Xiaoxia 309
Yong, Jianming 115

Z
Zhang, Guangquan 187
Zhang, Guijuan 309
Zhang, Ji 115
Zhang, Mengmeng 40
Zhang, Nan 261
Zhang, Xingping 309
Zhang, Xiyan 40, 135
Zhang, Yanchun 175, 283, 309
Zhang, Yi 187
Zhang, Yong 199, 213, 321
Zhao, Huiying 199
Zhao, Tao 213
Zhao, Xudong 40
Zheng, Wenkui 213, 321
Zhou, Xujuan 17

Printed in the United States
by Baker & Taylor Publisher Services